HEMOPHILUS INFLUENZAE

Proceedings of a Conference
on Antigen-Antibody Systems, Epidemiology,
and Immunoprophylaxis

April 24–25, 1972
Vanderbilt University Medical School
Nashville, Tennessee

Hemophilus Influenzae

SARAH H. W. SELL
Editor

DAVID T. KARZON
Associate Editor

1973
VANDERBILT UNIVERSITY PRESS
Nashville, Tennessee

Library of Congress Cataloguing-in-Publication Data
Main Entry under title:

Hemophilus influenzae.

"Proceedings of a conference on antigen-antibody systems, epidemiology, and immuno-prophylaxis, April 24-25, 1972, Vanderbilt University Medical School, Nashville, Tennessee."
Conference sponsored by Vanderbilt University and the Dept. of Pediatrics of the School of Medicine.
Includes bibliographies.
1. Hemophilus meningitis—Congresses.
2. Hemophilus influenzae—Congresses. I. Sell, Sarah H., 1913— ed. II. Karzon, David T., 1920— III. Vanderbilt University, Nashville. Dept. of Pediatrics. [DNLM: 1. Hemophilus infections—Congresses. 2. Haemophilus influenzae—Congresses.
QW 140 H489   1972]
RC376.H45   616.8'2   73-4557
ISBN 0-8265-1185-6

TO
MISS LILY PETER

But if we could break the code of the violent pathogens,
What gracious release from suffering this would bring.

—Lily Peter, "Meditations on an Electron Microscope," 1972

Table of Contents

SECTION IX

SECTION X

List of Illustrations

List of Tables

Foreword

Hemophilus influenzae, first described by Richard Pfeiffer in 1892 as the cause of influenza, has been a challenge to microbiologists and clinicians ever since. It is a small, Gram-negative, pleomorphic bacillus which requires special growth factors as enrichment for cultivation on artificial media. For this reason, it is a bacterial species which easily can be missed in the usual hospital routine cultures. Even though it is no longer considered to be the primary agent of clinical influenza, as Pfeiffer suggested, it is a leading etiological agent of serious infections, especially in infants and young children. Acute bacterial meningitis due to type b is the clinical condition of most concern to physicians attending children. Despite the lowered mortality from antibiotic and improved supportive therapy, nearly half of the survivors have been shown to have long-term sequelae of some detectable degree. For this reason, immunoprophylaxis, which has long been a dream of those who work with children, is being explored by modern techniques and methods. It is now possible to prepare large quantities of the purified capsular substance of type b, polyribophosphate, which is thought to be the important protective antigen.

The rapid explosion of research related to antigen-antibody systems and immunology of *H. influenzae* made it urgent to bring those together who were working independently in these areas. In addition, it was important to bring into the discussions others who were working in related spheres such as epidemiology, natural history, microbiology, and biochemistry. Through the generosity of Miss Lily Peter, an alumna of Vanderbilt University, such a conference was made possible, in April 1972. It was sponsored by Vanderbilt University and the Department of Pediatrics of the Vanderbilt School of Medicine, with the Children's Regional Medical Center chosen as the host site. Attendance was limited to forty people in order that all participants might actively engage in the discussions. It is hoped that this publication of the proceedings of the conference will reach a large audience, many of whom would have enjoyed attending in person.

The book contains two types of information. The first consists of the formal papers as chapters, each written by the authors in their own style and documented by tables, charts, and bibliography. They represent the leading edges of our knowledge at the present time. Of the twenty-six papers presented during the conference, that of Dr. Thomas H. Stoudt, Director of the Department of Applied Microbiology of Merck Sharpe and Dohme, was not available for publication. Dr. Stoudt spoke on "Capsular Antigen of *Hemophilus influenzae.*" The other chapters in this book consist of open and spontaneous discussions which include many helpful suggestions for further study. They were taped during the conference, corrected by the discussants, and referenced. The book is arranged in sections, so that a group of related subjects is followed by a chapter of discussion.

The mood prevailing at the conference was enthusiastic and co-operative. It is hoped that this exchange of ideas and experiences will hasten the realization of a safe and effective immunizing agent against *Hemophilus influenzae.*

SARAH H. SELL

Vanderbilt University School of Medicine
September 1972

SECTION I

CHAPTER 1

Natural Infections with *Hemophilus influenzae* in Children:
I. Types Identified

Sarah H. Sell
Dorothy J. Turner
Charles F. Federspiel

Even though *Hemophilus influenzae* was described as long ago as eighty years (Pfeiffer, 1892), the natural history of infections in children remains poorly understood. It has been accepted that type b is the important strain in meningitis and almost all serious infections (Sell, 1970; Turk and May, 1967). With the exception of acute epiglottitis, these tend to occur in infants and young children before school age. It has been assumed that immunity accrues with age by repeated experiences with infections which probably originate in the nasopharnx (Alexander, 1968). However, there have been no long-term studies of the natural history to elucidate the problem.

This report concerns a longitudinal study of 104 normal children, living at home with their families, followed for three to five years, with periodic histories, physical examinations, nasopharyngeal cultures for *H. influenzae,* and blood samples. The results of the cultures for *H. influenzae* at various ages will be presented in relation to the state of health of the children at the time of the observations.

Supported by United States Public Health Service Institute of Allergy and Infectious Disease, National Institute of Health, Bethesda, Maryland, Grant AI 06110.

Appreciation is expressed to Linda Arnold, Shirley Stansell, Ana Womack, Sharon Matthews, and Lucille Hampton for technical assistance during the study; to the physicians of the Pediatric House Staff of Vanderbilt University Hospital for assistance in patient care; and to Helen Johnson for typing the manuscript.

METHODS

Selection of patients and plan of study. From all infants delivered on the
Staff Service of Vanderbilt University Hospital during the period from June
1964 through October 1965, cord blood was collected at birth. Return visits to
the Well Baby Clinic were scheduled at age 4 weeks. All parents of normal babies
living in the Nashville area were interviewed. Those who agreed to bring their
child back at monthly intervals for 5 months and then quarterly thereafter for
three years were chosen for the study. Return visits were requested, additionally,
during respiratory illness and, also, one month after each culture in which *H.
influenzae* was identified. Each visit included an interval history, physical
examination, nasopharyngeal culture, and blood sample—as well as any indicated
therapeutic measures. Of the 140 subjects selected, all were in the lower
socioeconomic level; however, many of the parents were students. Eighty
percent were black; twenty percent were white.

For the purpose of data retrieval, the term *episodes of health* was selected to
describe clinical status at the time of the observations. For example, a regularly

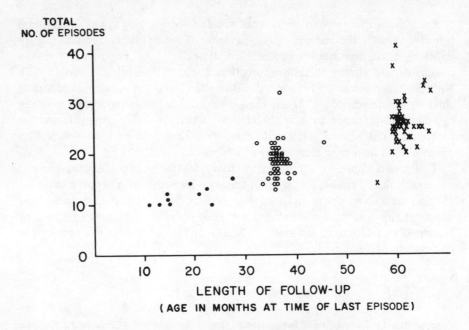

Fig. 1. *Hemophilus influenzae* in 104 children followed.

Legend: ● = subject followed for 1 to 2 years
          O = subject followed for 3 to 4 years
          X = subject followed for 5 years

scheduled check-up, when the child was considered to be well, was an "episode"; similarly, a bout of acute respiratory illness, during which time several visits were required for patient care, was considered as one "episode."

Figure I shows the numbers of subjects in the study, episodes observed, and total length of follow-up for each child. One hundred and four children were followed for the first year of life (36 dropped out within the first three months), 94 for three years and 44 for approximately five years. After the third year, 50 children were dropped.[1] Some of the 10 children who dropped out before the end of three years had as few as 10 observations, but, of those 44 who were followed for the entire five years, 43 were seen at least 20 times, with one child having 41 episodes. Altogether, there were 2,194 observed episodes of health.

Bacterial identification began in the treatment room with inoculation of fresh Levinthal's agar plates directly from nasopharyngeal swabs. After over-night incubation at 37°C, single colonies were picked for six-hour cultures which were typed by slide agglutination (Pittman, 1931). For those strains which failed to agglutinate immediately with only one of the six type-specific antisera (prepared in our laboratory by the method of Alexander, Leidy, and MacPherson, 1946), slides were prepared for the immunofluorescent techniques, previously described (Sell et al., 1963). Specificity of fluorescence was checked in each instance by blocking with the unlabelled antiserum in a duplicate set of slides.

The isolates were also tested to determine that X and V growth factors were required (Harris and Coleman, 1963).

Although identification of *H. influenzae* was our primary interest, pneumococci were also identified. Gram-positive cocci from 1- to 2-mm colonies which produced alpha hemolysis on sheep-blood agar and were inhibited by optochin discs were classified as pneumococci. No attempt at typing was made.

RESULTS

Differences by age. Table 1 shows the total rate of isolation of *H. influenzae* (all strains) during the first five years of life. The proportions of positives increased up to the third year and then decreased. The differences in the percentages positive for each period were statistically significant (P< .001), as was the trend indicated. Table 2 shows, by age, the rate of isolation for typable strains. Although the largest percentages of typable cultures were found in children in their fourth year of life, the differences in percentages positive by age groups were not statistically significant. There was a big drop in the fifth year, but the numbers were small.

1. Funding was originally available for the first three years, then later extended but too late for continuity for all the children.

TABLE 1

ISOLATION OF *H. INFLUENZAE* (all strains) DURING THE
FIRST FIVE YEARS OF LIFE

Age	No. Positive	% Positive
0 - 5 months	73/524	13.9
6 - 12 months	59/236	25.0
12 - 23 months	188/595	31.6
24 - 35 months	124/370	33.5
36 - 47 months	37/137	27.0
48 - 60 months	36/166	21.7
TOTALS	517/2028	25.5

Figure 2 shows the types which were identified. The height of each bar represents the percentage of positive cultures which were typable (also given in Table 2). In every year except the first, type b was found more frequently than any other type (56 isolates in all). Further, it can be seen that the proportion of positives which were type b increased through the fourth year, accounting in large part for the increased height of the bars. Type d, which was also found in all age groups, was recovered in 23 instances and was the predominate type during the first six months of age. Type e was also found in all age groups and was isolated 22 times. All six types were identified at one time or another.

Figure 3 shows the cumulative percentages of children with at least one positive culture. The lines in the figure show the ages at which the subjects had their first documented experience (positive cultures) with *H. influenze.* Half of the children had at least one positive culture by the time they were 10 months of age and almost 80% had by the time they were 2 years old. Based upon the

TABLE 2

ISOLATION OF TYPABLE STRAINS OF *H. INFLUENZAE* DURING
THE FIRST FIVE YEARS OF LIFE

Age	No. Typable	% Typable
0 - 5 months	16/73	21.9
6 - 12 months	11/53	20.8
13 - 23 months	43/188	22.9
24 - 35 months	37/123	30.1
36 - 47 months	16/37	43.2
48 - 60 months	5/36	13.9
TOTALS	128/510	25.1

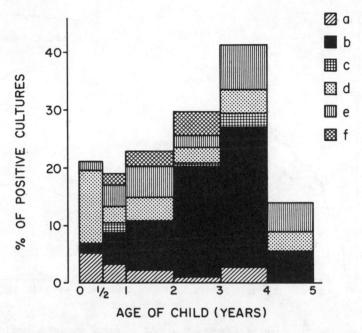

Fig. 2. Types of *Hemophilus influenzae* identified, percentage of positive cultures.

sampling used in the study, every child had experienced some strain of *H. influenzae* by age 5 years. Experience with type b, however, was rare before the age of one year. In less than 15% of the children were isolates identified by the age of two years and only in 38.5% by age 5. Thus, more than 60% of the children escaped type b, as identified in our sampling. The two cumulative distribution curves shown in Figure 3 reveal that, although experience with *H. influenzae* came rather early in life, the number of children who had experience with type b increased uniformly and gradually at a relatively slow rate. These data represent minimal figures, in that more frequent sampling might have yielded more isolates.

Correlation of H. influenzae *serotypes with clinical status.* Table 3 shows the results of cultures according to clinical status of the subject. The data are divided into three categories with respect to illness: ill at time of cultures, history of interim illness, and not ill. The percentages of positive cultures for these three groups were 40.8, 21.0, and 12.1, respectively. The differences in bacterial isolation rates vary significantly among the three categories of clinical status and clearly show the association between illness and the likelihood of a positive culture. The positive cultures, taken from children who were ill at the time of

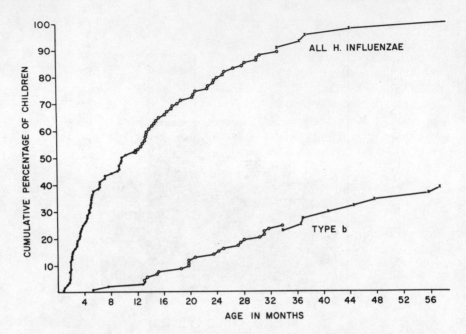

Fig. 3. Cumulative percentage of children with at least one nasopharyngeal culture positive for *H. influenzae*, by age.

Legend: Points on the graph are based on the 3 cohorts described in the test:
         ●—● = Cumulative percentages based on 104 subjects followed for 1 year.
         ○—○ = Cumulative percentages based on 94 subjects followed for 3 years.
         X—X = Cumulative percentages based on 44 subjects followed for 5 years.

TABLE 3

ASSOCIATION OF *H. INFLUENZAE* SEROTYPES WITH CLINICAL ILLNESS

	H. influenzae Cultures		Types Among Positives						
	Pos.	% Pos.	a	b	c	d	e	f	nt
III	341	40.8	10	47	3	17	15	9	233
Interim Illness	73	21.0	1	3	0	2	1	1	65
Not III	102	12.1	2	6	0	4	6	1	83
			(83)	(84)	(100)	(74)	(68)	(82)	(61)*
Degree of Illness									
Severe	38	44.2	1	3	0	3	1	2	26
Moderate	94	41.6	6	10	1	2	4	2	67
Mild	209	39.9	3	34	2	12	10	5	140

*   Numbers in parentheses are percentages of cultures of a given type isolated from children who were ill at time of cultures.

12

culture, are subclassified by severity of illness as severe, moderate, mild.[2] These percentages are all based on a relatively large number of cultures and, although the differences are small, they confirm an association between likelihood of a positive culture and severity of illness.

The right-hand side of Table 3 shows the results of typing of the positive cultures according to the illness classification. For each of the six types and the nontypable cultures, the percentage of cultures associated with illness is given in parentheses below. While 61% of the nontypable cultures were associated with illness, there were considerably higher percentages for typable strains. The difference between typable and nontypable cultures is highly significant, but the difference in percentages of cultures associated with illness for the six types is not. The percentage of cultures associated with illness is not significantly greater for type b than it is other identifiable types. Further, strains other than type b were associated with moderate and severe illness in a substantial number of instances.

OTITIS MEDIA

Of special interest to this conference are the culture results associated with acute otitis media. There were 155 observed episodes distributed among 68 of the 104 children in the study; 36 children had none; 26 had 1 episode; 22 had 2; 7 had 3; 7 had 4; 5 had 5; and 1 had 11 bouts. Twenty (29%) of the 68 subjects having otitis media accounted for 55% (85/155) of the episodes.

Figure 4 shows the culture results at time of otitis media by age. *H. influenzae* was identified in nasopharyngeal cultures in 43.2% (67/155) of the observed episodes. Of the positive cultures, only 28% (19/67) were typable, with 9% (6/67) being type b. All types except type c were identified, types b and e being the most common. During the first six months of life, *H. influenzae* was identified in only one fourth of the episodes of otitis media; during the second half year of life, 40%; and in the second, third, and fourth years of life, over half of the cases.

DISCUSSION

Our hope for immunoprophylaxis with capsular polyribophosphate from *H. influenzae*, type b, makes important any information which relates to infections

2. Definition of illness:

Mild $T = < 101°$ F. coryza, cough and/or conjunctivitis
Moderate $T = 101°$ to $103°$ F. with coryza, severe cough, and/or otitis media
Severe $T = 104°$ or greater and/or septicemia, meningitis, or pneumonia
Acute otitis = coryza and temperature $101°$ associated with bright red, bulging, or pearly
   media   tympanic membranes

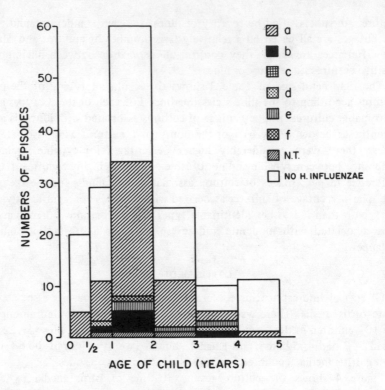

Fig. 4. Culture results at time of otitis media.

with this strain. The finding that type b was rarely isolated in the present longitudinal study from children under one year of age, the period of the most frequent sampling, is interesting. It was identified with increasing frequency thereafter up through the fourth year of life. These findings would indicate that natural immunization is delayed and that the artificial program should be started early in infancy.

Types a, c, d, e, and f were all isolated in significant numbers during the study, but type d was the most common type identified during the first year of life. It has been considered to be rare by some workers (Turk, Green, 1964).* However, in our experience, type d may not be stable, and promptness in typing is rewarded. Our routine primary cultures in Levinthal's agar, from which typical, irridescent colonies could be selected directly for typing, permitted

*D. C. Turk, 1972: personal communicaton.

identification from the first transfer. All types other than type b were associated with illness to the same degree as type b (see Table 3).

The significance of nontypable strains is not clear. However, if spontaneous mutations or transformations by suitable DNA could occur, *in vivo*, as suggested by Alexander, Leidy, and Hahn (1954), the large representation of these organisms might be more important than is now appreciated.

The nasopharyngeal cultures at time of otitis media are of interest in that type b was the msot prominent type-specific strain, even though the great majority of isolates were nontypable. We did not have simultaneous tympanocentesis cultures, but it is true that most of the patients came early in the course of their acute otitis, the period when the correlation is highest,* for identification of *H. influenzae* in both sites.

CONCLUSION

A longitudinal study of children followed from birth to 5 years of age with periodic nasopharyngeal cultures showed that 50% acquired the *H. influenzae* before age 6 months and all by age 5 years. Type b, the most frequently identified type, was rare before one year of age; less than 15% of the children had acquired it by age 2 and 38.5% by 5 years. All six types were identified at various ages, although the great majority of the strains were nontypable.

Cultures taken during episodes of illness yielded isolates of *H. influenzae* in 40.8%, while those from well children yielded this agent in 12.1% of episodes. Types b, d, and e, as well as nontypable strains, were associated with high illness rates.

There were 155 episodes of acute otitis media during the study. *H. influenzae*, in nasopharyngeal cultures, was associated with 43.2%. Of the strains of *H. influenzae*, 9% were type b. The great majority were nontypable.

*Virgil Howie, 1972: personal communication.

REFERENCES

Alexander, H. E. 1968. *"Hemophilus influenzae* Infections." In *Biologic Basis of Pediatric Practice,* edited by Robert E. Cook and Sidney Levin. New York: McGraw-Hill Book Co.

Harris, A. H., and M. B. Coleman. 1963. "Diagnostic Procedures and Reagents. Techniques for the Laboratory Diagnosis and Control of the Communicable Diseases." 4th edition. New York: American Public Health Assoc., Inc.

Pfeiffer, R. 1892. "Vorlaufige Mittheilungen uber die erreger der influenza." *Deutsche Med. Wchnschr.* 18:28.

Pittman, Margaret. 1931. "Variation and Type Specificity in Bacterial Species of *H. influenzae.*" *J. Exp. Med.* 53:471.

Sell, Sarah H. W. 1970. "The Clinical Importance of *Hemophilus influenzae* Infections in Children." *Ped. Clin. N.A.* 17:415.

Sell, Sarah H. W.; William J. Cheatham; B. Young; K. Welch. 1963. "*Hemophilus influenzae* in Respiratory Infections: I. Typing by Immuno-fluorescent Techniques." *Amer. J. Dis. Child.* 105:466.

Turk, D. C., and C. A. Green. 1964. "Measurement of Antibodies Reacting with Capsular Antigens of *Hemophilus influenzae.*" *J. Clin. Path.* 17:294.

Turk, David C., and J. Robert May. 1967. *Hemophilus influenzae: Its Clinical Importance.* London: The English Universities Press.

CHAPTER 2

Studies on *Hemophilus influenzae* Isolated from Otitis Media

Rachel Schneerson
J. B. Robbins
J. C. Parke, Jr.

Otitis media is a common disease in infants and in children. *Hemophilus influenzae* comprises 20% to 30% of the bacteria cultured from middle-ear exudates (Coffey, 1966; Gronroos et al., 1964; Dysart, 1967). Encapsulated *H. influenzae* organisms are classified into six groups according to their capsular polysaccharides. Those not possessing a detectable capsular polysaccharide by serological techniques are considered "nontypable." In cases of otitis media not associated with meningitis, most of the *H. influenzae* organisms were found to be nontypable (Bjuggren, Tunevall, 1952; Halsted et al., 1968), whereas the type b organisms are the etiological agent in most serious diseases caused by *H. influenzae* (Alexander, 1965; Turk and May, 1967).

The change from smooth to rough organisms which accompanies the loss of detectable type specificity occurs in the laboratory under unfavorable growth conditions, including incubation in-vitro with type-specific serum, as first noted by Dr. M. Pittman (1931). It has been recently suggested that some nontypable organisms may have lost most of their original capsule but may still be identified by more sensitive methods than the usual typing methods, such as by specific fluorescent antibody (Sell et al., 1968; Catlin, 1970).

This study of middle ear isolates of *H. influenzae* was undertaken in an attempt to study their type specificity by more sensitive methods and to search for additional antigens that would permit subgrouping of these bacteria. The organisms studied were 75 *H. influenzae* isolates collected from middle ear exudates by Dr. J. C. Parke, Jr., and two strains donated by Dr. Harry Feldman.

This work was done at the Developmental Immunology Branch of the National Institute of Child Health and Human Development, NIH, Bethesda, Maryland, and at the Department of Pediatrics, Charlotte Memorial Hospital, Charlotte, North Carolina.

13

14   *Hemophilus influenzae*

RESULTS

The age distribution of the patients in this study (see Fig. 1) is similar to that of bacterial and nonbacterial otitis media as found by other workers (Coffey, 1966; Gronroos et al., 1964; Halsted et al., 1968). This age distribution has a similar pattern to that of *H. influenzae*, type b, meningococcal and pneumococcal meningitis in infancy and childhood, indicating that acquired immunity to otitis media may occur (Fothergill and Wright, 1933; Goldschneider, Gotschlich, and Artenstein, 1969; Jonsson and Alvin, 1971). Anatomic factors,

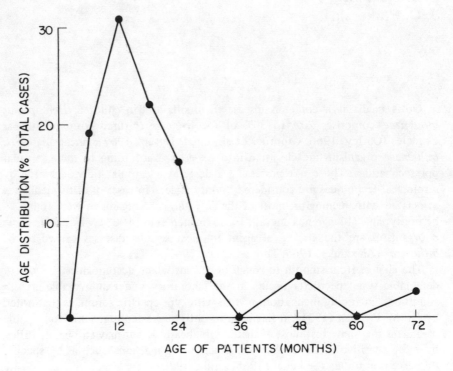

Fig. 1. Age distribution of patients with *Hemophilus influenzae* isolates from purulent otitis media.

such as obstruction of the Eustachian tubes, are commonly believed to be the basis for the high frequency of otitis media in infants and in children (Proctor, 1972). The age distribution of patients with otitis media, including those instances due to *H. influenzae*, suggests that lack of immunity may also be an important factor in the pathogenesis of this disease.

Of the 75 isolates examined in this study, only six (8%) were diagnosed as type b organisms by slide agglutination. Two of these were isolated from patients having had concomitant *H. influenzae*, type b, meningitis.

All of the 75 middle-ear organisms were tested by the antiserum agar technique (Petri, 1932; Bradshaw et al., 1971). The bacteria were streaked onto Levinthal agar plates into which *H. Influenzae*, type b, antiserum had been incorporated. Following incubation for 24 hours at 37° C, a halo forms (usually, not only at that time) around the individual *H. Influenzae*, type b, colonies due to the precipitation of the antiserum with the type b capsular antigen released into the media by the growing bacteria (Fig. 2). Halos of precipitation were observed around the six type b organisms; none were seen in the remaining 69 isolates.

Ten of these nontypable strains of *H. influenzae* were investigated more extensively for small amounts of the type b polysaccharide and also for other type-specific antigens. Immunodiffusion analysis was done on whole bacteria,

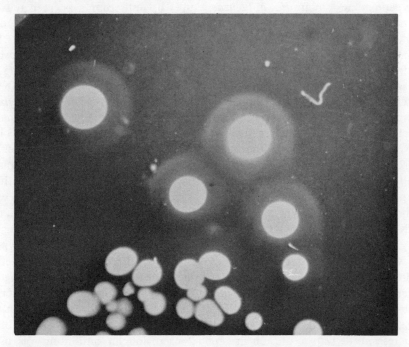

Fig. 2. *Hemophilus influenzae,* type b, grown on Levinthal-*Hemophilus influenzae*, type b, antiserum agar. Surrounding the individual bacterial colonies are "halos" formed by the precipitation of the type b polysaccharide antigen released into the media containing antiserum. Other encapsulated *H. influenzae* types (*a, c, d, e,* and *f*) do not yield this halo reaction with type b antiserum.

using either a six-hour growth in Levinthal media, or a suspension of a single colony in 0.1 ml of saline. The bacteria were reacted against the six *H. influenzae* typing antisera and no lines of precipitation were observed.

The ten nontypable middle-ear organisms were grown at 37° C to stationary phase in Levinthal broth. A polysaccharidelike material was obtained from the culture fluid by precipitation with cetyltrymethylammonium bromide (Cetavlon), reprecipitation with alcohol, and deproteinization with phenol. The yield of this material was very low: 2 to 3 mg per liter of culture fluid, as compared to about 20 mg of the type b polysaccharide (Strain "Rab"). These polysaccharidelike materials were reacted in concentration of 3 mg/ml with the *H. influenzae* typing sera in an immunodiffusion plate. No precipitation was observed. This serologic technique is capable of detecting 10 to 50 μg/ml of the type a, b, and d polysaccharides used as reference standards.

The ten middle-ear organisms were also tested for the type b polysaccharide reactivity with a fluorescent derivative of rabbit *H. influenzae* type b antibody. Hyperimmune rabbit *H. influenzae*, type b, antiserum was prepared by intravenous injection of whole encapsulated organisms (Strain "Rab") according to a published method (Alexander, Leidy, and McPherson, 1946). The fluorescent derivative was prepared by the method of Cebra and Goldstein (1965). The type b antibody concentration of the serum used for preparing the reagent was 2.8 mg/ml, and the final concentration of the fluorescent antibody used was 1.5 mg/ml of protein. Only one of the ten nontypable *H. influenzae*, Strain "Bar", did not react with this reagent (Table 1). The other nine organisms yielded faint but definite reactions with the fluorescent reagent. That this low level of fluorescence was due to non-type b antigens shared by other *H. influenzae*, was shown by the persistence of the reactivity of the nine organisms following complete absorption of the fluorescent antibody with the purified type b polysaccharide. Following absorption of the fluorescent antibody with whole *H. influenzae*, type a, organisms, the reactions with strains R.L., C.J., and S.K. were no longer observed. To remove all reactivity to the remaining six organisms, the fluorescent reagent had to be absorbed with *H. influenzae*, type f, as well. *H. influenzae*, type b, strain "Rab," yielded a bright, intense reaction with an unabsorbed reagent. Upon staining with the double absorbed reagent, there was a very slight diminution in the intensity of the staining. Absorption of the fluorescent reagent with type b organisms abolished all reactivity with the nontypable as well as the typable *H. influenzae*. As another control, a fluorescent derivative of human alpha-2-macroglobulin antiserum was used. There was no fluorescence using this fluorochrome with any of the organisms, under identical conditions of incubation and concentration of protein antibody.

Further to test the possibility that the type b or other type-specific polysaccharide was present in these organisms in concentrations too low to

TABLE 1

REACTION OF *HEMOPHILUS INFLUENZAE* NONTYPABLE EAR ORGANISMS
WITH FLUORESCENT *H. INFLUENZAE,* type b, ANTIBODY

Organism	Intensity of fluorescence (0-4+)		
	Unabsorbed	Absorbed with *H. influenzae* A	Absorbed with *H. influenzae* A+E
"Rab"	4	4	4
S.K.	0-1	0	0
C.J. R. Ear	0-1	0	0
L. Ear	0-1	0	0
NP	0-1	0	0
R.L.	0-1	0	0
R.Q. R. Ear	1-2	0-1	0
L. Ear	1-2	0-1	0
Bar.	0	0	0
Ch.S.	0*	0-1	0
H.L.	2	1	±
E.C.	1	0-1	0
Wi.	1-2	0-1	0
Sch.	0*	0-1	0

* A few organisms on each slide showed 1-2+ fluorescence upon
repeated examination.

permit detection by the previous methods, as well as to identify other antigenic components that could be used to distinguish the middle-ear organisms, antiserum against the ten middle-ear organisms was raised by intravenous injection of rabbits with *whole* formalinized bacteria. The resultant antisera reacted by precipitation in immunodiffusion plates with the homologous organisms but did not react against purified type b, a, and d, *H. influenzae* capsular polysaccharides. The levels of type b antibodies in these rabbits as measured by radioimmunoassay were within the low, natural range of unimmunized rabbits (0.23–1.95 µg/ml).

In another experiment devised to test the possibility that nontypable *H. influenzae* may represent rough variants of encapsulated organisms, it was attempted to reconstitute type-specific polysaccharide synthesis of the nontypable *Hemophili* by animal passage. This technique resulted in increased synthesis of other capsular polysaccharides such as *D. pneumoniae* (McLeod, 1972). Two strains of *H. influenzae* were used for these experiments: strain "Bar," which had no demonstrable reaction with the fluorescent antibody; and strain H.L., which had a relatively bright reactivity with the unabsorbed antibody. Both organisms were passed by intraperitoneal injection with gastric mucin, in two- to three-weeks-old mice, eight consecutive times. The LD 50 dose, which was 10^3 for strain "Bar" and 5×10^3 for H.L., was used for each passage. The organisms were isolated by culturing heart blood upon death or from live animals 48 hours after injection. The organisms recovered throughout the eight passages did not reveal the type b polysaccharide on antiserum agar plates. Following several animal passages, the colonies of the recovered bacteria seemed larger and smoother than the original. The type b and other type-specific polysaccharides were looked for by reacting saline suspensions of the bacteria recovered from the mice against the six *H. influenzae* typing sera. Following the fourth passage, multiple precipitin bands were observed between the bacterial suspensions and several of the typing sera. These bands were due to non-type-specific polysaccharide antigens as the antisera reacted in lines of nonidentity when the bacteria were tested next to purified polysaccharide preparations of *H. influenzae,* type a, b, and f, respectively. To identify these non-type-specific antigens in the bacteria isolated from animal passage as well as in the other eight middle-ear organisms, very dense bacterial suspensions were used. When reacted with the six typing sera, several patterns of precipitation were observed. Four *H. influenzae* ear organisms showed the same pattern of precipitation as shown in Figure 3. Three other patterns were seen among the remaining organisms. The difference between the most common and another pattern is shown in Figure 4.

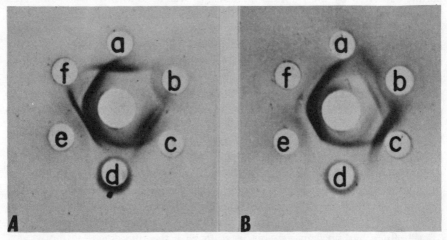

Figs. 3 and 4. Immunodiffusion analysis of whole bacterial suspensions of *Hemophilus influenzae* isolated from ear exudates. The central wells contain bacterial suspensions from (1) R.Q.R. ear and (2) Ch.S. The outer wells contain rabbit antiserum produced by intra-venous injection of representative *H. influenzae,* types *a, b, c, d, e,* and *f.*

Other investigators (Platt, 1937; Omland, 1964) have studied the multiple antigenic components of *H. influenzae* including nontypable organisms. The conclusion from their studies was that there was too varied an antigenic composition of noncapsular antigens to be useful in categorizing of *H. influenzae* organisms. However, this technique, using only ten organisms, has suggested that there are similar antigenic patterns and that antigenic analysis may be possible. Further studies using a larger number of strains are in progress. Also in progress are attempts to purify these antigens, the study of which may also help to understand the age-related acquisition of immunity. If such relationships can be established, these antigens may perhaps be used to induce immunity to otitis media by active immunization.

REFERENCES

Alexander, H. E. 1965. "The Hemophilus Group." In *Bacterial and Mycotic Infections of Man*, edited by R. J. Dubos and J. G. Hirsch, p. 724. 4th edition. Philadelphia: J. C. Lippincott.

Alexander, H. E.; G. Leidy; and C. F. C. McPherson. 1946. "Production of Types *A, B, C, D*, and *F, H. influenzae*, Antibody for Diagnostic and Therapeutic Purposes." *J. Immunol.* 54:207.

Bjuggren, G., and G. Tunevall. 1952. "Otitis Media in Childhood: A Clinical and Sero-bacteriological Study with Special Reference to the Significance of *Hemophilus influenzae* in Relapses." *Acta Otolaryng.* 42:311.

Bradshaw, M. W.; R. Schneerson; J. C. Parke, Jr.; and J. B. Robbins. 1971. "Bacterial Antigens Cross-Reactive with the Capsular Polysaccharide of *Hemophilus influenzae*, type b." *Lancet* 1:1095.

Catlin, B. W. 1970. "*Hemophilus influenzae* in Cultures of Cerebrospinal Fluid. Noncapsulated Variants Typable by Immunofluorescence." *Am. J. Dis. Child.* 120:203.

Cebra, J. J., and G. Goldstein. 1965. "Chromatographic Purification of Tetra-methylrhodamine-Immunoglobulin Conjugates and their Use in the Cellular Localization of Rabbit Gamma-globulin Polypetide Chains." *J. Immunol.* 95:230.

Coffey, John D., Jr. 1966. "Otitis Media in the Practice of Pediatrics: Bacteriological and Clinical Observations." *Peds.* 38:25.

Dysart, B. 1967. "Otitis Media and Complications." *Arch. Otolaryng.* 86:472.

Fothergill, L. D., and J. Wright. 1933. "The Relation of Age Incidence to the Bactericidal Power of Blood against the Casual Organism." *J. Immunol.* 24:273.

Goldschneider, I.; E. C. Gotschlich; and M. Artenstein. 1969. "Human Immunity to Meningococcus: I. The Role of Humoral Antibodies." *J. Exp. Med.* 129: 1307.

Gronroos, J. A.; A. E. Kortekangas; Leo Ojala; and M. Vouri. 1964. "The Aetiology of Acute Middle-Ear Infection." *Acta Otolaryng.* 58:149.

Halsted, C.; M. L. Lepow; N. Balassanian; J. Emmerich; and E. Wolinsky. 1968. "Otitis Media. Clinical Observations, Microbiology, and Evaluation of Therapy." *Am. J. Dis. Child.* 115:542.

Jonsson, M., and A. Alvin. 1971. "A Twelve-Year Review of Acute Bacterial Meningitis in Stockholm." *Scand. J. Infect. Disc.* 3:141.

McLeod, C. M. 1971. "The Pneumococci." In *Bacterial and Mycotic Infections of Man,* edited by R. J. Dubos and J. G. Hirsch, p. 396. Philadelphia: J. B. Lippincott.

Omland, T. 1964. "Serological Studies on *Hemophilus influenzae* and Related Species." *Acta. Path. Microbiol. Scand.* 62:89.

Petri, G. F. 1932. "A Specific Precipitin Reaction Associated with the Growth on Agar Plates of Meningococcus, Pneumococcus, and *B. Dysenteriae.* (Shiga)." *Br. J. Exp. Path.* 13:380.

Pittman, M. 1931. "Variation and Type Specificity in the Bacterial Species *Hemophilus influenzae.*" *J. Exp. Med.* 53:471.

Platt, A. E. 1937. "A Serological Study of *Hemophilus influenzae* and Related Species." *Acta. Path. Microbiol. Scand.* 62:89.

Proctor, B. 1972. "Etiology of Otitis Media." In *Otitis Media: Proceedings of the National Conference, Callier Hearing and Speech Center, Dallas, Texas,* edited by A. Gloric and K. C. Gerwin. Springfield, Illinois: Charles C. Thomas.

Sell, S. H. W.; W. J. Chatam; B. Young; and K. Welch. 1968. *"Hemophilus influenzae* in Respiratory Infections." *Am. J. Dis. Child.* 105:78.

Turk, D. C., and R. L. May. 1967. *Hemophilus influenzae: Its Clinical Importance.* London: English Universities Press.

CHAPTER **3**

Hemophilus influenzae Isolated from Children with Otitis Media

A. Lynn Harding
Porter Anderson
Virgil M. Howie
John H. Ploussard
David H. Smith

The availability of a nontoxic immunogen that stimulates the production of antibody activity in children (Peter, Anderson, and Smith, 1972) and adults (Anderson, Johnston, and Smith, 1972; Scheerson et al., 1971) has raised the possibility that active immunization might provide resistance against *Hemophilus influenzae,* type b, diseases. On the basis of previous studies of bacteria isolated from middle-ear exudates, it is known that *H. influenzae* is the second most common cause of childhood otitis media, producing up to 34% of cases. The state and type of encapsulation of the otitis *H. influenzae* has not been frequently evaluated, but most have been reported to be nontypable, while only 5 to 8% have been type b (Table 1). These findings differ strikingly from those reported for *H. influenzae* isolated from systemic lesions, in which essentially all isolates are type b. Since the antibody activity produced by PRP is bactericidal and opsonic for type b, but not for other *H. influenzae* types, it seemed important to re-evaluate the role of type b organisms in otitis media. Accordingly, the state of encapsulation of the *H. influenzae* isolated from middle-ear exudates and, in some instances, isolated from the nasopharynx of young children with otitis media in Huntsville, Alabama, has been studied.

This project is supported by Research Grant CC00511 from the Center for Disease Control, Atlanta, Georgia, and by Contract 71-2196 from the National Institute of Allergy and Infectious Diseases, Bethesda, Maryland.

21

TABLE 1

LITERATURE REVIEW OF BACTERIOLOGIC STUDIES OF
MIDDLE-EAR EXUDATES

Author	Year	No. of Cultures	*H. influenzae* (%)	*H. influenzae* Type b (%)	Location
Lahikainen	1951	--	3	--	Literature Review
Nielson	1945	811	16	--	Denmark
Bjuggren & Tunevall	1950	178	8	--	Sweden
Bjuggren & Tunevall	1952	131	17	--	Sweden
Lahikainen	1953	734	15	--	Finland
Mortimer & Watterson	1956	68	13	7.6	Ohio
VanDishoeck et al.	1959	306	34	--	Netherlands
Jones	1960	57	∿30	--	Iowa
Gronroos et al.	1964	563	18	5.9	Finland
Feingold et al.	1966	90	14	--	Massachusetts
Coffey	1966	267	27	--	Mississippi
Coffey et al.	1967	698	27	--	Mississippi
Dadswell	1967	113	16	--	England
Halsted et al.	1968	106	18	5	Ohio
Nilson et al.	1969	306	25	--	Maryland
Howie et al.	1970	858	24	--	Alabama

MATERIALS AND METHODS

Children of 3 years of age or younger with symptomatic, exudative otitis media were studied. Middle-ear exudate was collected as described previously (Howie and Ploussard,1969) and plated on appropriate bacteriological media in Huntsville. Isolates that appeared to be *H. influenzae* were tested for requirement of X and V factors for growth; each of several colonies of positive cultures were picked and streaked on a single chocolate agar slant and mailed to Boston. In some cases, a culture of the patient's nasopharynx was also performed in parallel; direct smears of certain of the middle-ear exudates were prepared on slides in a manner suitable for study by the fluorescent antibody method. In Boston, all cultures were subcultured on supplemented Brain Heart Infusion (BHI) agar (Anderson, Johnston, and Smith, 1972); several colonies were picked after an overnight incubation at $37°$ C and suspended in phosphate-buffered saline (PBS) to give $\sim 10^9$ organisms/ml. This suspension was used for slide agglutination tests and the preparation of subcultures in broth and solidified, supplemented BHI medium.

For slide agglutination, 0.01 ml of suspension was mixed at room temperature with antisera to each of six types of encapsulated *H. influenzae* (Massachusetts Biological Laboratories) and examined for macroscopic agglutination.

The growth of the second supplemented BHI agar subculture was resuspended in 0.2 ml sterile skim milk and stored in screw-cap vials at -70° C. (Subcultures are prepared from this stock by removing small aliquots of the frozen contents and plating on supplemented BHI agar. In our experience, this has been the simplest and most satisfactory method for prolonged storage of *H. influenzae.*)

An aliquot of the broth subculture was removed after 4 to 6 hours of agitated incubation in a 37° C water bath, centrifuged, and after the supernatant was removed, a portion of the cells was resuspended in 0.5 ml water. A loopful of this suspension was applied to a meticulously clean slide, air-dried, and fixed in absolute methanol for 10 minutes and stored at 4° C until stained. Type b specific rabbit serum with a hemagglutination titer of 1:64,000 was first absorbed with a PRP deficient *H. influenzea*, type b, strain to remove somatic antibodies and then conjugated by the method of Catlin and Tartagni, (1969). The gamma globulins were precipitated with saturated ammonium sulfate, removed by centrifugation, re-dissolved in PBS, and dialyzed overnight against 1/100 v/v PBS. Fluorescein isothiocyanate in carbonate buffer in saline, pH 9.5, was added to the dialysate at a concentration of 0.025 mg/mg protein and stirred 2 to 3 hours at 24° C. The protein-dye mixture was put onto a G25 Sephadex column and eluted with PBS. The leading three fourths of the first color peak was pooled and concentrated with polyethylene glycol to 25% original pool volume and stored at -20° C. Direct staining technique was employed. The conjugate was titered and tested with heterologous and blocked and unblocked homologous antigens. Test slides were coated with the conjugate, incubated at 37° C in a moist chamber for 30 minutes, washed in PBS 10 minutes, rinsed in distilled water, dried, and mounted with buffered glycerine. All slides were read on a Zeiss Fluorescent microscope, with a dark-field condensor, Osram HBO200 lamp, and BG38, BG12, 53/47 filters. No fluorescence was read as non-type b and a mixture of negative cells and cells with fluorescent embossments were read as probable type b.

Certain strains were also assayed for PRP by a hemagglutination inhibition method developed in this laboratory. An eighteen-hour broth culture (2.5×10^9 bacteria/ml) was sonified, centrifuged at 6,000 RPM for 10 minutes, and 25 μl of the supernatant fluid was incubated at 37° C for 30 minutes with a series of dilutions of rabbit anti-*H. influenzae,* type b, serum in microtiter trays; 25 μl of

PRP-sensitized sheep erythrocytes (Anderson, Johnston, and Smith, 1972) were added, mixed, and incubated at 37°C for 3 hours, at which time hemagglutination was read macroscopically. Supplemented BHI broth and 2.5 ng/ml PRP in supplemented BHI broth were run as the control. This method will detect as little as 2.5 ng of PRP/ml.

RESULTS

Of 300 *H. influenzae* isolates examined by agglutination, 249 were nontypable, 50 were type b, and 1 was type c. Of the 257 isolates examined by the HAI method, 229 were nontypable and 28 were type b. The FA technique gave results identical to those observed with the HAI method (Table 2). The false-positive results observed with agglutination almost certainly resulted from antibodies directed against somatic or noncapsular antigens of *H. influenzae*.

TABLE 2

H. INFLUENZAE ISOLATED FROM MIDDLE-EAR EXUDATES

Type	Agglutination	Typing Method HAI	FA
Nontypable	249	207	129
Not Done	------	42	120
Typable			
b	50	28	28
		22 Nontypable	22 Nontypable
c	1	ND	ND

The possibility that the organisms passed through the two subcultures were not representative of those causing the infection was evaluated by examining middle-ear exudate directly with anti-type b fluorescent antibody. In all but one of 49 specimens, the results of FA tests on the exudate were identical to those of the subcultured bacteria (Table 3).

Typable *H. influenzae* may "dissociate" *in vitro* to nonencapsulated strains. In order to determine whether the *H. influenzae* recovered from the inflammatory exudate in the middle ear have "dissociated" *in vivo* from type b strains, organisms isolated simultaneously from the nasopharynx and the middle ear were typed by the FA technique. *H. influenzae* were recovered from 44 paired naso-

TABLE 3

H. INFLUENZAE, type b, ISOLATED FROM OR DETECTED BY FA IN
MIDDLE-EAR EXUDATES

No. of Specimens	Exudates	Corresponding Isolates
2	b	b
1	Probable b	Non-b
46	Non-b	Non-b

pharyngeal and middle-ear exudate cultures. Four of the nasopharyngeal isolates were type b; three of the corresponding exudate isolates were type b; and the fourth was nontypable. The remaining paired nasopharyngeal and middle-ear isolates were nonencapsulated.

A review of the clinical records indicated that 40 of the children in this series (22%) had 76 recurrences of *H. influenzae* otitis, defined as a symptomatic, culture-proven episode separated by two weeks or more from an initial culture-proven, antibiotic-treated episode. Most of the children had only a single recurrence during the study period, but three children had four recurrences, and three had five separate episodes of *H. influenzae,* otitis. Nontypable bacteria generally caused the initial and subsequent infections. However, in four instances, infection caused by nontypable *H. influenzae* was followed by type b otitis; in four, type b otitis occurred after a previous type b otitis. Four of the 300 infections were followed by, or associated with, meningitis or septicemia. All four of these infections were caused by type b strains. Thus, four of 28, or 14% of type b middle-ear infections involved systemic infections.

DISCUSSION

The comparison of HAI and other typing methods indicates that *H. influenzae* can be typed accurately by slide agglutination or direct fluorescent antibody methods if properly prepared antisera are used. Typing serum must have a high titer of anticapsular antibodies and should be absorbed to remove antibodies directed against somatic antigens. Nonabsorbed serum will produce false positive results with nontypable *H. influenzae* that share somatic antigens with encapsulated types.

This study supports and extends earlier observations that most *H. influenzae* isolated from middle-ear exudates are nontypable. The selection and study of multiple colonies and the direct analysis of exudate by the fluorescent antibody method guaranteed that our observations were made from at least a majority population of *H. influenzae* in the exudate. Existing data therefore indicate that nonencapsulated *H. influenzae* are primary pathogens in otitis media. It is noteworthy that in parallel studies in the same patient population, nearly all pneumococci isolated from middle-ear exudates were encapsulated (Howie et al., 1972).

We, and others, have considered the possibility that nonencapsulated *H. influenzae* may be selected from encapsulated parent bacteria during the infection. The number of paired nasopharyngeal and exudate isolates studied were small, but our studies provide no support for this proposal. Furthermore, rough, agglutination-negative mutants isolated from the type b strains studied *in vitro* produce enough PRP to be detected by HAI (Anderson, Johnston, and Smith, 1972) and our fluorescent antibody (Anderson and Harding, unpublished data). Thus, the nontypable *H. influenzae* from middle-ear exudate differ from these isolated in the laboratory. These unpublished observations also raise questions about the absolute state of PRP production of the laboratory "variants" of encapsulated *H. influenzae*, which have been classically described to be nontypable and to have arisen by dissociation.

The frequency of repeated bouts of otitis media with *H. influenzae* emphasize the current paucity of information regarding host resistance to this disease, the immunogenicity of middle-ear infections, and the antigenic composition of nonencapsulated *H. influenzae* and the relationship of such antigens to those of encapsulated strains. Currently, we are analyzing acute and convalescent sera of these children and have initiated studies of the antigenic composition of nonencapsulated *H. influenzae* isolated from middle-ear exudate in an attempt to answer certain of these questions.

Finally, this study quantitates the concept, widely held but undocumented, that the child with type b otitis media is at high risk from systemic disease.

SUMMARY

H. influenzae isolated from middle-ear exudate of children with symptomatic otitis media were typed by agglutination, direct fluorescent antibody, and hemagglutination-inhibition methods. (Typing serum gave false positive results unless absorbed to remove antibodies directed against antisomatic antigens.) Ninety percent of the isolates were nontypable and 9% were type b. Direct studies of ear exudate with fluorescent antibody to PRP and typing of paired isolates from the nasopharynx and middle ear support the proposal that nonencapsulated *H. influenzae* are primary pathogens in otitis media. Review of clinical records indicated that 22% of the children had recurrent *H. influenzae* otitis, some of whom had multiple attacks. Of children with type b otitis, 14% had systemic infections.

REFERENCES

Anderson, P.; R. B. Johnston, Jr.; and D. H. Smith. 1972. "Human Serum Activities against *Hemophilus influenzae,* type b." *J. Clin. Invest.* 51:31.

Bjuggren, G., and G. Tunevall. 1950. "The Pfeiffer Bacillus in Otitis in Children: A Serobacteriological and Clinical Study." *Acta Otolaryng.* 38:130.

——— 1952. "Otitis in Childhood. A Clinical and Serobacteriological Study with Special Reference to the Significance of *Hemophilus influenzae* in Relapses." *Acta Otolaryng.* 42:311.

Catlin, B. W., and V. R. Tartagni. 1969. "Delayed Multiplication of Newly Capsulated Transformants of *Hemophilus influenzae* Detected by Immuno-fluorescence." *J. Gen. Microbiol.* 56:387.

Coffey, J. D., Jr. 1966. "Otitis Media in the Practice of Pediatrics: Bacteriological and Clinical Observations." *Ped.* 38:25.

Coffey, J. D., Jr.; A. D. Martin; and H. N. Booth. 1967. "Neisseria catarrhalis in Exudate Otitis Media." *Arch. Otolaryng.* 86:403.

Dadswell, J. V. 1967. "Bacteriological Findings in Acute Otitis Media. *Lancet* 1:243.

Feingold, M.; J. O. Klein; G. E. Haslam; J. G. Tilles; M. Finland; and S. S. Gellis. 1966. "Acute Otitis Media in Children: Bacteriological Findings in Middle Ear Fluid Obtained by Needle Aspiration." *Am J. Dis. Child.* 111:361.

Gronroos, J. A.; A. E. Kortekangas; L. Ojala; and M. Vvori. 1964. "The Aetiology of Acute Middle Ear Infections." *Acta Otolaryng.* 58:149.

Halsted, C.; M. L. Lepow; N. Balassanian; J. Emmerich; and E. Wolinsky. 1968. "Otitis Media: Clinical Observations, Microbiology, and Evaluation of Therapy." *Am. J. Dis. Child.* 115:542.

Howie, V. M., and J. H. Ploussard. 1969. "The 'In Vivo Sensitivity Test'—Bacteriology of Middle Ear Exudate during Antimicrobial Therapy in Otitis Media." *Ped.* 44:940.

Howie, V. M.; J. H. Ploussard; R. Austrian; A. J. Ammann; and R. B. Johnston. 1972. "Pneumococcal Serotypes and Antibody Responses in Otitis Media in Children." *Ped. Res.* 6:390.

Jones, M. 1960. "Comparison of Bacteria from Ear and Upper Respiratory Tract in Otitis Media." *Arch. Otolaryng.* 72:329.

Lahikainen, E. A. 1953. "Clinico-Bacteriologic Studies on Acute Otitis Media: Aspiration of Tympanum as a Diagnostic and Therapeutic Method." *Acta. Otolaryng. Suppl.* 107:1.

Laxdal, O. E.; R. M. Blake; T. Cartmill; and H. E. Robertson. 1966. "Etiology of Acute Otitis Media in Infants and Children." *Canad. Med. Assoc. J.* 94:159.

Mortimer, E. A., Jr., and R. L. Watterson, Jr. 1956. "Bacteriologic Investigation of Otitis Media in Infancy." *Ped.* 17:359.

Nielson, J. C. 1945. *Studies of Aetiology of Acute Otitis Media.* Copenhagen: Munksgaard.

Nilson, B. W.; R. L. Poland; R. S. Thompson; D. Morehead; A. Baghdassarian; and D. H. Carver. 1969. "Acute Otitis Media: Treatment Results in Relation to Bacterial Etiology." *Ped.* 43:351.

Peter, G.; P. Anderson; and D. H. Smith. 1973. "Immunization of Adults and Children with Polyribophosphate, the Capsular Antigen of *Hemophilus influenzae.*" Chapter 24, this volume.

Schneerson, R.; L. P. Rodriques; J. C. Parke; and J. B. Robbins. 1971. "Immunity to Disease Caused by *Hemophilus influenzae,* type b." *J. Immunol.* 107:1081.

VanDishoeck, H. A.; A. C. Derks; and R. Voorhorst. 1959. "Bacteriology and Treatment of Acute Otitis Media in Children." *Acta Otolaryng.* 50:250.

Discussion

David T. Karzon, Presiding

David T. Karzon: These three papers have set the stage and have indicated some of the problems of infection and disease. Efforts have been made in two laboratories, using much the same techniques, to find out whether the 90% of otitis and other noninvasive respiratory infections caused by nontypable strains represents infection with type b strains carrying a quantity of a capsular antigen which is not evident by ordinary techniques. It looks as if they have shown that these are, in fact, not type b strains. The floor is open for discussion.

Carl W. Norden: I would like to ask Miss Harding a question. I enjoyed the paper very much. You said that there were 50 isolates which typed as b by agglutination and only 28 by HAI. Was the agglutination test performed with absorbed sera or unabsorbed? Do you think there would have been only 28 if you had used absorbed serum?

A. Lynn Harding: The typing serum used was unabsorbed. If absorbed serum had been used, probably only the 28 strains would have been identified.

Sarah H. Sell: Did you try all six types of antisera at the same time?

Harding: Yes.

John B. Robbins: I would like to make two comments. First, there is a great variability of potency in typing sera that are commercially available. I make a plea that further attempts be made to have monospecific typing sera. Some are licensed products and some are very weak and have insignificant activity, and this should be appreciated. Second, I would like to make a plea for other laboratories to try to use the antiserum-agar techniques for surveys of *Hemophilus influenzae,* type b. There are limitations in its use in that the enrichment activity in the agar to sustain *Hemophilus influenzae* growth declines rather rapidly. Despite that limitation, it can be very helpful, because you can distinguish one organism from a mixed culture that yields this halo phenomenon and, therefore, obviates the necessity of scraping off each individual *Hemophilus* colony. I realize it is very expensive in terms of serum; but, at present, immunization of a large animal, such as a sheep or a burro, may not be more expensive than many small laboratory animals such as rabbits.

29

Sell: I would like to comment about typing. We found that, if the cultures which were taken from patients were typed using the first transfer, a higher percentage of type-specific strains could be identified than if multiple transfers took place. Many strains lost typability in 4 to 5 transfers. Types c and d were especially unstable, in our experience. In the instances where strains were identified in one center, then shipped to another for typing, I am afraid that many may have lost their type-specificity in the process. It would be far better to be able to type them promptly. The antiserum-agar method might help to simplify this problem. We have made our own typing sera being meticulous to use 6-hour cultures for antigens. After the first two weeks (3 injections per week) of formalin-killed bacterial suspensions, the rabbits subsequently received live bacteria freshly prepared immediately before use. Dr. Buddingh taught me to do this. Would you like to comment, Miss Leidy?

Grace Leidy: I found in this regard that conversion from S to R or mutation from S to R has varied with the strain. Some are very stable and some are unstable. Even in a few subcultures, one begins to see the intermediate types down to the nonirridescent type.

Sell: What is your experience with this, Dr. Buddingh?

G. John Buddingh: It should be emphasized that otitis media is essentially a surface infection. The sequence of events in its pathogenesis would explain why, in most instances, strains of *Hemophilus* are usually untypable at the time cultures are taken. These events can be followed in an experimental model following the introduction of *H. influenzae* on the surface of the chorio-allantoic membrane of 12- to 14-day-old embryonated eggs. In this environment, the micro-organisms proliferate rapidly and to prodigious numbers during the first 6 to 12 hours following initiation of the infection. During this time, which corresponds to the logarithmic phase in artificial culture, the majority of the microbial population is encapsulated and typable. This, however, is before much clinical manifestation is discernible. In the membranal infection, this period is marked by an inflammatory response leading to the accumulation of many phagocytes, macrophages, mononuclears, red cells, and thrombocytes on the membranal surface, in which the bacteria become enmeshed and for the most part segregated to the outer edges of the layer of exudate. Although considerable phagocytosis takes place, the majority of the bacterial population remains extracellular. The surface exudate usually functions as a barrier to the spread of the microbes into the underlying membranal tissue spaces and circulation. Degeneration of the inflammatory cells rapidly ensues, with coagulation, a shift to an acid pH, and eventual hyalinization. All of this occurs within 12 to 24 hours, creating an environment in which nutrients essential to maintaining virulence and/or capsules are dimished or absent. The majority, if not all, of the bacterial population is no longer encapsulated and thus untypable. This, in most instances, represents the state in the pathogenesis of this surface infection in which the clinical manifestations of otitis media are encountered. In some instances, in the experimental infection, the inflammatory exudate disintegrates instead of becoming hyaline, ulceration of ectodermal epithelium develops, and extension of proliferating bacteria into the membranal mesodermal intercellular fluids occurs, with invasion of the blood stream, followed by death of the embryo.

Leidy: In relation to some of the nontypable strains, this is sort of ancient history by now, but you may be interested in some of our early results. I worked with Dr. Hattie Alexander. We produced antisera to varied nontypable forms and tried to classify them by agglutination tests. We were unsuccessful in getting any indication of types. When we got into transformation and tried to convert many of those strains into typable strains, we were unsuccessful, even though we were able to confer streptomycin resistance in those populations which were competent. I'll tell you the history of one patient with type b meningitis. He was treated with streptomycin and subsequently relapsed. Type b, resistant to over 1,000 micrograms/ml, was isolated from the spinal fluid. The patient was subsequently cured with sulfonamide therapy. The interesting point was that, after the meningitis, *H. influenzae,* type b, resistant to streptomycin, of equally high degree was isolated from his nasopharynx. Subsequently a nontypable form up to a period of nine months, at several-month intervals, was isolated, but no type b was identified. Then we tried transformation. We took the culture, which we will call Rb, and tried transforming it, because we noted that, if we took an R strain from type b and exposed it to the six DNA containing fractions of all six types, we could transform Rb rarely to an ab type and readily to types b, c, and d. This was working with R strains derived from several type b's. If we used our Rd strain, we could transform it to all six types. Therefore, we took the nontypable strain from the patient and were able to transform it. It fitted the pattern of the Rb transformation experiments.

Sell: This is one of the reasons we were so interested in type d when we kept getting it from young children. This is a fascinating area, I think.

Virgil M. Howie: First, in regard to antibody impregnated plates, we tried that method about forty times. We found no halos when the plate was made directly from the ear exudate so that we were not able to increase our yield types. In connection with Dr. Buddingh's comment about the surface infection, we had 25 patients that had *H. influenzae* ear infections and were treated with a placebo consisting of kaopectate and tylenol. Over a four-day period, the *H. influenzae* failed to grow when the exudate was subsequently cultured. I think it is quite true that *H. influenzae,* perhaps, loses its capsule.

It certainly loses its viability with placebo treatment on occasion.

Roger A. Feldman: My comment does not relate to typing procedures, but rather to the population from which the cases were drawn. It is too easy to make generalizations from these three different samples about how much *H. influenzae* in untypable. As I understand it, Dr. Parke's isolates were probably from a group of black children in Charlotte, Dr. Howie's from a relatively poor county in Alabama, and I am not certain where Dr. Sell's families came from. I do not know that we can say that the frequency with which untypable isolates or type b isolates as found in otitis media in these three groups is going to be applicable to large groups elsewhere.

Karzon: An epidemiologist points out that his demographic outlook is important here.

Howie: The average income in Huntsville per family is $10,000. I am not too sure that is very poor.

Karzon: That portion of Alabama is special. Many studies show a high percentage of nontypable strains. The question raised is whether the proportion of nontypable strains in respiratory disease, and particularly otitis media, varies with socioeconomic circumstances.

Porter Anderson: I have a question for Dr. Buddingh. Do you think that the change you are seeing is from mutation and selection, or is this a change of phenotype? I just wondered whether, if the organisms are recultured and then typed, they still appear to be untypable. A second part of the question is, why is it that the inflammatory processes that go on are not active against the untypable or rough strains?

Buddingh: The inflammatory reaction is effective in overcoming the nonencapsulated (untypable) *Hemophilus.* It does not seem to me to involve mutation, but rather starvation. Were one able to obtain cultures within six to twelve hours after the infection started, most, if not all, of them would by typable. One gets involved here in the problem of the dynamics involving bacterial population composition as it relates to the relative proportion of virulent and avirulent elements.

Anderson: If one transferred bacteria to the Levinthal's agar from one of the membranes eight hours after the experiment started, would there be irridescent or nonirridescent colonies?

Buddingh: It is more likely that, if, from an untypable culture at this stage, either from the experimental or natural infection, 30 to 50 colonies (clones) were isolated in subculture on Levinthal's agar, a small proportion of them would produce irridescent colonies representative of the infecting strain.

Robbins: One problem is to decide whether the nontypable strains that cause otitis media are *Hemophilus* organisms that have lost their ability to synthesize capsules because of the host environment. This is a difficult problem to study, especially when one is studying the end product. Obviously, what is needed here is another genetically controlled marker which would permit identification of the type b organisms independent of the synthesis of polysaccharide. That marker is not currently available.

Karzon: Has anyone found any mixed cultures where individual clones of more than one potential are present?

Sell: Yes, we found types b and d in the same patient.

Karzon: Types b and d from the same ear? Same patient? Same NP culture?

Buddingh: Types b, d, e, and a. This would require subculturing many colonies and serotyping them. That is quite a task.

Karzon: The frequency of the individual types is sufficiently high that one would expect a certain incidence of two types (a nontypable and/or typable) which would give an opportunity for genetic exchange, I presume.

Buddingh: I have encountered an age-related sequence of infection with different types. Dr. Sell's experience with this is somewhat diffcrent from mine. We have the imprcssion that infection with type a precedes type d and then is followed by type b. I do not know exactly what this means, but I suspect it reflects the serological immune state of the adult population. It would be interesting to know, for instance, what proportion of adults have antibodies to type a, d, and others. I have no idea whether this would promote or prevent genetic exchange.

Sell: Did you find type a in very young children?

Buddingh: Yes, in those under 6 months of age—that is, from nasopharyngeal cultures.

Johnston: Dr. Buddingh's model is also an interesting one in regard to antibodies. What "chicken immunologists" call IgG is present early in fetal life, apparently from the mother. The ability to respond with antibodies, as I understand it, probably does not occur until about the time of hatching (day 20) or later. Thus, I guess what you are seeing here, Dr. Buddingh, is a full inflammatory response, including phagocytosis of encapsulated bacteria, with the aid of little if any specific antibody.

Buddingh: That is why the chick embryo provides such a good model for the study of the infectious process. In this, host reaction to and recovery from the infection takes place in the absence of conventional immunoglobulins.

Karzon: Would anybody like to discuss the other topic that has been mentioned? What is the relationship between non-b infection and disease? Are you implying on the basis of a temporal relationship that the non-b strains may cause disease?

Sell: All I can say is that the majority of our children were ill at the time we identified *H. influenzae.* Whether the bacteria were responsible for the illness, I am not prepared to say. Our data show the temporal relationship, however.

Howie: Children with non-b disease or with *H. influenzae,* any strain, in the middle ear may not be very ill as whole persons, but their ears are ill and the ears have exudate and pus in them. These children, as I have recorded previously, usually do not have much fever or pain, but they have an abnormal fluid in the middle ear, a localized disease. I think everybody here would like to say that they all come from type b because that would make it so simple, but I am not sure at all that that is true.

Buddingh: Types other than b very likely participate in the disease, but I rather doubt that they are effective by themselves. In my opinion, these are combined infections with bacteria superimposed on an initial virus infection; perhaps adenovirus or one of the parainfluenzas. I am not going into the problem of combined infections, but little children with respiratory illness will pick up any type under those circumstances.

Sell: We had a patient with type f meningitis recently. Type f was found in cultures of blood, cerebrospinal fluid, and tympanocentesis fluid. Types other than b do participate in the serious illnesses, but not very often. This has been known for many years, however.

Karzon: Although it's not one of Koch's postulates, I suppose that if one finds an organism in a parenteral site, it is certainly highly suspicious.

James C. Parke: I wonder what the relationship might be between the nasopharyngeal culture taken on the same side and the middle ear. It is my impression that when we culture type b from the nasopharynx, we recover type b from the middle ear at the same time. We very rarely see the type b from the ear without finding type b in the nasopharynx. I wonder if other people are finding this?

Buddingh: Yes, in general, that is so.

SECTION II

Detection of the Capsular Polysaccharide of *Hemophilus influenzae,* type b, in Body Fluids

David L. Ingram
Richard O'Reilly
Porter Anderson
David H. Smith

A number of species of encapsulated bacteria release soluble capsular antigen in the body fluids of the infected host. Immunologic detection of such antigens has been available for some decades as an adjuct to bacteriologic diagnosis. With *Hemophilus influenzae,* type b, there are some clinical situations in which detection of the polyribophosphate (PRP) capsular antigen would be of practical diagnostic use. In addition, a means for assay in body fluids will assist quantitation of the extent of antigenemia resulting from disease or immunization.

Alexander and associates (1958) layered test fluid onto antiserum and read a ring of visible precipitate at the interface as a positive result. This test is rapid and simple to perform. In our hands, its sensitivity is in the area of a few micrograms of PRP per ml of test fluid. We have therefore been evaluating two other techniques in search of greater sensitivity. The first, countercurrent immunoelectrophoresis (CIE), has recently been used to detect capsular polysaccharides in cerebrospinal fluid (CSF) or serum of patients with systemic

This work was done at the Infectious Disease Unit, Children's Hospital Medical Center, and Beth Israel Hospital, Department of Pediatrics, Harvard Medical School, Boston, Massachusetts.

Work was supported in part by Research Grant CC00511 from the Center for Disease Control, Atlanta, Georgia, and Training Grant T01-AI-00350 from the National Institute of Allergy and Infectious Diseases.

This paper is based on and includes much of the same material as that used by David L. Ingram, Porter Anderson, and David H. Smith in "Countercurrent Immunoelectrophoresis in the Diagnosis of Systemic Diseases Caused by *Hemophilus influenzae,* type b," *J. Ped.* 81 (1972):1156-1159 (submitted for publication before Nashville conference on *Hemophilus influenzae,* April 24-25, 1972).

meningococcal (Edwards, 1971; Greenwood, Whittle, and Dominic-Rajkovic, 1971) and pneumococcal (Dorff, Coonrod, and Rytel, 1971) diseases. The other, a latex-particle agglutination method, has been used to detect various types of antigens, including PRP (Newman, Stevens, and Gaafar, 1970).

METHODS

CSF, serum, subdural, and joint fluids were tested immediately after their collection or stored at -70°C until tested. CIE was performed with glass slides coated with 1% agarose in 0.075M sodium barbital buffer (pH 8.6). Wells 3 mm in diameter were cut in the agarose in parallel rows 6 mm apart. The well nearest the anode was filled with 0.005 ml of rabbit anti-*H. influenzae,* type b, serum and the well nearest the cathode was filled with 0.005 ml of the test fluid. The buffer system was 50mM sodium barbital (pH 8.6). After electrophoresis for 1½ hours at 4°C, 200 volts, and 30 milliamps, or at 25°C, 55 volts, and 11 milliamps, the agarose plate was examined in indirect light with a hand lens for the precipitin line which formed near the antibody well.

PRP concentrations in body fluids were determined by comparison with dilutions of purified antigen, which were mixed in normal body fluids of the same type (CSF or sera) being tested.

Cultures of *Diplococcus pneumoniae,* types 6, 15, and 29, and rabbit anti-*H. influenzae,* type b serum, prepared against strain Eagan and strain 62b, were obtained from Leslie H. Wetterlow, Biologic Laboratories, Massachusetts Department of Public Health. Sheep, burro, and three different preparations of rabbit and anti-*H. influenzae,* type b, strain Rab, sera and *Escherichia coli,* strain Easter and its purified capsular polysaccharide (EPS) from this strain were the gifts of Dr. John Robbins of the National Institute of Child Health and Human Development, Bethesda, Maryland. The purified PRP employed has been described previously (Anderson et al., 1971). *D. pneumoniae,* type 35, was obtained from the American Type Culture Collection, Rockville, Maryland. The supernatant fluid of overnight cultures of these organisms, grown in brain-heart infusion broth (BBL, Cockeysville, Maryland), were used as test fluids for CIE.

Anti-*H. influenzae,* type b, sera that cross-reacted with EPS or certain types of pnuemococci were absorbed (2 hours at 37°C and 48 hours at 4°C) with ten times the concentration of purified EPS that produced optimal precipitation, as determined by the method of Kabat (1967). The latex agglutination technique of Newman and colleagues (1970) was employed.

RESULTS

The sheep and burro sera migrated away from the antigen in CIE and therefore could not be used with these test conditions. Seven of the eight rabbit antisera tested reacted with PRP, but the sensitivity and specificity of the sera varied (Table 1). The least amount of PRP detected by the sera ranged from 30 to 1750 ng/ml. The sensitivity of the assay was identical for PRP diluted in buffer, normal CSF or serum. Since only 5 microliters of antigen solution was tested, as little as 150 pg of PRP could be detected by the best antisera.

TABLE 1

SENSITIVITY AND SPECIFICITY OF RABBIT ANTI-*HEMOPHILUS INFLUENZAE*, type b, SERUM IN CIE

Serum	Prepared vs. Strain	PRP (μg/ML) Detectable	Cross-Reactivity				
			Pneumo				E. Coli
			6	15	29	35	Easter
RI 9	6 2 B	0.03	0	0	0	0	+
H.A.	Rab	0.07	0	0	0	0	+
12	Rab	1.75	0	0	0	0	0
8A Com	Rab	0.35	0	0	+	0	+
8585	Eag	0.03	0	0	0	0	+
8547	Eag	0.03	0	0	0	0	0
Hyland	Rab	0.7	0	0	0	0	+
Difco	?	None (>170)	-	-	-	-	-

SOURCE: David L. Ingram, Porter Anderson, and David H. Smith, "Countercurrent Immunoelectrophoresis in the Diagnosis of Systemic Diseases Caused by *Hemophilus influenzae*, type b," *J. Ped.* 81 (1972): 1156-1159.

Pneumococcal polysaccharide types 6, 15, 29, and 35 (Alexander, 1958) and the K antigen of certain *Escherichia coli* (Bradshaw et al., 1971) have been reported to react with anti-*H. influenzae*, type b, serum. The cross-reactivities were thus looked for in CIE. Two of the rabbit antisera tested (one anti-Eag and one anti-Rab) did not react with antigens prepared from any of these "cross-reacting" bacteria; five of the sera (the anti-62b, one anti-Eag and 2 anti-Rab) reacted only with EPS, and one (anti-Rab) serum reacted with EPS and type 29 pneumococcal polysaccharide (Table 1).

J. B. Robbins* advised that the *E. coli* reactivity could be absorbed out with the purified EPS. Figure 1 shows the precipitin activity of rabbit serum RI 9 with EPS and with PRP. Absorption with either EPS or PRP eliminated all precipitin activity for the *E. coli* polymer. However, absorption with EPS reduced but did not eliminate the activity for PRP. The EPS absorption also eliminated the cross-reactivity with pneumococcus, type 29.

*1971: personal communication.

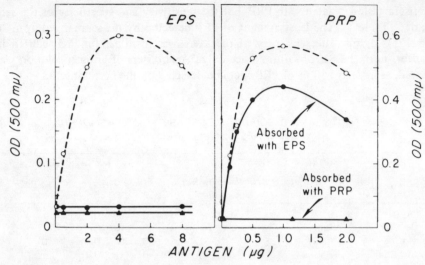

Fig. 1. Precipitin activity of rabbit serum RI 9.

One of the non-cross-reacting antisera, which detected as little as 30 ng PRP/ml, was used in the survey of clinical specimens (Table 2). No PRP was detected in the spinal fluid or serum of 41 children with fever and no meningitis, or in 12 children with aseptic meningitis. None was detected in 9 with culture-proven meningitis due to bacteria other than *H. influenzae,* type b; these were: pneumococci, two ; meningococci, four; group B streptococcus, one; and *Pseudomonas aeruginosa,* two.

TABLE 2

DETECTION OF PRP IN CSF AND/OR SERUM
BY COUNTERCURRENT IMMUNOELECTROPHORESIS

Clinical Diagnosis	No. of Patients	No. with PRP
Fever, no Meningitis	41	0
Aseptic Meningitis	12	0
Non-*H. Influenzae* Bacterial Meningitis	10	0
H. Influenzae, b Meningitis	14	11
Partially-treated Meningitis	10	4

SOURCE: David L. Ingram, Porter Anderson, and David H. Smith, "Countercurrent Immunoelectrophoresis in the Diagnosis of Systemic Diseases Caused by *Hemophilus influenzae,* type b," *J. Ped.* 81 (1972):1156-1159.

PRP was detected at the time of hospitalization in the spinal fluid or serum, or both, of 11 of the 14 children with culture-proven *H. influenzae*, type b, meningitis. Antigen concentrations in the spinal fluid ranged from 30 to 480 ng/ml and in sera from 30 to greater than 960 ng/ml.

CIE was positive in three children in whom the Gram stain of spinal fluid was negative, and the test was negative in one culture-proven case in which the Gram stain of the spinal fluid was reportedly positive. Follow-up samples were studied in two of these 14 patients: PRP was not detected in the serum of one child 15 hours after the onset of treatment with ampicillin (300 mg/kg/day), but it was still detectable in the serum of a second child 72 hours after the onset of the same therapy. Ten patients were studied who, prior to admission, had been treated for meningitis with antibiotics without a bacteriologic diagnosis (partially treated meningitis; see Table 2). PRP was detected in the serum or spinal fluid of four of the ten. The antigen was also detected in subdural fluid in two patients with culture-proven *H. influenzae,* type b, meningitis, and in the joint fluid of one patient with culture-proven septic arthritis.

More recently, we have begun to evaluate the latex agglutination method for assay of PRP in body fluids. In this method, the reaction of antibody and antigen is amplified for the eye by the addition of latex particles. The components are simply mixed at room temperature and read for agglutination after five minutes. Preliminary tests indicate that the method is much more sensitive than CIE. With the same antiserum that can detect 30 ng of PRP/ml, the latex test detects 1 ng/ml. The clinical specimens described above were retested with the second method. By the latex method, all 14 CSFs, culture positive for *H. influenzae,* type b, were positive. Moreover, the technique was able to demonstrate circulating antigen following subcutaneous immunization of healthy individuals with 25µg of PRP.

It was reported that certain spinal fluids and many sera give false-positive latex agglutination tests, and that these could be eliminated by heating the specimen at 100°C for 15 minutes (Newman et al., 1970). With our specimens, we found that this treatment reduces the sensitivity of the test in some spinal fluids and does not always prevent the false positives. We are presently engaged in devising a better means of preventing the nonspecific agglutination.

DISCUSSION

The present studies indicate that methods are available for the detection of the capsular antigen of *H. influenzae,* type b, in body fluids of patients with systemic diseases caused by that organism and of individuals immunized with PRP. The antiserum employed must be tested for specificity and for sensitivity before its routine use in identifying PRP. The results of studies of the precipitin activities of the tested sera for PRP and EPS indicate that the capsules of *H. influenzae*, type b, and certain *E. coli* share a common antigenic determinant, but that PRP has at least one nonshared determinant. Furthermore, the data presented indicate that EPS absorption eliminates cross-reactivity for the pneumococcus 29 antigen when tested by CIE. Thus, absorption of cross-reacting anti-*H. influenzae*, type b, serum with EPS produces a reagent satisfactory for routine laboratory use in the identification by CIE of PRP.

Specimens require no special preparation for CIE and all tests for PRP that are eventually positive without staining are visibly positive by one and a half hours. The sensitivity of the test would presumably be increased by staining the gels, but this would add several hours to the duration of the test. When performed as described, samples may be simultaneously tested for the capsular antigens of pneumococci, *H. influenzae*, type b, and meningococcus Groups A and C by using appropriate anti-sera.

If the current problems with the false-positive reactions can be eliminated, the latex agglutination method should prove to be more satisfactory than CIE for the detection of PRP and other bacterial polysaccharides. It is extremely rapid, simple, and sensitive, and when perfected, it should be useful to all diagnostic laboratories.

SUMMARY

Methods and reagents are available to detect minute quantities of the capsular polysaccharide of *Hemophilus influenzae*, type b, in body fluids of infected patients. Such an assay should be useful in diagnosis, particularly in partially treated meningitis, and in the assessment of the patient with *Hemophilus influenzae*, type b, meningitis who has a clinical relapse during therapy. The assay should also be useful in quantitating antigenemia in vaccination studies with PRP.

REFERENCES

Alexander, H. E. 1958. "The Hemophilus Group." In *Bacterial and Mycotic Infections of Man*, edited by R. J. Dubos, Chap. 22, p. 475. 3rd edition. Philadelphia: J. B. Lippincott Company.

Anderson, P.; G. Peter; R. B. Johnston, Jr.; L. H. Wetterlow; and D. H. Smith. 1972. "Immunization of Humans with Polyribophosphate, the Capsular Antigen of *Hemophilus influenzae*, type b." *J. Clin. Inves.* 51:39.

Bradshaw, W.; R. Scheerson; J. C. Parke, Jr.; and J. B. Robbins. 1971. "Bacterial Antigens Cross-reactive with the Capsular Polysaccharide of *Hemophilus influenzae*, type b." *Lancet* 1:1095.

Dorff, G. J.; J. D. Coonrod; and M. W. Rytel. 1971. "Detection by Immuno-electrophoresis of Antigen in Sera of Patients with Pneumococcal Bacteremia." *Lancet* 1:578.

Edwards, E. A. 1971. "Immunologic Investigations of Meningoccal Disease, Group-specific *Neisseria meningitidis* Antigens Present in the Serum of Patients with Fulminant Meningococcemia." *J. Immunol.* 106:314.

Greenwood, B. M.; H. C. Whittle; and O. Dominic-Rajkovic. 1971. "Counter-current Immunoelectrophoresis in the Diagnosis of Meningococcal Infections." *Lancet* 2:519.

Kabat, E. A. 1967. In *Experimental Immunochemistry,* edited by E. A. Kabat and M. D. Mayer, Chap. 2, pp. 22-90. 2nd edition. Springfield, Illinois: Charles C. Thomas.

Newman, R. B.; R. W. Stevens; and H. A. Gaafar. 1970. "Latex Agglutination Test for the Diagnosis of *Hemophilus influenzae* Meningitis. *J. Lab. Clin. Med.* 76:107.

Discussion

Sarah H. Sell, Presiding

John R. Robbins: I would like to compliment Drs. Anderson, Ingram, and Smith. I have some questions and suggestions regarding their work. Have you been able to detect any *Hemophilus influenzae,* type b, antigen other than PRP by these techniques? Have you tried using your internally labelled PRP to add as a carrier to the body fluids that you study so that you can use radio-autography? This procedure may reveal antibodies or antigens that have not been previously identified. Another technique, which is used in the study of poliovirus antibody reactions, utilizes an antiglobulin to the reaction which accentuated the precipitation and makes the autography a little more sensitive. Just one other suggestion: in the latex particle agglutination, perhaps some of your false positives might be due to the fact that hyperimmune rabbit serum prepared by intravenous injection of bacteria very frequently has rheumatoid factor, and it might be worthwhile to see if you could absorb out that rheumatoid factor by insoluble IgG. With this procedure, you might eliminate some false positives. The last thing is really only open for discussion: many of us tried to evaluate, in indirect ways, the protective role of type b antibody. One of the very indirect truths or indirect pieces of evidence we are using is that patients with invasive *Hemophilus,* type b, disease have no detectable type b serum antibodies during the acute phase of their disease. Now, your findings that the antigen is present urge us to go back and examine this problem considering that we have a circulating inhibitor of antibody detection.

Sarah H. Sell: This is very interesting. Dr. Anderson, please comment.

Porter Anderson: The particular set-up of the countercurrent electrophoresis, I think, predisposes toward missing antigen-antibody systems which are not being sought. They might tend to wind up in the well together or might tend to move away from one another. The answer is that no other antigens were seen. Even simpler means of amplifying the detection of the precipitate have not been tried yet. For example, they were not stained or were not tanned to bring out the precipitate and the next level of using radioactive label has not been used; in fact, interest in the latex system more or less cut off the

44

working time that Dr. Ingram applied to the countercurrent system. I am sure that sensitivity could be amplified by using radio-autography; whether it will be worth the trouble will depend on whether we can iron out the latex test which, if the false-positive problem could be worked out, would seem to be the method of choice.

We will take to heart the possibility that it is rheumatoid factor. My guess about many of the false positives is that they will disappear if the test material is merely deproteinized. This has proved to be true in preliminary tests where we have used simple means to deproteinize. I cannot definitely say, however, that this does not lower sensitivity. It is very much a work in progress. I think the important question is: What is the implication for detection of antibody where there is evidence of circulating antigen? I think certainly the issue of how much antibody, on a molecular basis, there might be present but not free to react in a detection system is an issue that we must consider. An accompanying question is: What is the extent of persistence of the antigenemia or the persistence of the possible binding of the antibody by the antigen?

I have an anecdotal result to report in that vein. We have received from Dr. Wilkins some samples, following immunization with PRP, taken at fairly close time intervals. One can almost titrate the appearance of the presence of antibody activity and the disappearance of detectable antigen. One sees drops in pre-existing antibody and the presence of free antigen; and then, when the antigen disappears, one begins to see antibodies. This is anecdotal and is not a significant survey, but I think it shows the promise of the method being applied, so far as dissecting out some of the immunobiology of this antigen.

Richard B. Johnston, Jr.: You have already alluded to this, but the timing of the appearance of the PRP is germane to Dr. Robbins's questions regarding the usefulness of antibody studies. In vaccination circumstances, when did the PRP appear and how long did it last? Was it, perhaps, gone? It seems to be that the reticulo-endothelial system is going to clear rather rapidly; and perhaps, when we start measuring it, antibody in fact does interfere.

Anderson: This is just anecdotal information. We had samples of serum drawn at three days, seven days and 14 days. Antigenemia did not consistently appear, but where it appeared it was generally at three to seven days, particularly at three days.

David T. Karzon: If we draw analogy from antigenemias in virology where viremias might be persistent chronically, the problem resolves itself, not in the presence of antigen or antibody, but in the mixture and therefore circulating complexes. It has been found useful to use antibody directed against immunoglobulin to detect the complex and therefore the antigen and antibody. Has this been tried?

Anderson: Not by me, no.

Karzon: The complex may be the major form in which it is present.

Robert H. Alford: Dr. Jack Bennet has used the latex agglutination test, as I
think everyone knows, for detecting cryptococcal polysaccharide. He reported also false positives due to rheumatoid factor in human sera and reported that this effect could be removed simply by heat inactivation of sera. I
do not know whether or not this would be helpful.

SECTION III

Serologic Relationship between *Hemophilus influenzae,* type b, Capsular Polysaccharide and Polyribitol Teichoic Acids of Gram-Positive Bacteria

Meir Argaman

In this publication, we report preliminary findings which show that the capsular polysaccharide of *H. influenzae,* type b, shown by Rosenberg and Zamenhof (1961) to contain ribose-phosphate, serologically cross-reacts with extracts of gram-positive bacteria that contain polyribitol-phosphate teichoic acids. *H. influenzae,* type b, capsular polysaccharide was also shown (Bradshaw et al., 1971) to cross-react with the Kf147 antigen of some *E. coli* strains.

Baddiley and his colleagues (Armstrong et al., 1958; Archibald, Baddiley, and Buchanan, 1961; Sharp, Davison, and Baddiley, 1964; Davison and Baddiley, 1963; Adams et al., 1969) reported that teichoic acids were either attached to or formed an integral component of the cell wall and the cell membrane of numerous gram positive bacteria. While all cell-membrane-teichoic acids tested by these workers were shown to be composed of a polyglycerol-phosphate backbone, the cell-wall-teichoic acids of certain bacteria consisted of a polyribitol-phosphate backbone connected by a phosphodiester bond with 1, 5 linkage (Baddiley, 1968). The polyribitol-phosphate teichoic acids of the various bacteria differed in their side chains that contained different monosaccharides or muramic acid peptides. It is of interest that the ribitol-phosphate teichoic acids were found in bacteria of wide distribution in nature, including those of the human gastrointestinal tract. Of these polyribitol-phosphate-teichoic-acid-containing organisms, the enteric bacteria, Bacillus and Lactobacillus, are nonpathogenic for humans.

We chose the following strains of bacteria for our study: *Staphylococcus aureus,* var. copenhagen, previously characterized by Strominger (1959); *Bacillus subtilis,* designated strain Sh-18, isolated in our laboratory from neonatal rabbit stool; *Lactobacillus plantarum* was obtained from Dr. Wolin of the University of Illinois; Group D *Streptococcus faecium* was isolated from a patient by Dr. Viola

49

Young of the Baltimore Health Center. The cross-reacting substances were purified by precipitation of the whole fluid culture with cetavlon followed by deproteinization with phenol.

Hyperimmune burro sera were obtained by intravenous injections of formaldehyde-treated micro-organisms. The first antiserum designed B-132 was prepared by injecting *H. influenzae,* type b, strain "Rab". The other, designated B-139, was prepared by injecting *E. coli,* strain "Easter." The sera were heated to 56°C for thirty minutes before use. D-ribitol-5-phosphate was synthetized by Dr. Darrel Liu, of the Brookhaven Laboratories, who also performed the gas-chromotographic analysis of the alkali-treated, alkaline-phosphatase-digested polysaccharides from the *H. influenzae,* type b, meningitis isolated strains "Rab," "Eagen," and "Johnson." The Eagen strain was obtained from Drs. P. Anderson and D. Smith, Boston, and the epiglottitis strain "Carbone" was obtained from Dr. Fred Cantor, Yale University. All the type b capsular poly-

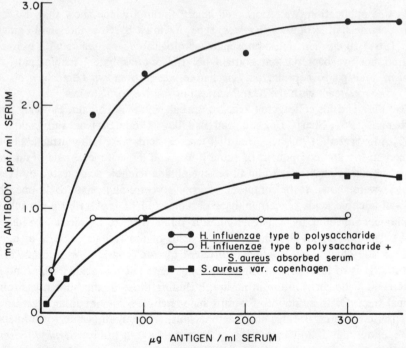

Fig. 1. Representative precipitation curves of hyperimmune burro serum (prepared against *H. influenzae,* type b, strain Rab) and the same serum absorbed with *S. aureus,* var. copenhagen polysaccharide reacting with *H. influenzae,* type b, and with *S. aureus,* var. copenhagen polysaccharides.

saccharides tested were found to contain ribitol. A representative precipitation analysis of B-132 serum with the "Rab" type b polysaccharide and with poly-ribitol-phosphate containing extracts of four gram-positive bacteria is shown in Figure 1. *Staphylococcus aureus* and *Bacillus subtilis* precipitated 45% of the total antibody reactive with the type b polysaccharide. Smaller amounts were pre-cipitated by *Lactobacillus plantarum* and by group D *Streptococcus faecium* (not shown on Fig. 1). No precipitate was detected with a polyglycerol phos-phate containing extracts from *Bacillus pumilis* or with the polysaccharide of *H. influenzae,* type a.

A precipitation curve formed by these polysaccharides with B-139 serum (Fig. 2) shows that *S. aureus* and *B. subtilis* polysaccharides precipitated 33% of the total anti-type b antibody. This difference between the *H. influenzae,* type b, and *S. aureus* indicates that the cross-reaction between *E. coli,* strain

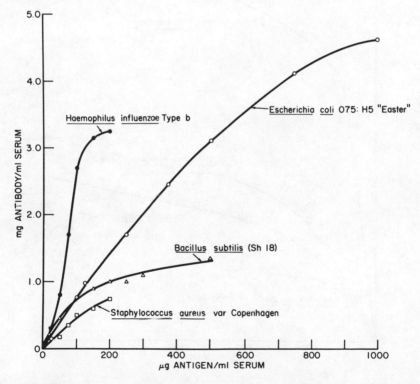

Fig. 2. Precipitation curves of hyperimmune burro serum (prepared against *E. coli* 075:H5, strain Easter) with polysaccharides from *H. influenzae,* type b; *E. coli* 075:H5, strain Easter; *B. subtilis* (Sh-18); and *S. aureus,* var. copenhagen.

"Easter," and *H. influenzae,* type b, strain "Rab," differs from the reaction observed with the gram-positive bacteria. The nature of this difference is now under study.

Immunodiffusion studies, using the same reagents, showed that more antigenic sites were revealed by B-139 serum with *H. influenzae,* type b, polysaccharide than observed for *B. subtilis* (Sh-18) and *S. aureus* polysaccharides. Following absorption with the *H. influenzae,* type b, polysaccharide, the B-139 anti-*E. coli* serum would no longer react with either the *B. subtilis* or *S. aureus.* Conversely, absorption of the anti-*E. coli* B-139 serum with the *S. aureus* polysaccharide did not completely remove the antibodies to *H. influenzae,* type b, thus

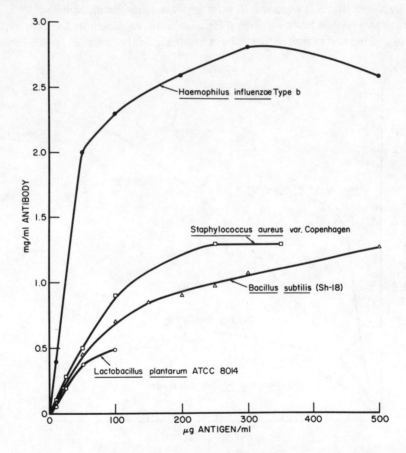

Fig. 3. Precipitation curves of hyperimmune burro serum (prepared against *H. influenzae,* type b, strain Rab) with *H. influenzae,* type b; *S. aureus,* var. copenhagen; *B. subtilis,* (Sh-18); and *Lactobacillus plantarum* (ATCC 8014) polysaccharides.

indicating that, while all three polysaccharides share antigenic determinants, they are not serologically identical. More detailed studies of the reaction between the polysaccharides of the *S. aureus* and of the *H. influenzae*, type b, when reacting with anti-type b B-132 serum, were carried out (Fig. 3). While *H. influenzae*, type b, polysaccharide precipitated 2.8 mg antibody per ml serum, only 1.25 mg were precipitated by the *S. aureus* polysaccharide. Following absorption of the anti-type b, B-132 serum with the *S. aureus* polysaccharide, the type b polysaccharide precipitated only 0.9 mg antibody per ml serum. This figure also shows that the curve formed by the type b polysaccharide and the unabsorbed serum can be described as a composition of two curves while the curve with the absorbed serum is a homogenous one. Here, as in other experiments, we have observed that the precipitation with *H. influenzae*, type b, polysaccharide and its antiserum suggests at least two antigenic determinants and raises the possibility that two different types of molecules are present in the *H. influenzae*, type b, polysaccharide preparations. These results are consistent with inhibition data (Fig. 4), where *S. aureus* polysaccharide absorbed and un-

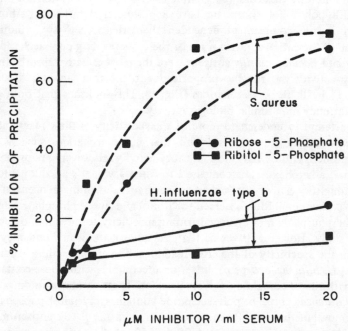

Fig. 4. Representative inhibition of precipitation of hyperimmune burro serum (prepared against *H. influenzae*, type b, strain Rab, polysaccharide) with *S. aureus*, var. copenhagen and *H. influenzae*, type b, strain Rab, polysaccharides by ribose-5-phosphate and ribitol-5-phosphate.

absorbed *H. influenzae,* type b, B–132 antiserum was used. A significant inhibition of precipitation between the type b polysaccharide and its antiserum occurs
by the addition of either ribose-5-phosphate or ribitol-5-phosphate. Ribose-
5-phosphate was slightly more effective in this system than ribitol-5-phosphate,
inducing a 22% inhibition as contrasted to 18% inhibition by ribitol-
5-phosphate. It is most likely that these two inhibitors interact with the same
antibody site, as no additive effect was seen using both of them together. Both
of these monosaccharides phosphate esters were far more effective in inhibiting
the precipitation of the *S. aureus* polysaccharide by the B-132 serum. In this
case, ribitol-5-phosphate seemed to be a more effective inhibitor, yielding slightly higher inhibition and achieving maximal inhibition at a lower concentration.
No inhibition was induced either by ribose-5-phosphate or by ribitol-
5-phosphate upon the B-132 serum previously absorbed with *S. aureus* polysaccharide. This latter finding indicates that only one portion of the anti-type b
antibodies present in the *H. influenzae,* type b, B-132 antiserum were cross-
reactive with the *S. aureus,* and it is this cross-reactive population of antibodies
that is inhibited by these monosaccharide esters. These absorptions of the B-132
serum with polyribitol phosphate have a biological significance. About 50%
reduction in the complement dependent bactericidal activity is induced by
absorption of the antiserum with some of the cross-reacting polysaccharides. The
S. aureus and *Bacillus subtilis* antigens were the most effective absorbents as the
inhibitory activity was roughly proportional to the total amount of antibody
precipitated by these polysaccharides (Fig. 1). This indicates that both populations of antibody have similar biologic activity.

In an attempt to understand more of the specificity of these reactions, other
inhibitors were studied. It was found that monosaccharides such as ribose,
ribitol, and deoxyribose have no inhibitory activity. However, a phosphate ester
of fructose, a ketohexose, as compared to ribose, which is an aldopentose, did
exhibit inhibitory activity at higher concentrations than the concentrations inducing maximum inhibition observed for ribitol and ribose phosphate esters. The
role of the phosphate moiety in confirming specificity to these monosaccharides
is under study. However, it seems that the phosphate ester bond may be important in the specificity of the cross-reactions. The cross-reactions studied here
show that *H. influenzae,* type b, antiserum precipitates with ribose-containing as
well as with ribitol-containing polysaccharides. These serologic findings suggest
that *H. influenzae,* type b, polysaccharide contains polyribitol phosphate. The
partial removal of the precipitating antibodies from the B-132 antiserum by the
polyribitol phosphate indicates that 30 to 45% of the antibodies in the serum
react with polyribitol phosphate.

Some chemical data suggest that the type b antigen is not entirely composed
of polyribose phosphate. Quantitative analysis of pentose in the *H. influenzae,*

type b, polysaccharide, by the orcinol reaction (Drury, 1948) revealed a lower proportion of ribose than predicted from the dry weight and phosphorous content. We, and others (Anderson et al., 1972), found values lower by 30 to 40% of the expected pentose contents. We suggest that this discrepancy is due to polyribitol phosphate that will not be detected in the orcinol reaction and that this polyribitol phosphate is the antigen common to the cross-reacting polysaccharides studied. As mentioned above, ribitol has been found in the polysaccharides of the *H. influenzae* strains studied by Dr. Liu and in the polysaccharides of *Diplococcus pneumoniae,* types 29 and 34, reported previously to cross-react with *H. influenzae,* type b (Turk & May, 1967), as studied by Roberts, Buchanan, and Baddiley (1962) and by Rao et al. (1968). Of interest is the observation that the ribose phosphate, ribitol phosphate, and fructose phosphate share some degree of cross reactivity, as shown by the inhibition experiments.

REFERENCES

Adams, J. B.; A. R. Archibald; J. Baddiley; H. E. Coapes; and A. L. Davidson. 1969. "Teichoic Acids Possessing Phosphate-Sugar Linkages in Strains of Lactobacillus Plantarum." *Biochem. J.* 113:191.

Anderson, P. G.; R. B. Johnston; L. H. Wetterlow; and D. H. Smith. 1972. "Immunization of Humans with Polyribosephosphate, the Capsular Antigen of *Hemophilus influenzae*, type b." *J. Clin. Invest.* 51:39

Archibald, A. R.; J. Baddiley; J. G. Buchanan. 1961. "The Ribitol Teichoic Acid from *Lactobacillus arabinosus* Walls: Isolation and Structure of Ribitol Glucosides." *Biochem. J.* 81:124.

Armstrong, J. J.; J. Baddiley; J. G. Buchanan; B. Carss; and G. R. Greenberg. 1958. "Isolation and Structure of Ribitol Phosphate Derivatives (Teichoic Acids) from Bacterial Cell Walls." *J. Chem. Soc.* 4344.

Baddiley, J. 1968. "Teichoic Acids and the Molecular Structure of Bacterial Walls." *Proc. Roy. Soc. B.* 170:331.

Bradshaw, M. W.; R. Schneerson; J. C. Parke; and J. B. Robbins. 1971. "Bacterial Antigens Cross-Reactive with the Capsular Polysaccharide of *Haemophilus influenzae,* type b." *Lancet* 1:1095.

Davison, A. L., and J. Baddiley. 1963. "The Distribution of Teichoic Acids in Staphylococci." *J. Gen. Microbiol.* 32:271.

Drury, H. F. 1948. "Identification and Estimation of Pentoses in the Presence of Glucose." *Arch. Bioch.* 19:455.

Rao, E. V.; M. J. Watson; J. G. Buchanan; and J. Baddiley. 1969. "The Type-Specific Substance from Pneumococcus, Type 29." *Biochem. J.* 111:547.

Roberts, W. K.; J. G. Buchanan; and J. Baddiley. 1962. "The Specific Substance from Pneumococcus Type 34 (41)." *Biochem. J.* 88:1.

Rozenberg, E., and S. Zamenhof. 1961. "Further Studies on Polyribosephosphate." *J. Biol. Chem.* 236:2845.

Strominger, J. L. 1959. "Accumulation of Uridine and Cytidine Nucleotides in *Staphylococcus aureus*, Inhibited by Gentian Violet." *J. Biol. Chem.* 234:1520.

Sharpe, M. E.; A. L. Davison; and J. Baddiley. 1964. "Teichoic Acids and Group Antigens in Lactobacilli." *J. Gen. Microbiol.* 34:333.

Turke, D. C., and J. R. May. 1967. *Haemophilus influenzae: Its Clinical Importance.* London: English Universities Press.

CHAPTER 6

Escherichia coli Antigens Cross-Reactive with the Capsular Polysaccharide of *Hemophilus influenzae,* type b

Richard L. Myerowitz
Zeev T. Handzel
Rachel Schneerson
John B. Robbins

Serum antibodies to *Hemophilus influenzae,* type b, are present in most adults and are passively transferred to the newborn. As shown first by Fothergill and Wright (1933), the absence of serum antibody, which occurs approximately between the ages of six months and three years, is inversely related to the high incidence of *H. influenzae,* type b, meningitis during this age period. Asymptomatic carriage of the homologous bacterium does not appear to be the only antigenic stimulus for this "natural" immunity, since the carrier rate of *H. influenzae,* type b, is very low (Turk, 1963). A similar pattern of age-related acquisition of natural immunity to *H. influenzae,* type b, has been observed in rabbits in the absence of detectable *H. influenzae,* type b, (Schneerson and Robbins, 1971). One possible antigenic source for natural immunity may be cross-reacting structures present on bacteria in the normal flora of the gastrointestinal tract (Springer, Horton, and Forbes, 1959).

Incorporation of precipitating antiserum to the capsular polysaccharide of *H. influenzae,* type b, into the agar medium used for cultivation, as shown in Figure 1, results in the formation of an immunoprecipitin halo around the bacterial colony after overnight growth (Petrie, 1932). This "antiserum-agar technique"

This work was done at the Developmental Immunity Branch, National Institute of Child Health and Human Development, National Institutes of Health, Bethesda, Maryland.

The authors wish to thank David Rogerson for his help in preparation of the *E. coli* antigens and Dr. George Hermann of the Center for Disease Control, U.S. Public Health Service, Atlanta, Georgia, for serotyping the *E. coli* isolates.

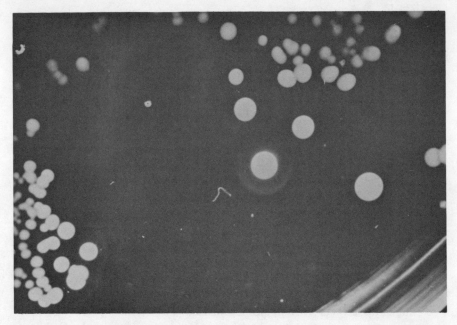

Fig. 1. Antiserum-agar technique: Precipitin halo around the colony of *Hemophilus in-fluenzae,* type b, grown on Levinthal's agar medium containing 15% (v/v) sheep antiserum to *H. influenzae,* type b.

can be used to identify bacteria cross-reacting with the type b capsular poly-saccharide, since these colonies will also form a precipitin halo (Bradshaw et al., 1971). The specificity of this precipitin reaction is confirmed by prior absorp-tion·of precipitating activity from the incorporated antiserum with the type b capsular polysaccharide and by the failure of cross-reacting strains to yield a halo on agar medium containing hyperimmune serum not specific for *H. influenzae,* type b.

Using the antiserum-agar technique, a survey of stool and throat cultures from humans and other animals was made (Bradshaw et al., 1971). A large number of bacteria of a variety of species was found which cross-reacted with *H. influenzae,* type b. *Escherichia coli* was chosen for further study because it is ubiquitous in the gastrointestinal tract and is usually nonpathogenic when confined there. The present study was undertaken to examine the frequency of cross-reacting structures in *E. coli,* as well as to define the nature of the cross-reactive antigen.

MATERIALS AND METHODS

Serologic. Antisera were raised in sheep by intravenous immunization with formalinized whole bacteria according to a reported schedule (Alexander, Leidy, and MacPherson, 1946). Immunodiffusion was carried out in 1.2% (w/v) agarose gels made up with phosphate-buffered saline and incubated for 48 hours at 4° C. Immunoelectrophoresis was carried out in 1.2% agarose gels using 0.05M veronal acetate buffer, pH 8.6 (Scheiddeger, 1955). Quantitative precipitin analyses were carried out as described (Kabat and Mayer, 1961). Immonuflourescence using a flourescein isothiocyanate derivative of sheep anti-*H. influenzae*, type b, antibody was prepared and utilized as described (Cebra and Goldstein, 1965).

Bacteriologic. All studies with *H. influenzae*, type b, organisms or antisera utilized strain "Rab" kindly donated by Miss Grace Leidy. Bacteria were studied for cross-reactivity by use of the antiserum-agar technique (Petrie, 1932), which was modified for study of cross-reaction to *H. influenzae*, type b (Schneerson, et al., 1972). Cross-reacting *E. coli* were serotyped by the Enterobacteriology Unit of the Center for Disease Control.

Biologic. Dr. Sam Formal of the Walter Reed Army Research Institute performed two bioassays of enteropathic virulence; the guinea-pig eye test for invasiveness (Formal, et al., 1971), and the ligated rabbit ileum assay for enterotoxin production (Smith and Halls, 1967). Mucin-enhanced mouse protection assays (Fothergill, Dingle, and Chandler, 1937) and complement-dependent bacterial reactions (Landy, Michael, and Whitby, 1962) were performed as described.

Chemical. *E. coli* cross-reactive antigens from five strains (designated as "Easter," "89," "10," "BCH," and "Kf147") were isolated from broth culture supernatants by ethanol precipitation and deproteinization with phenol (Schneerson, et al., 1972). Tentative identification of monosaccharides liberated by acid hydrolysis (1N sulfuric acid at 100°C for one hour) of polysaccharide was done by descending paper chromatography in ethyl acetate: pyridine: water (12:5:4).

RESULTS

Various human and animal sources provided 1607 strains of enteric bacteria which were studied for cross-reactivity (Table 1). These included at least one representative of every known serologically defined *E. coli*, *Salmonellae*, *Citrobacter*, and *Klebsiella* from the reference collections of the World Health Organization and the Center for Disease Control. Also included were *E. coli* strains from infants with diarrheal disease, strains isolated from patients with urinary tract infection, and strains isolated from normal human feces. Twenty-five *E.*

TABLE 1

SURVEY OF *ESCHERICHIA COLI* POSSESSING
CROSS-REACTING ANTIGENS TO THE
POLYSACCHARIDE OF *HEMOPHILUS INFLUENZAE,* TYPE b

Origin of Micro-organisms	No. of Organisms Tested	No. and Serotype of Micro-organisms with Cross-Reacting Antigen
I. Reference collections with defined serotypes	306	1 *E. coli* 075a,b:H5 (CDC) 1 *E. coli* 07:H5 (#10) 1*E. coli* 075:H4 (#89) 1 *E. coli* 0120:K?:H6,35w (WHO)
II. *E. coli* of human origin: Urinary tract	426	11 *E. coli* 075a,b:H5 1 *E. coli* 075:K2:H5 1 *E. coli* 07:H5 1 *E. coli* 02a,2b 14:H5 (Shigella Group D) ±BCH 58272) 1 Shigella Oundetermined:NM
Stool	390	4 *E. coli* 075a,72b:H5
Blood	9	0
Wounds and Abscesses	23	0
Routine Hospital Specimens	322	3 *E. coli* 075a,75b:H5
III. *E. coli* from animal milk and stool	131	0
Total	1607	26 (1.5%)

coli strains were found which cross-reacted with the capsular polysaccharide of *H. influenzae,* type b, representing a variety of O and H serotypes. Nineteen of the 25 strains were of the serotype 075:H5, although not all isolates of this serotype were cross-reacting. The most frequent source of cross-reacting *E. coli* were isolates from the urinary tract. None of the strains isolated from blood, spinal fluid, abscesses, or from the stools of patients with infantile diarrhea had cross-reactivity. Five strains of cross-reacting *E. coli* were examined for entero-pathic virulence characteristics including invasiveness and enterotoxin production. None of the strains were positive by either assay.

The frequency of cross-reacting *E. coli* in human bacterial flora was studied by consecutive mixed bacterial cultures of a variety of in-patients at the Char-

TABLE 2

SURVEY OF MIXED BACTERIAL CULTURES UTILIZING THE
"ANTISERUM-AGAR" TECHNIQUE FOR CROSS-REACTING ORGANISMS
TO *HEMOPHILUS INFLUENZAE,* type b

Source	#Positive/ Total Cultures	Site and Organism	
Normal newborn	4/336	1—umbilical cord	*E. coli**
		1—rectal	*E. coli**
		1—skin	*E. coli**
		1—urine	*E. coli**
Adult G-U Clinic	0/20		
Pediatric OPD	3/77	1—urine	*E. coli**
		2—rectal	*E. coli**
Nasopharyngeal and Rectal swabs from 20 immunized infants	9/119†	9—rectal	*E. coli**
Normal 4-day-old infants	2/88	2—rectal	*E. coli**

* All *E. coli* were serotype 075:H5.
†There were 9 positive cultures from 4 patients.

lotte (North Carolina) Memorial Hospital utilizing the "antiserum-agar" technique. These cultures were kindly performed by Dr. James C. Parke. Table 2
shows that 18 isolates from 640 cultures (2.8%) were cross-reacting. All cross-
reacting isolates were *E. coli* 075:H5.

The *E. coli* cross-reactive antigen was isolated from five strains. In each instance, the antigen was a polysaccharide whose immune reactivity was not destroyed by heating at 100° C for two hours. Analysis of the monosaccharide
components of these polysaccharide antigens (Fig. 2) revealed that three strains
(Easter, BCH, and Kf147) had multiple components including ribose. However,
four of five antigens contained ribitol and strains 89 and 10 yielded only ribitol
after acid hydrolysis. Cross-reacting *E. coli* strains, when stained with flourescein
labelled anti-*H. influenzae,* type b, antibody, bound the flourochrome reagent
exterior to the cell wall. Immunoelectrophoretic analysis of the antigens at pH
8.6 (Fig. 3) revealed each to migrate strongly toward the anode. All polysaccharides including the *H. influenzae,* type b, polysaccharide displayed marked
electrophoretic heterogeneity.

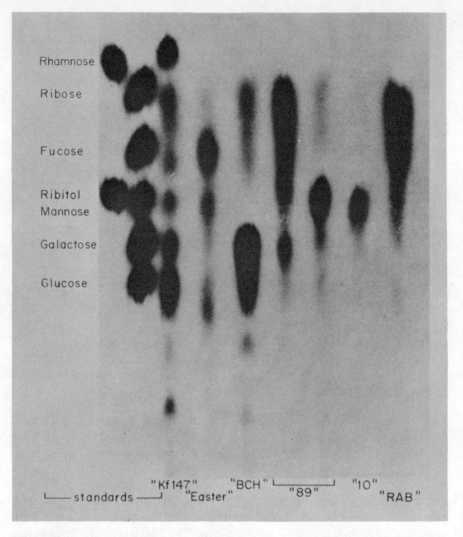

Fig. 2 Descending chromatography in ethyl acetate: Pyridine: H_2O. *H. influenzae*, type b (Rab) polysaccharide compared with cross-reacting *E. coli* polysaccharides.

Quantitative precipitin analysis using sheep antiserum to *H. influenzae*, type b, (Fig. 4) revealed that each of the cross-reactive antigens precipitated about 40 to 50% of the antibody precipitated by the type b capsule. However, the antigen from *E. coli* strains 89 and 10 were the most antigenically active as the equivalence zone was reached with only 200 μg of these polysaccharides in contrast

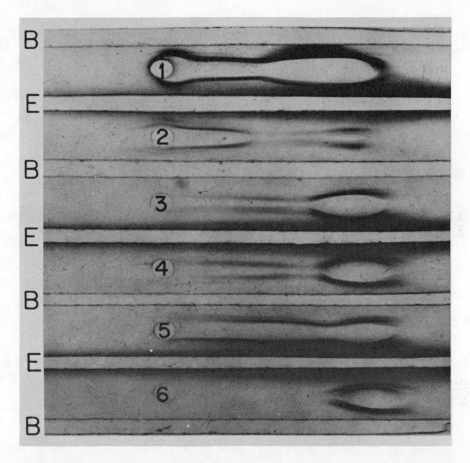

Fig. 3. Immunoelectrophoretic analysis of *Hemophilus influenzae,* type b, and *E. coli* cross-reacting capsular polysaccharides (1.0 mg/ml). Sample wells contain: (1) *H. influenzae,* type b, capsular polysaccharide; (2) Kf147; (3) 89; (4) Easter; (5) BCH; (6) 10. Troughs labelled *B* contain sheep antiserum to *H. influenzae*, type b, and those labelled *E* contain sheep antiserum to *E. coli,* strain Easter.

to 500 μg of the other three polysaccharides required for maximal precipitation. Antisera were raised with three cross-reacting *E. coli* strains (Easter, 89, and 10). Quantitative precipitin analysis of these antisera revealed that all reacted with the type b capsule with precipitin curves similar to that observed with *H. influenzae,* type b, antiserum. Immunodiffusion analysis (Fig. 5) revealed that the type b capsular polysaccharide yielded a reaction of partial identity with *E. coli* antigens when reacted with *H. influenzae,* type b, antiserum. The cross-reacting

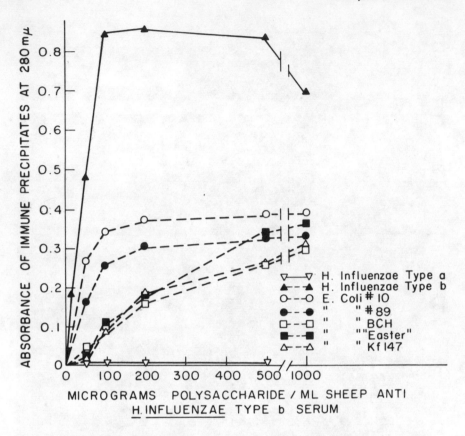

Fig. 4 Immune precipitation induced by polysaccharides and sheep anti-*Hemophilus influenzae,* type b, serum (#815).

moiety of all *E. coli* antigens were immunologically identical using this antiserum. Using antiserum to one cross-reacting *E. coli* (Fig. 6), the *E. coli* antigens were partially identical with the type b antigen.

Antiserum to *E. coli*, strain Easter, has marked bactericidal and mouseprotective activity toward *H. influenzae*, type b. As shown in Table 3, based upon their content of precipitating anti-type b antibody, *H. influenzae*, type b, antiserum and *E. coli* antiserum had comparable bactericidal and mouseprotective activity. *E. coli*, strain Easter, was resistant to the complementdependant bactericidal effect using anti-*E. coli* serum, and these reagents failed to protect mice as well from mucin-enhanced infection with this *E. coli* strain. *E. coli*, strain 89, was, however, susceptible to killing by antibody and complement which also protected mice from lethal infection with *E. coli*, 89. Antisera to two other cross-reasting *E. coli* strains also had high levels of bactericidal and mouse-protective activity toward *H. influenzae*, type b.

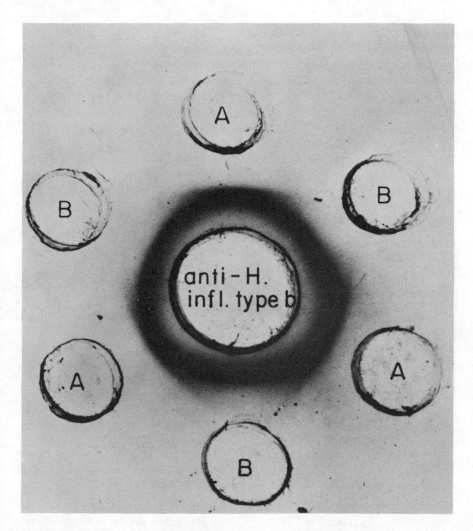

Fig. 5. Immunodiffusion analysis using sheep antiserum to *Hemophilus influenzae*, type b. Samples are: (a) *H. influenzae*, type b (Rab), capsular polysaccharide (1.0 mg/ml); (B) *E. coli*, strain 89, antigen (1.0 mg/ml).

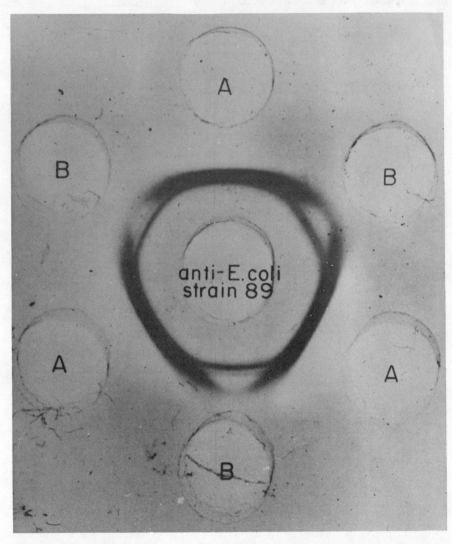

Fig. 6. Immunodiffusion analysis using sheep antiserum to **E. coli**, strain 89. Samples include: (A) **E. coli**, strain 89, antigen (1.0 mg/ml); (B) **H. influenzae**, type b (Rab), capsular polysaccharide (1.0 mg/ml).

TABLE 3
BIOLOGIC ACTIVITIES OF SHEEP *H. INFLUENZAE*
type b, AND *E. coli* ANTISERA

Specificity of Sheep Antiserum	Antibody Content (mg protein/ml)* Antigen		Reciprocal Titer					
			Complement—Dependant Bactericidal Reaction			Mouse—Protection Assay		
	H. inf. type b (Rab)	*E. coli* (Easter)	*H. inf.* type b (Rab)	*E. coli* (Easter)	*E. coli* (#89)	*H. inf.,* type b (Rab)	*E. coli* (Easter)	*E. coli* (#89)
H. inf., type b (Rab)	1.60	0.54	6400	0	8000	100	0	1
E. coli (Easter)	1.20	3.81	6400	0	4000	50	0	5

*Determined by quantitative precipitin analysis.

DISCUSSION

In this study, 1.5% of the enteric bacteria were shown to contain an antigen which cross-reacts with the capsular polysaccharide of *H. influenzae*, type b. All cross-reactive strains were members of the species *E. coli*. Cross-reacting *E. coli* were also commonly found among random cultures of human bacterial flora. The cross-reacting antigen is a thermostable, acidic polysaccharide, present on the outer portion of the bacterial cell and is associated with a variety of O and H serotypes. It has, therefore, been tentatively designated as a K or capsular antigen of the A type.

Cross-reaction of *E. coli* K antigens with the capsular polysaccharides of pathogenic bacteria have been previously described, including *E. coli* K antigens with pneumococcal polysaccharide types 30, 42, and 85 (Heidelberger, et al., 1968), and *E. coli* K1 with the group B meningococcus (Grados, and Ewing, 1970). Although these antigens cross-react with encapsulated pathogens, the *E. coli* cross-reactive antigens in this study did not appear to be associated with enteropathic virulence characteristics.

The chemical basis for cross-reactivity for at least some of these antigens appears to be through their content of ribitol. Differences were observed among the five cross-reacting *E. coli* strains that were studied most intensively. These five strains appear divisible into two groups. One group is exemplified by strain 89, which is susceptible to the killing effect of antibody and complement and which has a cross-reactive antigen that is almost pure polyribitol and antigenically very active. The second group, exemplified by strain Easter, is not susceptible to the killing effect of antibody and complement and contains a cross-reactive antigen with a heterogenous monosaccharide composition which is therefore, less antigenically active on a weight basis. The immunogenicity of these cross-reactive antigens has been confirmed by the biologic activity of *E. coli* antisera toward *H. influenzae,* type b.

We suggest that gastrointestinal bacteria with cross-reactive structures may, indeed, be an antigenic source for natural immunity to *H. influenzae,* type b. Further, the possibility is raised that deliberate neonatal colonization of the gastrointestinal tract with a nonpathogenic cross-reacting *E. coli* may provide a way of stimulating the production of natural immunity at an earlier age than expected.

ABSTRACT

An *Escherichia coli* antigen was shown to be cross-reactive with the capsular polysaccharide of *Hemophilus influenzae,* type b. The cross-reactive antigen was identified as a thermostable acidic capsular polysaccharide consistent with its designation as *E. coli* K antigen (type a). Antibodies raised by intravenous injection of formaldehyde-treated *E. coli* possessing the cross-reactive antigen precipitated with the *H. influenzae,* type b, capsular polysaccharide and had protective activity against *H. influenzae,* type b, in biologic assays. The cross-reactive antigen was identified in *E. coli* with various O and H serotypes and did not appear to be associated with pathogenicity.

REFERENCES

Alexander, H. E.; G. Leidy; and C. F. C. MacPherson. 1946. "Production of Types A, B, C, D, E, and F *Hemophilus influenzae* Antibody for Diagnostic and Therapeutic Purposes." *J. Immunol.* 54:207.

Bradshaw, M. W.; R. Schneerson; J. C. Parke; and J. B. Robbins. 1971. "Bacterial Antigens Cross-Reactive with the Capsular Polysaccharide of *Hemophilus influenzae,* type b." *Lancet* 1:1095.

Cebra, J. J. and G. J. Goldstein. 1965. "Chromatographic Purification of Tetramethylrhodamine-Immune Globulin Conjugates and their Use in the Cellular Localization of Rabbit Gamma Globulin Polypeptide." *J. Immunol.* 95:230.

Formal, S.B.; H. Dupont; R. B. Hornick; J. Labonati; and E. H. LaBrec. 1971. "Experimental Models in the Investigation of the Virulence of Dysentery Bacillus and *Escherichia coli." Ann. N.Y. Acad. Sci.* 176:190.

Fothergill, L.D.; J. H. Dingle and C. A. Chandler. 1937. "Studies of *Hemophilus influenzae:* I. Infection of Mice with Mucin Suspensions of the Organisms." *J. Exp. Med.* 65:721.

Fothergill, L. D. and J. Wright. 1933. "Influenzal Meningitis: The Relationship of Age Incidence to the Bactericidal Power of Blood against the Causal Organism." *J. Immunol.* 24:273.

Grados, O. and E. H. Ewing. 1970. "Antigenic Relationship between *Escherichia coli* and *Neisseria meningitidis.*" *J. Inf. Dis.* 122:100.

Heidelberger, M.; K. Jann; B. Jann.; F. Orskov; I. Orskov; and O. Westphal. 1968. "Relations between Structures of Three K Polysaccharides of *Escherichia coli* and Cross-Reactivity in Antipneumococcal Sera." *J. Bact.* 95: 2415.

Kabat, E. A., and M. M. Mayer. 1961. *Experimental Immunochemistry.* Springfield, Illinois: Charles C. Thomas.

Landy, M.; J. G. Michael; and J. L. Whitby. 1962. "Bactericidal Method for the Measurement in Normal Serum of Antibody to Gram-Negative Bacteria." *J. Bact.* 83:631.

Petrie, G. F. 1932. "A Specific Precipitin Reaction Associated with the Growth on Agar Plates of Meninococcus, Pneumococcus, and B. dysenteriae (Shiga)." *Brit. J. Exp. Path.* 13:380.

Scheiddeger, J. J. 1955. "Une Micro-Methode de l'immunoelectrophorese." *Int. Arch. Allerg. and Appl. Immunol.* 7:103.

Schneerson, R.; M.W. Bradshaw; J. K. Whisnant; R. L. Myerowitz; J. C. Parke; and J. B. Robbins. 1972. "An *Escherichia coli* Antigen Cross-Reactive with the Polysaccharide of *Hemophilus influenzae,* type b: Occurrence among Know Serotypes, and Immunochemical and Biological Properties of *E. coli* antisera toward *H. influenzae,* type b." *J. Immunol.* In press.

Schneerson, R., and J. B. Robbins. 1971. "Age-Related Susceptibility to *Hemophilus influenzae,* type b, Disease in Rabbits." *Infect. and Immun.* 4:397.

Springer, G. F.; R. E. Horton; and M. Forbes. 1959. "Origin of Anti-Human Blood Group B Agglutinins in White Leghorn Chick." *J. Exp. Med.* 110:221.

Smith, H. W. and S. Halls. 1967. "Studies on *Escherichia coli* Enterotoxin." *J. Path. Bact.* 93:536.

Turk, D.C. 1963. "Naso-Pharyngeal Carriage of *Hemophilus influenzae,* type b." *J. Hyg.* 61:247.

CHAPTER 7

Gastrointestinal Colonization of Neonatal Rabbits with Cross-Reacting *Escherichia coli:* An Approach to Induction of Immunity toward *Hemophilus influenzae,* type *b*

Zeev T. Handzel
Richard L. Myerowitz
Rachel Schneerson
John B. Robbins

Several *Escherichia coli* strains have been shown to have a K antigen which cross-reacts with the capsular polysaccharide of *H. influenzae,* type b (Schneerson et al., 1972). When injected intravenously as formalinized organisms, these cross-reactive antigens are capable of stimulating biologically active antibodies toward *H. influenzae,* type b. Cross-reacting enteric bacteria, such as these *E. coli,* may act as an antigenic stimulus for the age-related acquisition of "natural" immunity toward *Hemophilus influenzae,* type b. Since these cross-reacting *E. coli* strains did not reveal enteropathic virulence characteristics, the possibility that neonatal gastrointestinal colonization of animals and humans by these cross-reacting bacteria might stimulate "natural" immunity toward *H. influenzae,* type b, at an earlier age than expected, was investigated in laboratory rabbits.

Gastrointestinal colonization of human newborn infants by *E. coli* 083 has been accomplished without ill effect by R. Lodinova and her colleagues. They demonstrated that this colonization results in the production of serum and copro-antibodies to the O antigen at an earlier age than expected for these antibodies (Lodinova, Jouja, and Laue, 1967).

The authors wish to thank Mr. Patrick Crarey for excellent technical assistance and Dr. George Hermann for serotyping the *E. coli* isolates.

METHODS

Newborn rabbits (NZW strain) were fed a saline suspension of freshly prepared live *E. coli* within 24 hours after birth. All members of a litter were fed an identical number of bacteria. Gastrointestinal colonization was detected by weekly rectal and throat swabs, using Levinthal's agar medium containing antiserum to *H. influenzae,* type b (Bradshaw et al., 1971). Organisms yielding a halo reaction were checked for specificity by subculturing on normal serum-agar and indentified by the Enterobacteriology Unit for the Center for Disease Control, Atlanta, Georgia. As controls, newborn animals were fed an equal volume of a sterile saline solution. Serum antibody to *E. coli* K antigen was determined by passive hemagglutination of polysaccharide-coated, glutaraldehyde-fixed, group O-negative erythrocytes (Bing, Weyand, and Stavitsky, 1967). Serum bactericidal activity toward *H. influenzae,* type b (strain Rab), was carried out as described (Landy, Michael, and Whitby, 1962; Schneerson et al., 1971). Serum antibody to the type b capsular polysaccharide was determined by a modified Farr assay with I^{125} labelled capsular polysaccharide (Gotschlich, 1971).

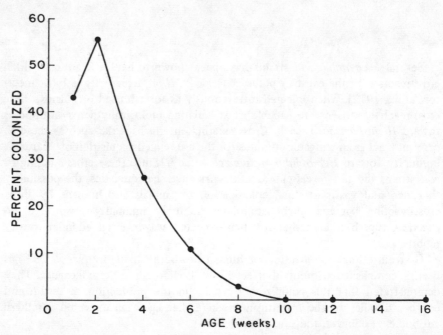

Fig. 1. Percentage of animals colonized with *E. coli,* strain Easter, as a function of age. Note the exponential decline in the proportion of fed animals that yielded the cross-reacting *E. coli* in stool or throat culture.

RESULTS

Two colonization experiments were performed with two *E. coli* 075 strains. *E. coli*, strain Easter, was fed in the first experiment. All members of a litter were either colonized or not. One of the two litters fed 10^9 bacteria per animal, one of the two litters fed 10^6 bacteria per animal, and the one litter fed 10^3 bacteria per animal were colonized. None of the control animals yielded a cross-reacting organisms at any time during the experiment. No *H. influenzae*, type b, isolates were detected at any time from either experimental or control animals.

The number of deaths within the first week of life and the rate and absolute amount of weight gain were not significantly different for experimentals or controls. Figure 1 shows that colonization was only transient: the cross-reacting *E. coli* was not isolated from any rabbit after the eighth week of life.

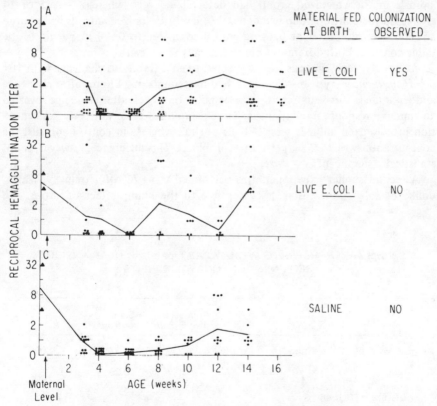

Fig. 2. Reciprocal hemagglutination titers measuring antibody to *E. coli,* strain Easter, K antigen as a function of age. Each point represents the value for an individual animal. Values are plotted on a scale of log base two. The unbroken line in each panel connects the geometric mean titer for each weekly set of measurements.

Serum hemagglutinating antibody response to the *E. coli* K antigen is shown in Figure 2. All animals had undetectable levels of antibody by age six weeks. At eight weeks of age, detectable antibody was observed in colonized animals at a constant level through week fourteen. Controls did not reach this level until the twelfth week. The average titer of colonized animals from weeks eight through fourteen was significantly greater than control animals (P< .005) due primarily to the differences observed at weeks eight and ten. Although the number of animals is small, the pattern of response in animals fed *E. coli* but not detectably colonized appeared similar to the colonized animals.

Serum antibody response to the type b capsular polysaccharide is shown in Table 1. All animals had undetectable antibody levels (< 0.1 μg antibody protein/ml serum) from weeks six through twelve. At 14 weeks of age, 14 of 17 animals in the colonized group had detectable levels, whereas only 5 of 14 animals in the control group had detectable levels. Colonized animals had a mean antibody concentration of 0.47 μg per ml compared to 0. 29 μg per ml in the saline controls. Both differences are statistically significant.

At week fifteen, animals were subjected to an intravenous challenge with 10^7 live *H. influenzae*, type b. All animals had bacteremia at 24 hours after challenge and all animals survived. Serum samples taken one week after challenge revealed an immune response in all animals. The mean anticapsular antibody concentration in colonized animals was 24.0 μg per ml, whereas in control animals, the concentration was 14.2 μg per ml (see Table 1). This difference, however, is not statistically significant.

A second similar experiment was performed using *E. coli*, strain 89, which, unlike *E. coli*, strain Easter, is susceptible to the killing effect of anti-*E. coli*

TABLE 1

SERUM ANTI-*HEMOPHILUS INFLUENZAE*, type b, CAPSULAR ANTIBODY
RESPONSE OF NEONATAL RABBITS

		Animals fed live *E. coli*	"Saline" controls	P
Animals with detectable antibody at 14 weeks		14/17	5/14	<0.005
Antibody level* (μg/ml) (mean and range)	14th week	0.47 (<0.1-2.0)	0.29 (<0.1-1.6)	<0.005
	Post Challenge	24.0 (2.3-50.0)	14.2 (7.4-30.0)	>0.05

*Farr assay, minimum detectable = 0.1 μg antibody/ml serum.

antibody and complement and, which has a cross-reactive antigen with greater precipitating activity (Schneerson et al., 1972). The *E. coli* were fed to 11 newborn rabbits from three litters at a dosage of 10^9 bacteria per animal. Ten other animals from two litters received sterile saline. Since, in the previous experiment, the greatest differences in serum-immune response between experimental and control animals appeared to be at eight and ten weeks of age, all animals in this experiment were challenged at eight weeks with 5×10^7 intravenously administered live *H. influenzae*, type b.

Unlike the previous experiment, not all members of a single litter were colonized. Four of the four animals in litter A, one of three in litter B, and two of four in litter C were colonized. Colonization with the cross-reacting bacteria was again transient as all animals failed to reveal the cross-reacting *E. coli* in stool culture by the eighth week of age. No animal in the control group yielded a cross-reacting organism, nor were any *H. influenzae*, type b, organisms isolated from any animal. No harmful effects of colonization were detected as judged by perinatal mortality and weight gain.

The serum-immune response of fed and control animals is shown in Table 2. At 8 weeks of age, hemagglutinating activity toward the *E. coli* K antigen was detectable in all animals, but the geometric mean titer was higher in the animals

TABLE 2
IMMUNE RESPONSE OF NEONATAL RABBITS FED
E. COLI (STRAIN 89) AT BIRTH

	8 weeks old		5 days post-challenge	
	E. coli 89	Saline	*E. coli* 89	Saline
Reciprocal anti-*E. coli* haemagglutination titer (geom. mean)	3.4	2.7	5.7	4.9
Reciprocal bactericidal titer ("rab")	N.D.‡	N.D.	4.5	4.2
No. with detectable antibody	10/11	1/10†	11/11	10/10
Anticapsular antibody concentration in μg/ml (mean and range)	0.08 (0.06-0.19)	<0.06	1.60 (0.07-8.0)	0.59* (0.06-2.14)

*P <0.01
†P <0.005
‡Not detectable

fed *E. coli*, although this difference was not statistically significant. Serum bactericidal activity was not detected in either experimental or control animals at this time. However, ten of eleven experimental animals, as compared to one of ten control animals, had anticapsular antibody concentrations detectable by radioimmunoassay at 8 weeks of age. The lower limit of detection by the radio-immunoassay at this time was 0.06 µg antibody per ml serum.

After challenge with live organisms, all animals were bacteremic at 24 hours and all animals survived. By the fifth post-challenge day, blood cultures were negative in all animals. By hemagglutination, bactericidal, and radio-immunoassay, the level of antibody was greater in the animals fed *E. coli* than in the control group (see Table 2). The mean anticapsular antibody concentration was 1.60 µg per ml in the animals fed *E. coli*, as compared to 0.59 µg per ml in the control animals. This difference is statistically significant.

DISCUSSION

Gastrointestinal colonization of neonatal rabbits by cross-reacting *E. coli* was accomplished in two experiments without harmful effect. In both experiments, about 60% of fed animals were detectably colonized. The success of colonization did not appear to be related to the dosage of bacteria fed at birth. The method of detection, weekly rectal culture plated on a single solid medium, may not have detected all colonized animals. The similarity of the immune response of colonized animals to those fed *E. coli*, but not detectably colonized, suggests that colonization may have been successful for all fed animals.

The reason for the disappearance of detectable cross-reacting *E. coli* in colonized animals by the eighth week of age is not known. However, the possibility that this disappearance follows a local immune response is presently under investigation.

The serum anti-type b capsular antibody concentration in both experimental and control animals was undetectable by assay of bactericidal activity toward *H. influenzae*, type b. Using the sensitive radioimmunoassay, however, the earlier appearance of low levels of anti-capsular antibody could be observed in fed animals, as compared to controls. No protective effect of the anticapsular antibody could be demonstrated, since both experimentals and controls survived the challenge with live *H. influenzae*, type b. This result may be due to insufficient numbers of bacteria used for challenge (Schneerson and Robbins, 1971).

Analysis of the immune response following challenge revealed rapid production of anticapsular antibody. However, antibody concentrations in fed animals were higher than in controls in both experiments, suggesting that neonatal colonization had resulted in primary sensitization of the experimental animals.

From one of the animals fed *E. coli*, strain 89, a *Bacillus* strain (designated Sh 18) was isolated from rectal culture, which also cross-reacted with *H. influenzae*, type b. This animal had the highest anticapsular antibody response of all animals after feeding. This intriguing observation may indicate that other cross-reacting bacteria, such as those of the *Bacillus* or *Lactobacillus* species, should be studied for their ability to induce immunity to *H. influenzae*, type b, after gastrointestinal colonization. Neonatal gastrointestinal colonization by nonpathogenic, cross-reacting bacteria may provide active immunization against *H. influenzae*, type b, disease that resembles "natural" immunity.

ABSTRACT

Neonatal rabbits were fed *Escherichia coli* cross-reactive with *Hemophilus influenzae*, type b, at birth. Gastrointestinal colonization was accomplished in 60% of the animals and no harmful effects of feeding were observed. Feeding appeared to stimulate a primary immune response toward *H. influenzae*, type b, although the protective effect of this response could not be demonstrated. Neonatal colonization by nonpathogenic cross-reacting bacteria may provide active immunization that resembles "natural" immunity against *H. influenzae*, type b, diseases.

REFERENCES

Bradshaw, M. W.; R. Schneerson; J.C. Parke, Jr.; and J. B. Robbins. 1971. "Bacterial Antigens Cross-Reactive with the Capsular Polysaccharide of *Hemophilus influenzae*, type b." *Lancet* 1:1095.

Bing, D. H.; J. G. M. Weyand; and A. B. Stavitsky. 1967. "Hemagglutination of Aldehyde-Fixed Erythrocytes for Assay of Antigens and Antibody." *Proc. Soc. Exp. Biol. Med.* 124:1166.

Gotschlich, E. C. 1971. "A Simplification of the Radioactive Antigen-Binding Test by a Double-Label Technique." *J. Immunol.* 107:910.

Landy, M.; J. G. Micheal and J. L. Whitby. 1962. "Bactericidal Method for the Measurement in Normal Serum of Antibody to Gram-Negative Bacteria." *J. Bact.* 83:631.

Lodinova, R.; V. Jouja; A. Laue. 1967. "Influence of the Intestinal Flora on the Development of Immune Reactions in Infants." *J. Bact.* 93:797.

Schneerson, R.; M. W. Bradshaw; J. K. Whisnant; R. L. Myerowitz; J. C. Parke, Jr.; and J. B. Robbins. 1972. "An *Escherichia coli* Antigen Cross-Reactive with the Capsular Polysaccharide of *Hemophilus influenzae*, type b: Occurrence among known Serotypes and Immunochemical and Biological Properties of *E. coli* antisera toward *H. influenzae*, type b." *J. Immunol.* In press.

Schneerson, R., and J. B. Robbins. 1971. "Age-Related Susceptibility to *Hemophilus influenzae,* type b, Disease in Rabbits." *Infect. and Immun.* 4:397.
Schneerson, R.; L. P. Rodrigues; J. C. Parke, Jr.; J. B. Robbins. 1971. "Immunity to Diseases Caused by *Hemophilus influenzae*: II. Specificity and Some Biologic Characteristics of Natural, Infection-Acquired, and Immunization-Induced Antibodies." *J. Immunol.* 107:1081.

Discussion

Sarah H. Sell, Presiding

Carl W. Norden: I wanted to ask, to be sure I understood: You observed hemagglutinating activity against *E. coli* in rabbits prior to challenge, is that correct? Did you not observe bactericidal activity?

Richard L. Myerowitz: No bactericidal activity was detectable in experimental or control rabbits prior to challenge. Hemagglutinating antibody to the *E. coli* K antigen was detectable prior to challenge.

Norden: Do you have any thoughts as to why this discrepancy occurs? I thought your slide also showed hemagglutinating activity against *H. influenzae,* type b.

Myerowitz: Anti-type b capsular antibody was measured by the radio-immunoassay. We did actually perform the hemagglutinating assays for anti-type b antibody and it, too, was undetectable prior to challenge. The bactericidal and hemagglutination activities were thus parallel. I presume that the poor sensitivity of these assays (relative to radio-immunoassay) is responsible for the apparent, though not real, lack of response in experimental animals.

Norden: Did you observe any protection?

Myerowitz: No, protection could not be demonstrated as all animals (experimental and controls) survived challenge. However, this result is probably due to insufficient dosage of bacteria used for challenge.

Sarah H. Sell: Any other comments?

Richard B. Johnston, Jr.: This is an obvious question, but it has not been asked yet: Would it be more effective to spray the antigen into the nasopharynx, the most likely site of invasion for this particular bacterium?

Sell: We will get into this later; I think it is a great idea. Dr. Anderson, did you want to make a comment?

Porter Anderson: The question is to Dr. Myerowitz about an interpretation of the statement that polyribitol phosphate and polyribose phosphate are present. I wonder if you envision that what you have is a mixture of two polymers, or is it a polymer that contains both kinds of sugars, or would you rather not say? I am inviting you to guess if you do not know.

Sell: Who will answer that question?

79

John B. Robbins: We would also like to know. There is no answer, yet.

Norden: I would like to ask Dr. Robbins's group what they think are the possibilities of immunization. Although they can detect the antibodies by the Farr
technique, they cannot show protection following challenge with live bacteria.
Why do they feel that this program would be potentially useful?

Robbins: We did not show protection, but it may be a function of the numbers
of bacteria injected. In other words, the controls did not die from our challenge because our challenge dosage just was not high enough.

Sell: Do you think it was dose-related?

Robbins: We were basing it on the data of Dr. Schneerson, who has studied this
relation in rabbits that had not been experimentally manipulated. She has
shown that four-week-old animals do not have detectable antibody and, like
young infants, appear to be susceptible to septicemia. If challenged with the
right dose of bacteria, a significant proportion get bacteremia and die. We
tried to do this experiment with the *E. coli*-fed and control animals by
injecting 10^7 *H. influenzae,* type b. We plan to increase this challenge dosage
to compensate for the fact that the anti-type b response induced by the *E.
coli* was observed at eight to fourteen weeks. I do think that if antibody is
detectable, protection could be demonstrated if the challenge dosage were
sufficient. However, if one uses a high dose (10^9-10^{10}) they are all going to
die, probably, because this amount of bacteremia is toxic in itself.

Sell: Yes, I agree with that.

Anderson: About animal protection: it is worthwhile checking, rather than just
assuming, that the virulence in an animal system of *Hemophilus influenzae,*
type b, is really increased by the encapsulation. I found, in trying to use the
mouse system, that there really was not a very good correlation between type
b encapsulation of strains and the virulence, as if other factors than that were
responsible for the virulence. This is an experience with just one strain of
mouse. It may not be true in all. I think that the human analogy is not
necessarily true with all animals' systems. Perhaps I would ask whether this
was studied with infant rabbits or mice.

Robbins: One of the observations made by Dr. Alexander and Miss Leidy was
that repeated mouse passage did not result in increasing encapsulation as
observed for pneumococcus, for instance. To illustrate the limitation of the
mouse-protection test as a bioassay which utilizes gastric mucin, consider
myself as an experimental animal. If you perform the equivalent of the
mouse-protection test on me, you would have to inject me intraperitoneally
with seven liters of something which has the consistency of chewed bubble
gum to induce an infection. Thus, I think that Dr. Anderson's comments
about the relationship between animal models and human disease is a valid
one.

The other point here is that the feeding experiments are different from active immunization intravenously. The colonization experiments were done to mimic natural immunity, which can be a very slow process. It occurs in normal and control animals at a slower rate, as was shown in the fed animals. The colonization study has limitations in that ultimately most adult rabbits become immune, fed or not.

Sell: Miss Leidy, would you like to make any comments about this? You have had a great deal of experience in animal tests for protection against *H. influenzae* infection.

Grace Leidy: Mostly the mouse-protection tests. But I agree with Dr. Anderson: it is more than just the presence of the capsule, because in transformation experiments where we transformed Rb to b and Rd to b, unfortunately the Rd strain was so virulent that you could not bring out the difference between the transformed or the Sd types. The Rb strain was not quite so virulent as Sb. These are natural, and the Rb, and the nonencapsulated derived from it, so that there was a slight difference in the virulence, but it was not dramatic. These were bacteria suspended in mucin. We also tried nonmucin, but it did not work very well.

Thomas H. Stoudt: Even in the case of pneumococcus, there is not correlation between encapsulation and the virulence in the mice. Even though there is a need for encapsulation, the amount of the capsulation has no correlation. As a matter of fact, if one isolates *in vitro* organisms which have capsules of much greater than normal size, and test these in mice, they are nonvirulent. There certainly must be other factors.

John K. Whisnant: I would like to ask Dr. Anderson if the mice used were inbred and, if so, what strain?

Anderson: These are not inbred. I do not know what strain; we just ordered mice.

Whisnant: The reason I ask is that there are strain differences in hosts, as well as bacteria. We have been interested in this and have some very preliminary data to suggest that the susceptibility to infection may be host-related as well as strain-related. If one injects multiple inbred strains with *H. influenzae,* type b, from the same culture, some animals die, and some do not. The pattern of genetics is not clear yet, but the results are encouraging.

Kenneth McIntosh: How do you explain the apearance of anti-type b polysaccharide antibody in the control rabbits?

Robbins: It is probably related to cross-reacting bacterial antigens that induce "natural" antibodies. If one just waits long enough, the "natural" antibodies develop in both groups. There are, of course, other strains with cross-reacting antigens, in addition to the ones we have identified. In humans, if one waits till the age of four years, most children will be immune to *Hemophilus* and this could be analogous to the rabbit.

Myerowitz: I think Dr. Robbins will go into more detail about this tomorrow, but we might mention that the technique used for detecting gastrointestinal cross-reacting bacteria only tests a very small portion of the bacteria flora that are residing in the gastrointestinal tract. We do not use culture media necessary for some of the other enteric bacteria that have special metabolic needs and that do not grow on these plates. Furthermore, we did not look for cross-reacting anaerobic bacteria. Therefore, the fact that we did not find bacteria with cross-reacting structures in the control animals who develop natural immunity, anyway, is not surprising. There may be antigenic stimuli for the acquisition of natural immunity other than the ones we are proposing.

Robbins: We have not looked for any anaerobes for cross-reacting antigens. Also, two more comments: First, we looked very carefully for *Hemophilus influenzae,* type b, in rabbits, and, while we are not very good microbiologists, I think probably our deficiencies are made up by the antiserum agar technique. To date, we have failed to find *Hemophilus influenzae,* type b, in about 1,000 rabbits of various ages. So at least this bacterial species, as recognized in man, does not exist in rabbits as we detect it, but rabbits do make *H. influenzae,* type b, antibodies. The antiserum technique is not good for all bacteria that contain known cross-reactions. The halo effect, especially with lactobacillus, is not that sharp, clear precipitation reaction which is found with *E. coli.* The antigen diffuses rapidly and forms a large halo that is difficult to detect, especially in stool culture, when there is a heavy growth. The polyribitol phosphate, which we think is giving the cross-reaction, is low in molecular weight so that it diffuses into the media and gives a slight halo.

Anderson: As long as Dr. Robbins is warmed up, I would like to ask how much leeway there is between an antiserum concentration in the agar that will reveal the halo and one which will inhibit the bacteria. Might this differ from strain to strain of *Hemophilus?*

Robbins: I do not know what causes the inhibition, but Dr. Anderson is certainly correct in that it occurs. If one uses a high concentration of antiserum, hardly anything grows and if too little, the halo is not visualized. Goat serum is not very good for the antiserum agar technique and, we presume, this is due to the high NADase activity which may inactivate one of the growth factors for *H. influenzae.* We do have some quantitative data about what seems to be the optimum concentration: that is, in a fifteen-ml aliquot for a single plate, 1.5mg of antibody seems to permit growth and yield halo formation. However, we have not tested large numbers of *Hemophilus* strains to see whether this is universal. If there are rabbit strains of *Hemophilus* that are more inhibited by the antiserum than strains isolated from humans, we would miss *H. influenzae,* type b, by this technique.

Anderson: Not only rabbit strains, but possibly there are some human strains that conceiveably might be missed. Do you think you are picking up all the human strains?

Robbins: We have worked with three strains. In a series of experiments, *Hemophilus influenzae*, type b, was mixed into cultures in known amounts and then replated on agar, using Levinthal's media and the antiserum agar technique. The antiserum agar did not give as large colonies as did the Levinthal's agar without the antiserum, but quantitative recovery experiments showed that we did not lose colonies. However, we have not tested a wide variety of strains and perhaps we should. That is a good suggestion.

John Witte: Have you tried colonizing germ-free animals with *E. coli* strains and then challenging them with *H. influenzae*, type b?

Robbins: Yes, we tried two experiments. We have done mouse experiments, and the sera are being analyzed. In the first experiment, we stopped at four weeks of age because the cleaning woman kicked the mice out of our bathtub. At this time, our radio-immunoassay was detecting 0.4 micrograms/ml of antibody. After four weeks, we could not detect any antibody in colonized or uncolonized animals. All animals fed the *E. coli* were colonized, and none of them died. The second experiment we have taken out to six weeks and have not finished the data yet. It does not seem to be a virulent procedure for germ-free mice. We treated them for three days after birth with *E. coli* in the drinking water. At the fourth day, we changed their drinking water, and the colonization was 100%.

SECTION IV

Methodology in Detection of Human Serum Antibodies to *Hemophilus influenzae,* type b

Porter Anderson
Richard B. Johnston, Jr.
David H. Smith

Our laboratory has used, modified, or devised a number of methods for measuring serum antibodies to *H. influenzae,* type b. The intent has been to establish a framework with which to evaluate the role of humoral antibodies in host resistance. Some of the methods are similar to those used by other workers, including several present here; the details of our tests are documented or described in the Appendix to this paper.

Earlier studies concluded that the PRP capsular antigen was the key to virulence of this organism (summarized in Alexander, 1958), so our initial efforts have been concentrated on anti-PRP antibodies. Human adults immunized with a few micrograms of purified PRP generally have a prompt and long-lasting antibody response. The data outlined in Table 1 are based upon sera of several individuals who had a good response and who had had undetectable or very low values before immunization.

Precipitating antibody is detectable if micromethods are used. Values obtained at equivalence are in the general area of 100 μg Ab/ml serum. At equi-

This work was done at the Infectious Disease Unit, Childrens' Hospital, Medical Center, and Beth Israel Hospital, Department of Pediatrics, Harvard Medical School, Boston, Massachusetts.

Supported by grants from the Milton Fund, the Medical Foundation, Inc., the Hood Foundation, the Maternal and Child Health and Crippled Children's Services Program of the Massachusetts Department of Public Health, by contract 71-2196 from the National Institute of Allergy and Infectious Diseases, Bethesda, Maryland, and Grants AI-05877 and 1-F03-AI46905 from the National Institute of Allergy and Infectious Disease.

TABLE 1

ASSAYS FOR HUMAN SERUM ANTIBODY TO PRP

Assay	Limit, μg/ML*	Comment
Precipitation	20	
Passive Hemagglutination, 37°C	0.5	Activity of IgM $\gg$ IgG. IgA?
Passive Hemagglutination, 4°C	0.1	IgG Activity Increases
Farr Test, Using 20 μl Serum	0.01	Depends on S.A. of Radioantigen
Farr Test, Using 100 μl Serum	0.003	Depends on S.A. of Radioantigen
H. Influenzae b Bactericidal	1	Activity of IgM $\approx$ IgG
		Requires Complement through C3
		Not PRP-specific
H. Influenzae b Opsonizing	20	Not PRP-specific

*Based on precipitating antibody content of reference postimmunization sera

valence, about 50 μg of antibody is precipitated by 1 μg of the antigen. This suggests a relatively high multiplicity of antigenic determinants per molecule. The values we have seen in human post-immunization sera do not greatly exceed the practical limits of the assay. The precipitin technique is thus not suitable for study of sera of lower activity. It does provide an approximate reference value by which the sensitivity of other techniques can be calibrated.

PRP binds very strongly to erythrocytes; fixing and tanning are not necessary. Such cells can be used for passive hemagglutination and hemolysis assays. Relative to precipitation, passive hemagglutination is a considerably more sensitive test, having a limit of about 0.5 μg Ab/ml. As previously described (Anderson, Johnston, and Smith, 1972), the test is done at 37° C. Under these conditions, purified IgM fractions from human sera are roughly 100-fold more active than IgG (Johnston et al., 1972). We've not yet tried to evaluate purified IgA. The strong IgM bias of this assay, then, makes it unsuitable for measurements such as placentally transmitted antibodies or of antibodies in the standard therapeutic gamma globulin. It was useful in evaluating the antibody response to purified PRP in a large number of adults (Anderson et al., 1972), but is insufficiently sensitive for use with young children.

We have recently found that passive hemagglutination becomes even more sensitive when incubated at 4°C. The increased sensitivity appears to be entirely due to an increased activity of IgG antibody. This version of the assay has permitted the detection of antibody responses in infected children and in PRP-immunized children that were not detectable with the 37° C test.

The passive-hemagglutination method must be used with careful attention to the possibility of a nonspecific agglutination; non-PRP-sensitized cell control tests should be run with every serum. (The use of glutaraldehyde-fixed erythrocytes, although convenient, caused an increased frequency of nonspecific reactions with our sera.) For the 4° C test, the sera must be preabsorbed for removal of cold hemagglutinins. Children, particularly infected children, often have high titers of anti-I hemagglutinins.

The Farr test, which measures binding of radio-labeled antigen to the ammonium sulfate-precipitable globulins, is less subject to non-specific interference; and with an antigen of sufficiently high specific activity, it can be even more sensitive than passive hemagglutination. We have used PRP endogenously labeled with tritium as the antigen, and the double-label technique of Gotschlich (Gotschlich, 1971; Gotschlich et al., 1972) to determine the extent of binding. Dr. Robbins and colleagues have also been using the Farr test, and we agreed to begin using their reference serum (from S. Klein) as a standard so as to facilitate comparison of results. For calibration, the reference serum (whose precipitin content is known) is tested in a wide range of dilutions with each of a series of antigen concentrations. Plotting percent binding vs. dilution thus generates a series of overlapping curves (Fig. 1). The test serum is assayed undiluted with the series of antigens. The percent binding, obtained from the most appropriate

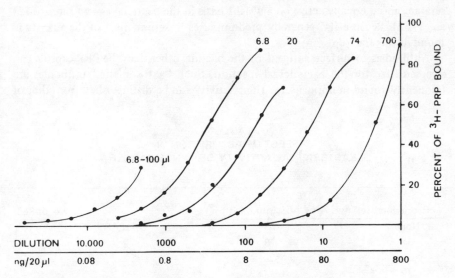

Fig. 1. Calibration of the ria with serum of S. Klein.

antigen concentration, is then equated to a dilution of the reference serum and hence to an antibody concentration. We quote the values as "ng Ab per ml serum," but strictly speaking, this should be quoted as "equivalent in binding capacity to so many nanograms of S. Klein precipitating antibody per ml."

With the increased sensitivity of the Farr test, we have detected weak and sometimes transient antibody responses in infected and in immunized children not detectable even with the $4°$ C passive hemagglutination test.

Serum bactericidal activity has been viewed as an important criterion of humoral resistance since the classic studies of Fothergill and colleagues (Fothergill and Wright, 1933; Ward and Wright, 1932; Wright and Ward, 1932). We do the assay by incubating test serum, a source of complement, and exponential phase bacteria—then plating for viable count. The test serum can be diluted, giving a cidal titer. In many sera, however, activity is not detectable at a dilution of one half or greater, but can be found with an incubation mixture containing 80 to 85% test serum. This is particularly true of sera of children. The reaction, if it occurs at all, is complete within minutes; prolonged incubation times tend to obscure weak activity due to growth of the survivors. When a serum deficient in C3 was used as the fresh-serum source, activity was much diminished, suggesting that this component is a necessary factor. For the antibody requirement, antibodies to PRP are sufficient. They are active against all of the dozens of b strains so far tested. The sensitivity in terms of precipitating antibody is about 1 μg/ml, just slightly less than the passive hemagglutination test. In contrast to the passive hemagglutination assay, however, IgG and IgM from adult immunized sera are about equally active on a weight basis in the bacterial assay (Johnston et al., 1972). Because IgG generally predominates in serum, most of the activity is found in this fraction.

Antibodies to surface antigens of the bacillus other than the PRP capsule can also sensitize for the bactericidal reaction. Such "anti-somatic" antibodies are frequently found in normal sera. Their activity can be distinguished from that of

TABLE 2
EFFECT OF ABSORPTION ON
BACTERICIDAL ACTIVITY OF 14 NORMAL SERA

Representative Titers After Absorption with:			No. of Sera
None	U-1	U-1+PRP	
64	8	<2	8
32	<2	<2	3
32	8	8	3

anti-PRP antibodies in the same serum by absorption studies. Table 2 summarizes for a group of 14 normal sera the effect on bactericidal titer against strain b-Rab of absorption with the PRP-negative, untypable strain U-1, which has somatic antigens in common with b-Rab. In eight normal sera, activity was reduced by U-1 absorption and the remaining activity was eliminated by absorption with purified PRP (indicating that both antisomatic and anti-PRP were present). In three, activity was eliminated by U-1. In three, activity was reduced by U-1 but not further reduced by PRP (indicating that more somatic antigens than one are involved and that not all are present on U-1).

The somatic antigens vary among b strains, and therefore b strains may differ in susceptibility to the bactericidal antibodies of particular sera (Table 3). Thus the outcome of a survey of the prevalence of type b bactericidal antibodies will

TABLE 3

THE BACTERICIDAL ACTIVITY OF NORMAL ADULT SERA
AGAINST TWO STRAINS OF *HEMOPHILUS INFLUENZAE,* type b

STRAIN	Cidal Titer vs Strain Eagan		Cidal Titer vs Strain Rabinowitz	
	−PRP	+PRP	−PRP	+PRP
JP	4	<2	8	4
AN	8	2	64	64
BL	<2	<2	32	32
SF	2	<2	16	16
SJ	4	4	64	64
JL	8	8	32	32

be affected by the choice of test strain. The nature of these antigens is presently undefined. In conjunction with Dr. Robbins' group, we are assembling a collection of strains and antisera with which to define their number and distribution.

Antibodies to *H. influenzae,* type b, can also be detected by opsonization *in vitro,* in which test serum and exponential phase bacteria are incubated with peripheral phagocytes. Dr. Johnston will fully describe this system later in the program; I shall just make two points about it. The mechanics of the assay are different from the bactericidal assay, so that the sensitivites of the two cannot be fairly compared. Thus the figure of 20 μg/ml in Table 1 should not be interpreted as saying that a 20-fold higher antibody concentration is required for opsonization than bacteriolysis. Second, antibodies directed both to PRP and to "somatic" antigens are active, so the antigen specificity may be the same as for the bactericidal assay (Anderson, Johnston, and Smith, 1972).

The methods described above were used in the work being reported by Drs. Smith and Peter, and this presentation should give an idea of the classes and amounts of antibodies underlying the titers they report. Correlation of serum activities to immunity are still being evaluated. It is evident that the Farr test detects anti-PRP antibody far below the concentration at which antibacterial activity is detectable. But it may be important that the Farr test can distinguish between nonresponse and a scanty antibody response to PRP in young children. Thus, exposures to the antigen in infection and in immunization that could be interpreted as nonimmunogenic or toleragenic by less sensitive methods have been shown to be merely weakly immunogenic.

APPENDIX: SEROLOGIC METHODS

Quantitative precipitin determination. Formation and washing of specific precipitates was done according to Kabat and Mayer (1961); 0.1 to 20 μg of PRP in saline (volumes equalized to 0.1 ml) was used with 1-ml samples of serum. Protein in the washed precipitates was quantitated with the Folin phenol reagent (Lowry et al., 1951) or—for the values quoted here—by the method employed in Dr. Robbins's laboratory: dissolving in 1% sodium lauryl sulfate, determining optical density at 280 nm, and using (per Miller and Metzger, 1965) the extinction coefficient of

$$E_{1\,cm}^{1\%} = 14.3.$$

Passive hemagglutination. Type O, Rh negative human erythrocytes from fresh blood were washed in phosphate-buffered saline, pH 7.3 (PBS), sensitized by incubation in 0.25 μg PRP/ml at a cell density of 1.2% (v/v), rewashed, and suspended at 0.6%. For the 37°C test, pairs of twofold serial dilutions (25 μl) of test serum in PBS containing 0.25% bovine albumin were made in U-bottom microtiter wells, and 25 μg of sensitized or unsensitized erythrocyte suspension was added. The wells were sealed, incubated three hours at 37° C, and read for agglutination by tipping 90 degrees. Further details are given by Anderson et al. (1972). For the 4° test, sera were absorbed one hour at 0-4° C on an equal volume of the washed erythrocytes. The test was completed as described above except for the lower incubation temperature.

Farr test. PRP was endogenously labeled by culturing *H. influenzae*, type b, in the presence of ^{3}H-glucose. The stock antigen for the results reported here had a specific activity of about 5 x 10^4 d.p.m./ng. For the weakest sera, the stock was used at a concentration of 6.3 ng/ml; for stronger sera,[3] H-PRP was used at the same concentration but was mixed with unlabeled PRP to give the total concentrations shown in Figure 1. The antigen was dissolved in borate buffer (Farr, 1958) containing 0.15 μC of $Na^{36}Cl$/ml, which served as a volume marker. Twenty μl of antigen solution was mixed with 20 or 100 μl of test serum in a small conical polypropylene centrifuge tube and incubated one hour at 4° C. Saturated (at 4° C) ammonium sulfate, 40 or 120 μl respectively, was added, incubation was continued one hour, the mixtures were centrifuged, and the supernatant withdrawn—all at 4° C. The precipitate was dissolved with water and suspended by the use of Protosol (New England Nuclear Corp., Boston) in a toluene-based scintillation fluid (4 g PPO, 0.05 g POPOP/1 toluene). A liquid scintillation spectrometer was adjusted so that one channel counted ^{36}Cl at an approximate efficiency of 75% and ^{3}H at 0.03% and the second channel counted ^{36}Cl at 1.5% and ^{3}H at 15%. Calculation of the percentage antigen-bound was done as described by Gotschlich (1971) and of the antibody concentration as described by Gotschlich et al. (1972).

Bactericidal assays. For the dilution test, serial dilutions (25 μl) of test serum were made in 1 ml wells in a transparent plastic tray held on ice; the diluent was PBS containing 0.25% bovine albumin, 0.5mM $MgSO_4$, and 0.15mM $CaCl_2$. To each well was added 25 μl of a mixture containing, in the same diluent, about 400 bacteria from an exponential-phase broth culture and a sufficient proportion, generally one fourth, of antibody-negative fresh serum (stored at-70° C to preserve complement). The tray was transferred to a 37° C incubator for one hour, 0.8 ml of transparent agar medium (at 45° C) was added to the wells with thorough mixing, and the 37° C incubation was continued overnight. The dilution endpoint was > 50% reduction in viable count. Further details are given by Anderson, Johnston and Smith (1972).

The proportion of complement source necessary was determined for each test strain by dilution tests in presence and absence of a minimal antibody source. The most useful complement sources have been serum from a human X-linked agammaglobulinemic and from a calf denied colostrum (provided by Dr. Robbins). Guinea pig serum has been used, but its activity appeared to deteriorate at an unacceptable rate in storage at -70° C. When normal adult or infant rabbit serum was used, titers of human antisera were about 100-fold greater than with other complement sources, although the rabbit serum by itself lacked cidal activity. When rabbit serum absorbed at 0° C on test bacteria was used, the antiserum titers had the expected values. This phenomenon has not yet been analyzed; it is mentioned to illustrate the hazards that can be encountered in using normal sera as a complement source.

For the test with a higher serum concentration, the method previously described (Anderson, Johnston and Smith, 1972) has been simplified: 65 μl of unheated test serum, 10 μl of antibody-negative fresh serum, and about 800 exponential-phase bacteria in 5 μl diluent were mixed in a small conical tube on ice. A 20 μl sample was spread on an agar plate, the tube was incubated 30 minutes at 37° C, and a second 20 μl sample was spread. Proportional change in viable count was compared to that in an incubation containing 65 μl of diluent instead of test serum (generally a 10 to 30% increase).

REFERENCES

Alexander, H. 1958. "Hemophilus influenzae." In *Bacterial and Mycotic Infections of Man*, edited by R. J. Dubos. Philadelphia: J. B. Lippincott.

Anderson, P.; R. B. Johnston, Jr.; and D. H. Smith. 1972. "Human Serum Activities against *Hemophilus influenzae*, type b." *J. Clin. Invest.* 51:31.

Anderson, P.; G. Peter; R. B. Johnston, Jr.; L. H. Wetterlow; and D. H. Smith. 1972. "Immunization of Humans with Polyribophosphate, the Capsular Antigen of *Hemophilus influenzae*, type b." *J. Clin. Invest.* 51:39.

Farr, R. S. 1958. "A Quantiative Immunochemical Measure of the Primary Interaction between I*BSA and Antibody." *J. Infect. Dis.* 103:239.

Fothergill, L.D., and J. Wright. 1933. "Influenzal Meningitis. The Relation of Age Incidence to the Bactericidal Power of Blood against the Causal Organism." *J. Immunol.* 24:273.

Gotschlich, E. C. 1971. "A Simplification of the Radioactive Antigen-binding Test by a Double-Label Technique." *J. Immunol.* 107:910.

Gotschlich, E. C.; M. Rey; R. Trian; and K. J. Sparks. 1972. "Quanitative Determination of the Human Immune Response to Immunization with Meningococcal Vaccines." *J. Clin. Invest.* 51:89.

Johnston, R. B., Jr.; P. Anderson; F. S. Rosen; and D. H. Smith. 1972. "Characterization of Human Antibodies to Polyribophosphate, the Capsular Antigen of *Hemophilus influenzae*, type b." (Submitted for publication).

Kabat, E. A., and M. Mayer. 1961. *Experimental Immunochemistry*. Springfield, Illinois: Charles C. Thomas.

Lowry, O. H.; N. J. Rosebrough; A. L. Farr; and R. J. Randall. 1951. "Protein Measurement with Folin Phenol Reagent." *J. Biol. Chem.* 193:265.

Miller, F., and H. Metzger. 1965. "Characterization of a Human Macroglobulin. I. The Molecular Weight of its Subunit." *J. Biol. Chem.* 240:3325.

Ward, H.K., and J. Wright. 1932. "Studies on Influenzal Meningitis: I. The Problems of Specific Therapy." *J. Exp. Med.* 55:223.

Wright, J., and H. K. Ward. 1932. "Studies on Influenzal Meningitis: II. The Problem of Virulence and Resistance." *J. Exp. Med.* 55:235.

CHAPTER 9

Antibody Production Following
Hemophilus influenzae Meningitis

Carl W. Norden
Richard H. Michaels

The immunologic response to *Hemophilus influenzae,* type b, meningitis has not been well studied in the past, but it is now the subject of much interest. This paper reports findings in 29 children from Rochester, New York, with *H. influenzae* meningitis and in 26 additional children from Pittsburgh, Pennsylvania, with meningitis due to this organism. A distinct age-related difference in antibody response is noted in both groups.

METHODS

Study population. Twenty-nine children from Rochester, New York, with meningitis due to *H. influenzae,* type b, were studied during 1969 and 1970. There were 21 boys and 8 girls, ranging in age from 3 months to 11 years. Twenty-six children from Pittsburgh, Pennsylvania, also with meningitis due to *H. influenzae,* type b, were studied over a six-month period starting in the fall of 1971. Eighteen were boys and eight were girls, ranging in age from 2 months to 13 years.

The initial sera (acute) were obtained during the first five hospital days, and the second sera (convalescent) on the eleventh day or later.

This work was done in the Departments of Medicine and Pediatrics, University of Rochester, School of Medicine and Dentistry, Rochester, New York, and the Departments of Medicine and Pediatrics, University of Pittsburgh School of Medicine, Pittsburgh, Pennsylvania.

Work was supported by PHS/GRSG Research Grant Number FR 05403 and by Research Grant CC 00613 from the Center for Disease Control, Atlanta, Georgia.

Serologic tests: Assay for bactericidal activity. These studies were performed as previously described by Norden et al. (1972), with the following modifications for the sera obtained from the Pittsburgh children. The bacterial suspension was diluted 1 to 10,000 in phosphate buffered saline and thus about 7×10^2 colony forming units were added to each well. Since a more dilute inoculum was used, the contents of each well were streaked onto Levinthal's agar plates with a standard milk loop calibrated to deliver 0.01 milliliters.

Hemagglutination assay. This procedure was performed as previously described by Norden et al. (1972).

RESULTS

Antibody response: Rochester children. Twenty-two of 29 children showed no rise in either bactericidal (BA) or hemagglutinating (HA) antibody titers, while seven patients had fourfold or greater antibody rises. Among the latter, five had increases in both HA and BA, one HA only and one BA only. No differences were observed between the two groups (those with antibody response and those without) in the frequency of bacteremia, peak white blood cell counts, spinal fluid glucose levels, duration of symptoms before institution of antibiotic therapy, and duration of antibiotic therapy. The only striking difference between the two groups was in their ages. Among 22 children less than 24 months of age, only one had an antibody response, whereas six of seven more than 24 months responded. The mean age for the nonresponders was 11 months, while for the responders it was 57 months.

Antibody response: Pittsburgh children. Out of 26 children studied, 5 showed a fourfold rise in either HA or BA. Three children (ages 35 months, 5 years, 13 years) showed rises in both HA and BA. One child, age 22 months, had a rise in BA only and one child age 16 months, had a rise in HA only. Thus, of 3 children aged 24 months or older, all had fourfold or greater antibody responses, while only 2 of 23 children less than 2 years of age had an initial antibody response. The mean age of the nonresponders was 11 months and for the responders it was 57 months.

Two children without an initial antibody response showed subsequent evidence of antibody formation. One 10-month-old child with no antibodies in the first convalescent specimen obtained 18 days after admission to the hospital developed an HA titer of 1 to 16 in another convalescent specimen obtained 30 days after the onset of illness; no bactericidal activity was detected in either specimen. A 7-month-old child developed bactericidal activity detected only in the undiluted serum three months after the onset of illness; an earlier convalescent serum had no bactericidal activity.

DISCUSSION

These preliminary findings, from children with *H. influenzae* meningitis in Pittsburgh, Pennsylvania, are strikingly similar to those reported from Rochester, New York. The majority of children with meningitis due to this organism failed to produce either bactericidal or hemagglutinating antibodies to this organism and those children who did show an antibody response were almost invariably more than 2 years of age. This finding has also been reported from Boston, Massachusetts, by Greenfield et al. (1972) and from Los Angeles by Reid et al. (1972).

The reasons for the age-related difference in antibody responses remain unclear. In our initial publication from Rochester, New York (Norden et al., 1972), we raised several hypotheses in an attempt to account for this difference. Since that time, there has been very little new data to support or refute any of these speculations.

One distinct possibility is that the technique for measuring antibodies to *H. influenzae,* type b, which were employed in these studies are too insensitive to detect small quantities. Further studies will be required to test this hypothesis, but it can be stated with certainty that the quantitative antibody responses between younger and older children is strikingly different.

If PRP remains in the serum as a persistent source of antigen, this could interfere with the assays for antibody. This could certainly explain the failure to detect antibodies in the acute serum, but it seems less likely in the convalescent, and extremely unlikely in serum obtained six to 23 months after the acute illness (such sera were obtained in the Rochester series).

Another possible explanation is that the test organism selected for study of bactericidal activity could be unusually resistant to serum bactericidal activity (Norden, 1972). However, we have employed two different organisms in these studies with identical results, and we had previously shown that the sera from 5 children, when tested against the organism isolated from their own cerebrospinal fluid, gave identically negative results.

The possibility that "immune paralysis" could develop in the younger children was extensively discussed in an earlier publication by Norden et al. (1972). The best method to test this hypothesis would be to immunize these children who failed to show an initial antibody response with an optimal dose of polysaccharide. Such studies have not yet been reported.

Dr. M. South (1972), in an editorial, has offered one other explanation which was not discussed in our initial publicaton. She has pointed out that there is evidence for sequential development of the recognition system for immune responsiveness and cited as an example the fact that the neonate, when given typhoid vaccine, develops a good antibody response to the H antigen, but no response to the O antigen. She suggests that the immunologic unresponsiveness of the small child to *H. influenzae* could be explained by the assumption that the antigens of this organism have a late position in the sequence of the immune system's ability to recognize them.

There are some earlier studies, in the area of streptococcal infections, which also shows a definite relationship between age and the immune response. Kevy and Lowe (1961) studied 11 children with streptococcal pneumonia and emphysema. The two youngest children (both less than 2 years of age) showed the poorest antibody response, as measured by antistreptolysin-O titer. Rantz, Maroney, and DiCaprio (1951) also noted this phenomenon in studies with streptococcal pharyngitis, in that they found that children under the age of 2 years had either no rise or only a small rise in antistreptolysin-O titer. No explanation for these age-related differences in streptococcal antibody formation were given, although there was a suggestion from some of this work that the development of these antibodies required frequent infections with the streptococcus.

It may be that the younger child is making a primary immune response to *H. influenzae*, type b, which is weak or nondetectable. In contrast, the older child may be already sensitized, either by prior contact with *H. influenzae*, type b, or with other organisms which have cross-reacting antigens, so that the immune response seen may be a brisk, secondary response.

It is clear that older children and younger children do not respond immunologically in the same manner to *H. influenzae*, type b, meningitis. It is equally clear that further studies are required to elucidate the reasons for this difference.

REFERENCES

Greenfield, S.; G. Peter; V. Howie; J. Ploussard; and D. H. Smith. 1972. "Acquisition of Type-Specific Antibodies to *Hemophilus Influenzae*, type b." *J. Ped.* 80:204.

Kevy, S., and B. Lowe. 1961. "Streptococcal Pneumonia and Empyema in Children." *New Eng. J. Med.* 264:738.

Norden, C. 1972. "Variable Susceptibility of *Hemophilus influenzae*, type b, Strains to Serum Bactericidal Activity." *Proc. Soc. Exptl. Biol. Med.* 139:59.

Norden, C.; M. Melish; J. C. Overall; and J. Baum. 1972. "Immunologic Responses to *Hemophilus influenzae* meningitis." *J. Ped.* 80:208.

Rantz, L.; M. Maroney; and J. DiCaprio. 1951. "Antistreptolysin O Response Following Hemolytic Streptococcus Infection in Early Childhood." *Arch. Int. Med.* 87:360.

Reid, A.; D. Ivler; J. Leedom; A. Mathies; and P. Wherle. 1972. "Serologic Response in *Hemophilus influenzae* Meningitis." *Clin. Res.* 20:272.

South, M. 1972. "Lack of Immune Response to *H. influenzae.*" *J. Ped.* 80:348.

CHAPTER **10**

Opsonization and Phagocytosis of
Hemophilus influenzae, type b

Richard B. Johnston, Jr.
Porter Anderson
Simon L. Newman

Alexander (1958) noted that therapeutic administration of rabbit antiserum to children with *H. influenzae,* type b, meningitis was accompanied by a subsequent increase in the number of bacteria found inside spinal fluid phagocytes. She suggested that the capsule of type b, *H. influenzae,* might be antiphagocytic, like that of the pneumoncoccus, and that enhancement of phagocytosis (opsonization) by anticapsular antibody might play a major role in immunity to this organism. This proposal remains unproven. In this presentation, we review some previously reported work and present new findings directed toward gaining an understanding of the nature of the serum elements which promote the phagocytosis of *H. influenzae,* type b, and the role of phagocytosis in defense against infection by this bacterium.

MATERIALS AND METHODS

Opsonization assay. Enhancement of phagocytosis by serum was studied using previously described methods (Anderson, Johnston, and Smith, 1972), except that the buffer used was Hank's balanced salt solution (Grand Island

This work was done in the Departments of Pediatrics and Microbiology, University of Alabama Medical Center, Birmingham, Alabama, and the Department of Pediatrics, Harvard Medical School, Children's Hospital Medical Center, Boston, Massachusetts.

This investigation was supported by Grants AI-10286, AI-05877, AI-41657, RR-05300, and RR-05349 of the National Institutes of Health, and by the Tara Soper Fund.

We gratefully acknowledge the technical assistance of Susan Sawyer and Bryson Waldo and the helpful suggestions of Dr. Fred S. Rosen and Dr. David H. Smith.

Biological Company) containing 0.2% glucose. The test sera were handled to preserve complement activity and thus served as their own complement source. The extent of phagocytosis in this assay was measured by the reduction of nitroblue tetrazolium (NBT) dye (Johnston et al., 1969). The result was expressed as ΔOD at 515 nm, which was determined by subtracting the result (OD) achieved in the absence of serum (usually about 0.060) from that achieved in the presence of the test serum. Serum from a patient with X-linked agammaglobulinemia or fresh guinea pig serum (GPS), 0.12 ml/assay mixture, was used as a complement source when purified IgG or antibody were tested. In this case, the ΔOD was determined by subtracting the OD obtained with the complement source alone from that obtained with both the complement and the antibody sources. In some experiments, results were compared to those achieved with a standard high-titered reference serum obtained from an adult immunized with polyribophosphate (PRP), as previously described (Anderson et al., 1972).

Uptake of radio-labeled H. influenzae. The NBT assay was performed as described above, except that the bacteria were cultured in 10 ml of broth containing 10 μC of ^{14}C-1-glycine (New England Nuclear Corporation) for 15 hours, and the reaction was stopped with 4 ml chilled saline and the tubes immediately centrifuged in the cold at 250g for ten minutes. The centrifuged leukocytes were washed twice in 4 ml saline, resuspended, then trapped on the surface of a cellulose membrane (Millipore Corporation, 25 mm diameter, 0.45 μ diameter pore size) by filtration. After drying the filter in a counting vial, 10 ml of scintillation cocktail (toluence and Fluoralloy Mix TLA, Beckman Instruments, Incorporated) was added, and radioactivity was determined in a liquid scintillation counter. Bacteria left in the supernate after separation of leukocytes were centrifuged at 7,000g for 20 minutes in conical tubes, dried in the tubes, solubilized in 0.5 ml NCS (Amersham/Searle Corporation), and transferred to vials for determination of radioactivity.

Bactericidial (BC) and passive hemagglutination (PHA) assays. The assays for BC and PHA antibodies used in the experiments reported here were those previously described (Anderson, Johnston, and Smith, 1972).

Separation of immunoglobulins and purification of antibody. The separation of IgG and IgM from postvaccination serum and purification of IgG$_1$ antibody to PRP by immunoabsorption have been previously described (Johnston et al., 1972). The subclass of the IgG antibody was identified using antisera to human myeloma proteins generously donated by Dr. P. H. Schur.

Complement requirements for opsonizing activity. Serum specifically deficient in C2 was obtained from a healthy adult man homozygous for an hereditary deficiency of this complement component (Klemperer, Austen, and Rosen,

1967). Serum specifically deficient in C3 was obtained from a child with chronic membranoproliferative glomerulonephritis (Gotoff et al., 1965). Serum from $B_{10}D_2/Sn$ "old line," AKR/J and A/J strains of mice, deficient in C5, and from $B_{10}B_2/Sn$ "new line," CBA/J, and Balb/cJ strains of mice with normal C5 (Rosenberg and Tachibana, 1969; Cinader, Dubiski, and Wardlaw, 1964) were obtained from Jackson Laboratories, Bar Harbor, Maine. Mouse serum was used as a complement source with an additional source of antibody, which was 0.16 ml of the standard antiserum heated to 56° C for 30 minutes. Reaction volumes were equalized with 0.15 M NaCl. Hemolytic complement activity was compared for the normal and C5-deficient mouse sera by a modification of the method of Mayer (1961) in which two-fold dilutions of sera were tested. Glycyl-l-valine, glycyl-l-leucine, and glycyl-l-tyrosine were obtained and prepared as previously described (Johnston et al., 1969).

Phagocytic bactericidal activity. A modification of the method of Quie was used, as previously described (Baehner and Johnston, 1971), except that the distilled water in which samples of the reaction mixture were diluted contained 0.5% bovine serum albumin, and leukocytes were disrupted at both dilutions by sonication in a "cup horn" (Heat Systems-Ultrasonics, Incorporated) for two minutes at 60 w. One-tenth ml of the second dilution, delivered by micropipet (Bolab, Incorporated), was spread on the surface of chocolate agar, and colonies were counted the next day.

RESULTS

In the experiments reported here, quantitation of phagocytosis was achieved by the spectrophotometric measurement of nitroblue tetrazolium (NBT) dye reduced to a blue color inside phagocytes after ingestion of bacteria. When pneumococci are used in the assay, dye reduction has been shown to occur in direct proportion to the number of bacteria ingested (Johnston et al., 1969). In order to compare the extent of dye reduction and the uptake of *H. influenzae*, type b, ^{14}C-labeled bacteria were used in the NBT assay and phagocytes were separated from uningested bacteria after the phagocytic reaction had been terminated. Phagocyte–associated radioactivity achieved in the presence of two pools of normal adult sera were both 51% of that achieved with the high-titered postvaccination serum, after correction for the minimal radio-activity achieved in the absence of serum. NBT dye reduction (ΔOD) in the presence of the two pools of sera were 54% and 48% of that obtained with the postvaccination serum. Radioactivity counts remaining in the supernates were the converse of phagocyte-associated counts and thus reflected the removal of radio-labeled bacteria by phagocytosis.

Fresh sera from 32 normal adults and five individuals with congenital pan-hypogammaglobulinemia (prior to their treatment with gamma globulin) were tested in the NBT assay for their ability to promote the phagocytosis of viable type b, *H. influenzae* (data presented in part by Anderson, Johnston, and Smith, 1972). Results for sera from four representative normal adults and an agamma-globulinemic child are shown in Figure 1. Among the four normal sera, opsoniza-

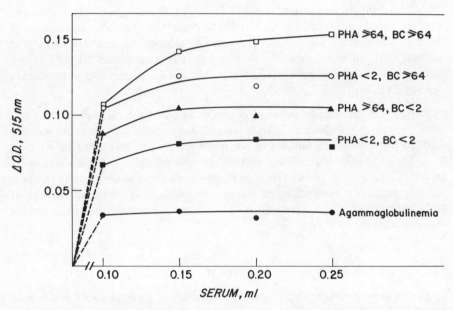

Fig. 1. Opsonization of *H. influenzae*, type b, by normal and agammaglobulinemic sera. Reciprocals of passive hemagglutination (PHA) and bactericidal (BC) titers are shown. (From P. Anderson, R. B. Johnston, Jr., and D. H. Smith, "Human Serum Activities against *Hemophilus influenzae*, type b," *J. Clin. Invest.* 51 (1972):31, with permission of the publishers.)

tion was greatest by that serum with a high titer in both the bactericidal (BC) and passive hemagglutination (PHA) assays and lowest by the serum which had undetectable levels in both assays. In general, opsonization correlated fairly well with BC activity and much better with BC than with PHA activity. However, there was not a quantitative relationship between results in the BC and opsoniza-tion assays. All of the normal sera tested, including four with BC and PHA titers both <1:2, had greater opsonizing activity than four of the five agamma-globulinemic sera. (One eight-year-old boy with X-linked agammaglobulinemia had low-normal opsonizing activity and a BC titer of 1:8, but no PHA activity.)

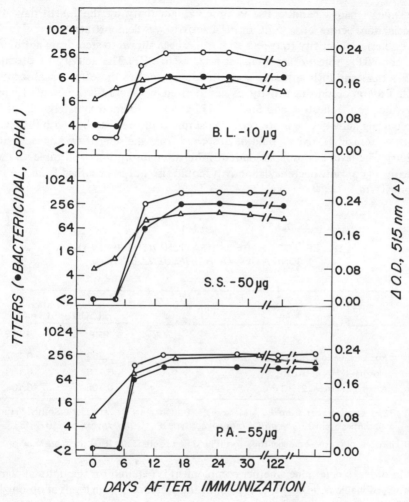

Fig. 2. The kinetics of response in PHA, BC, and opsonizing activities following immuniza-tion of three normal adults with 10, 50, or 55 μg PRP. Reciprocals of PHA and BC titers are plotted. (From P. Anderson, G. Peter, R. B. Johnston, Jr., L. H. Wetterlow, and D. H. Smith, "Immunization of Humans with Polyribophosphate, the Capsular Antigen of *Hemo-philus influenzae,* type b," *J. Clin. Invest.* 51(1972):39, with permission of the publishers.)

When serum from adults vaccinated with PRP was studied in the opsonization assay, a prompt and sustained increase in opsonizing activity could be demon-strated (Anderson et al., 1972). This increase correlated closely with that in the PHA and BC assays, as shown for three individuals in Figure 2. Two of these individuals had a definite rise in opsonizing activity by the fourth day after vaccination, before a rise in BC or PHA activity was demonstrated.

Bactericidal activity to type b strains has been shown to stem from antibodies to non-PRP, "somatic" antigens, as well as to PRP. The activity of opsonins other than anti-PRP antibody was studied by testing the effect of absorption with PRP on opsonizing activity, as summarized in Table 1 (data presented in part by Anderson, Johnston, and Smith, 1972). Although approximately half of the opsonizing activity of a postvaccination serum could be absorbed with PRP, very little opsonizing activity could be absorbed from the sera of two unvaccinated adults. The level of opsonization remaining after absorption of all three sera was clearly significant. Bactericidal activity could also not be absorbed from the two normal sera.

TABLE 1

THE EFFECT OF PREINCUBATION WITH PRP ON THE
OPSONIZATION OF *H. INFLUENZAE*, type b

Serum*	Opsonization (ΔOD at 515 nm)	
	–PRP	+PRP
Postvaccination (PHA 320, BC 160)	0.253	0.117
Normal (PHA 8, BC 16)	0.116	0.108
Normal (PHA <2, BC 64)	0.105	0.104

SOURCE: Data in part from P. Anderson, R. B. Johnston, Jr., and D. H. Smith, "Human Serum Activities against *Hemophilus influenzae*, type b " *J. Clin. Invest.* 51 (1972):31.

*Reciprocals of passive hemagglutination (PHA) and bactericidal (BC) titers are shown.

In order to determine whether complement is required for the optimal phagocytosis of viable *H. influenzae,* type b, in the presence of high levels of opsonizing antibody activity, enhancement of phagocytosis by the high-titered antiserum was compared before and after heating it to 56° C for 30 minutes. As shown in Figure 3, heated serum retained opsonizing activity. However, the extent of phagocytosis achieved with fresh serum was greater at every concentration at which the sera were compared, and the final level of phagocytosis reached in the presence of fresh serum was over twice that obtained with the heated sample. In contrast, the ability of the antiserum to promote the phagocytosis of an unencapsulated strain of *H. influenzae* did not decline after heating. Heating the serum did not diminish its antibody activity as measured by hemagglutination or, in the presence of added complement, bactericidal activity.

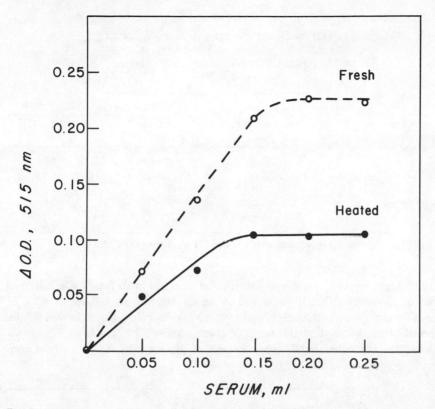

Fig. 3. A comparison of the extent of phagocytosis of *H. influenzae,* type b, achieved in the presence of fresh or heated antiserum, plotted as a function of the volume of serum in the reaction mixture.

Preparations of immune IgG and IgG_1 antibody to PRP purified by immuno-adsorption from postvaccination sera were tested for their ability to promote phagocytosis of *H. influenzae,* type b, with and without added complement. As shown in Table 2, there was enhancement of phagocytosis by the IgG and purified antibody preparations alone and a consistent further enhancement on the addition of complement. Opsonization was not achieved with IgM in concentrations equivalent to those found in normal human adult serum (Johnston et al., 1972).

The role of complement components C2 and C3 in the enhancement of phagocytosis was examined by comparing results obtained with varying amounts of normal serum and sera specifically deficient in C2 or C3 (Fig. 4). Levels of hemagglutinating and bactericidal antibody activity were comparable in the complement-deficient sera and the normal serum chosen for comparison (hemag-

TABLE 2

ENHANCEMENT OF PHAGOCYTOSIS OF *H. INFLUENZAE,* type b,
BY IMMUNE IgG AND ANTI-PRP IgG$_1$ IN THE
PRESENCE OR ABSENCE OF COMPLEMENT

Preparation	Amount Tested	Opsonizing Activity*	
		Without C	C Added
	mg	%	%
IgG	2.0	34	64
	4.0	46	83
Anti-PRP IgG$_1$	0.023	7	11
	0.046	11	18

* (ΔOD with test preparation/ΔOD with standard reference serum) x 100%

glutination titer 1:4 or 1:8 and bactericidal titer 1:4 in all three). The maximal
level of phagocytosis (ΔOD) achieved by serum which contained less than 5% of
the normal C2 concentration (Klemperer, 1969) was below that achieved by the
normal serum but within the range of levels obtained by sera from 32 normal
adults. On the other hand, enhancement of phagocytosis by the serum con-

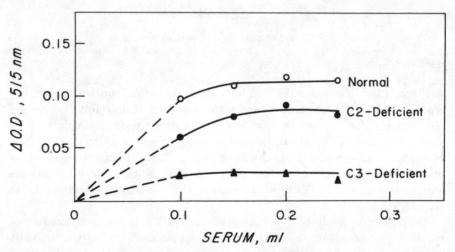

Fig. 4. A comparison of the extent of phagocytosis of *H. influenzae,* type b, achieved in the
presence of normal, C2-deficient, and C3-deficient fresh human sera, plotted as a function
of the volume of serum in the reaction mixture.

taining approximately 15% of the normal C3 concentration was clearly subnormal.

In order to ascertain whether the peptidase activity associated with C3 (Cooper and Becker, 1967; Johnston et al., 1969) might be necessary for the ingestion of encapsulated *H. influenzae,* enhancement of phagocytosis by fresh antiserum was tested in the presence of varying concentrations of glycyl-l-tyrosine, a known substrate for this enzyme (Cooper and Becker, 1967) and glycyl-l-valine and glycyl-l-leucine, employed as controls. When glycyl-l-tyrosine in concentrations greater than 7×10^{-4} M was present in the phagocytic system, inhibition of phagocytosis occurred (Fig. 5). There was no inhibition of phagocytosis by glycyl-l-valine (Fig. 5) or glycyl-l-leucine in the same concentration.

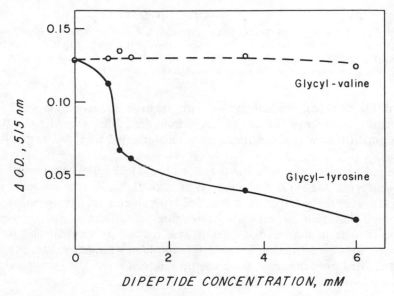

Fig. 5. A comparison of the extent of phagocytosis of *H. influenzae,* type b, achieved in the presence of 0.2 ml antiserum and varying concentrations of glycyl-l-tyrosine and glycyl-l-valine, plotted as a function of the concentration of dipeptide in the reaction mixture.

When serum from the $B_{10} D_2 /Sn$ "old-line" strain of mice with an inherited deficiency of C5 was compared to serum from the normal $B_{10} D_2 /Sn$ "new-line" strain, there was slightly less enhancement of phagocytosis by the C5-deficient serum at almost every concentration at which the sera were compared (Fig. 6, left). However, there was no difference in phagocytosis when serum from a second C5-deficient strain (A/J) and a second normal strain (Balb/cJ) were com-

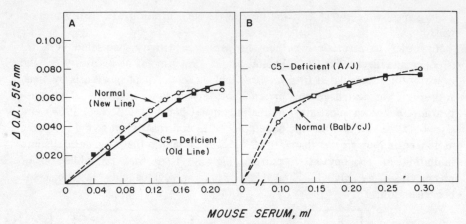

Fig. 6. A comparison of the extent of phagocytosis of *H. influenzae,* type b, achieved in the presence of 0.16 ml decomplemented antiserum and varying concentrations of serum from (A) $B_{10}D_2$/Sn "new line" and "old line," and (B) A/J and Balb/cJ mouse strains, plotted as a function of the volume of mouse serum in the reaction mixture.

pared (Fig. 6, right). The hemolytic activity of strain A/J serum was <20% that of strain Balb/cJ serum. Results with sera from the C5-deficient AKR/J and the C5-normal CBA/J strains confirmed the results achieved with A/J and Balb/cJ sera.

In order to determine if human peripheral blood leukocytes have the capacity to phagocytize and kill *H. influenzae,* type b, viable bacilli were incubated with phagocytes in the presence of antiserum heated to eliminate complement activity (and thus bacteriolysis). After 30 minutes of incubation, the number of viable bacteria in the reaction mixture was reduced to one-half and by 60 minutes, to one-third that of the original innoculum. When phagocytes or serum were omitted from the assay, there was no appreciable reduction in the number of viable bacteria.

DISCUSSION

The role of antibody and complement in the enhancement of *H. influenzae* phagocytosis has not been well examined in the past, at least in part because it has been difficult to apply available *in vitro* techniques to the study of this bacterium. Using a recently described spectrophotometric assay, it has been clearly demonstrated that antibody to capsular PRP will effectively promote the phagocytosis of type b, *H. influenzae.* Specifically, vacination with PRP elicited a prompt and sustained rise in opsonizing activity (Anderson et al., 1972). When postvaccination serum was absorbed with PRP, opsonizing activity was reduced to prevaccination levels. IgG_1 antibody purified from postvaccination sera by immunoadsorption with PRP contained opsonizing activity (Johnston et al., 1972).

Like bactericidal activity, however, opsonizing activity may not always require the presence of antibody specific for capsular PRP, in that significant opsonizing activity remained after absorption of sera with PRP. Moreover, opsonizing activity was appreciable in six sera which contained no detectable anti-PRP activity in the PHA assay.

It would appear from the studies reported here that, in the presence of high levels of antibody activity, phagocytosis of type b, *H. influenzae* (as well as *N. meningitidis* [Roberts, 1970]) can occur in the absence of complement.[1] However, it is clear that optimal opsonization of *H. influenzae* and pneumococci by immune or normal serum requires the fixation of C3 to the bacteria. Fixation of C3 to the pneumococcus may occur through the activity of specific antibody and complement components C142 (Johnston et al., 1969) or through the newly defined alternate pathway for C3 activation, which bypasses C142 (Shinn, Smith, and Wood, 1969; Winkelstein, Shinn, and Wood, 1972). The role of the alternate pathway in opsonization of type b, *H. influenzae*, remains to be elucidated. The finding of normal levels of phagocytosis in the presence of C2-deficient serum suggests that opsonization of *H. influenzae* may occur through this pathway. This mechanism could explain the opsonizing activity of normal sera which cannot be attributed to anti-PRP antibody.

The role of C5 in the ingestion of pneumococci was investigated by Shinn, Smith, and Wood (1969), who found opsonization by C5-deficient mouse serum to be slightly less effective than by serum from coisogenic normal mice. Using sera from these same coisogenic mouse strains, phagocytosis of *H. influenzae* was slightly better with serum of the normal strain. However, when sera from other C5-deficient and C5-normal strains were compared, there was a distinct difference in hemolytic activity, but no difference in opsonizing activity. It would seem likely that reagents other than mouse sera will be required to define clearly the role of C5 in the process of phagocytosis.

The enhancement of phagocytosis of *H. influenzae*, type b, by purified IgG_1 anti-PRP antibody could be demonstrated in the absence of complement, but there was definite further enhancement on the addition of complement. This is consistent with the recent observation that erythrocytes specifically coated with Rh antibodies or myeloma proteins of the IgG_1 or IgG_3 (but not IgG_2 or IgG_4) subgroups adhered to the surface of monocytes to form rosettes (Abramson et

---

1. In contrast, using the same assay system, phagocytosis of pneumococci fully sensitized with specific antibody was minimal in the absence of complement (Johnston et al., 1969).

al., 1970) and with the observation that rosette formation and phagocytosis of IgG-coated red cells could be enhanced by the addition of purified complement components 1, 4, 2, and 3 (Huber et al., 1968).

In contrast to the findings of Fothergill, Chandler, and Dingle with spinal fluid phagocytes (1937), it would appear that peripheral blood leukocytes can kill *H. influenzae*, type b, within minutes. In order to demonstrate this effect, we found it necessary to use decomplemented (heated) immune serum as the opsonin source, since in the presence of fresh serum it was difficult to separate the bactericidal effect of serum and phagocytes from that of serum alone. (See also Ward and Wright, 1932). Although this technical difficulty can undoubtedly be overcome, as it has been with enterobacteria, the relative importance of bacteriolysis and phagocytosis in defense against this bacterium will remain an unanswered question until these mechanisms can be separated *in vivo*. Since current knowledge of host defense against other extracellular bacteria strongly suggests that these organisms must be cleared by phagocytosis, it would seem important to continue to study opsonization and phagocytosis of *H. influenzae* until this question has been resolved.

SUMMARY

In vitro studies of the opsonization of *H. influenzae*, type b, by sera from normal and agammaglobulinemic individuals and sera from normal adults vaccinated with capsular PRP indicate that antibody to PRP will effectively promote the phagocytosis of this bacterium. Opsonization can also be achieved by serum lacking such antibody, perhaps through the activity of antibody to somatic antigen(s), or through the alternate pathway for C3 fixation, or both. Some opsonization can be achieved by specific antibody in the absence of complement; but it would appear that there is a strict requirement for C3, and apparently for the peptidase activity of bound C3, for the optimal phagocytosis of *H. influenzae*, type b. Although it was possible to demonstrate *in vitro* that peripheral blood phagocytes can ingest and rapidly kill *H. influenzae*, it has been difficult to separate both *in vitro* and *in vivo*, the bactericidal effect of serum and phagocytes from that of serum alone, and the role of opsonization and phagocytosis in defense against this bacterium remains to be defined.

REFERENCES

Abramson, N.; E. W. Gelfand; J. H. Jandl; and F. S. Rosen. 1970. "The Interaction between Human Monocytes and Red Cells. Specificity for IgG Subclasses and IgG Fragments." *J. Exp. Med.* 132:1207.

Alexander, H. E. 1958. *"Hemophilus influenzae."* In *Bacterial and Mycotic Infections of Man*, edited by R. J. Dubos, p. 470. Philadelphia: J. B. Lippincott.

Anderson, P.; R. B. Johnston, Jr.; and D. H. Smith. 1972. "Human Serum Activities against *Hemophilus influenzae*, type b." *J. Clin. Invest.* 51:31.

Anderson, P.; G. Peter; R. B. Johnston, Jr.; L. H. Wetterlow; and D. H. Smith. 1972. "Immunization of Humans with Polyribophosphate, the Capsular Antigen of *Hemophilus influenzae*, type b." *J. Clin. Invest.* 51:39.

Baehner, R. L., and R. B. Johnston, Jr. 1971. "Metabolic and Bactericidal Activities of Human Eosinophils." *Brit. J. Haemat.* 20:277.

Cinader, B.; S. Dubiski; and A. C. Wardlaw. 1964. "Distribution, Inheritance, and Properties of an Antigen, MuBl, and its Relation to Hemolytic Complement." *J. Exp. Med.* 120:897.

Cooper, N. R., and E. L. Becker. 1967. "Complement-Associated Peptidase Activity of Guinea Pig Serum: I. Role of Complement Components." *J. Immunol.* 98:119.

Fothergill, L. D.; C. A. Chandler; and J. H. Dingle. 1937. "The Survival of Virulent *H. influenzae* in Phagocytes." *J. Immunol.* 32:335.

Gotoff, S.P.; F. X. Fellers; G. F. Vawter; C. A. Janeway; and F. S. Rosen. 1965. "The Beta-1C Globulin in Childhood Nephrotic Syndrome: Laboratory Diagnosis of Progressive Glomerulonephritis." *N. Eng. J. Med.* 273:524.

Huber, H.; M. J. Polley; W. D. Linscott; H. H. Fudenberg; and H. J. Müller-Eberhard. 1968. "Human Monocytes. Distinct Receptor Sites for the Third Component of Complement and for Immunoglobulin G." *Science (Washington). 162:1281.*

Johnston, R. B., Jr.; M. R. Klemperer; C. A. Alper; and F. S. Rosen. 1969. "The Enhancement of Bacterial Phagocytosis by Serum. The role of Complement Components and Two Cofactors." *J. Exp. Med.* 129:1275.

Johnston, R. B., Jr.; P. Anderson; F. S. Rosen; and D. H. Smith. 1972. "Characterization of Human Antibody to Polyribophosphate, the Capsular Antigen of *Hemophilus Influenzae*, type b." *Clin. Immunol. Immunopath.* In Press.

Klemperer, M. R.; K. F. Austen; and F. S. Rosen. 1967. "Hereditary Deficiency of the Second Component of Complement (C'^2) in Man. Further Observations on a Second Kindred." *J. Immunol.* 98:72.

Klemperer, M. R. 1969. "Hereditary Deficiency of the Second Component of Complement in Man. An Immunochemical Study." *J. Immunol.* 102:168.

Mayer, M. M. 1961. "Hemolytic Assay of Complement." In *Experimental Immunochemistry* by E. A. Kabat and M. M. Mayer, p. 135. Springfield, Illinois: Charles C. Thomas.

Roberts, R. B. 1970. "The Relationship between Group A and Group C Meningococcal Polysaccharides and Serum Opsonins in Man." *J. Exp. Med.* 131:499.

Rosenberg, L. T., and D. K. Tachibana. 1969. "On Mouse Complement. Genetic Variants." *J. Immunol.* 103:1143.

Shinn, H. S.; M. R. Smith; and W. B. Wood, Jr. 1969. "Heat Labile Opsonins to Pneumococcus: II. Involvement of C3 and C5." *J. Exp. Med.* 130:1229.

Ward, H. K., and J. Wright. 1932. "Studies on Influenzal Meningitis: I. The Problems of Specific Therapy." *J. Exp. Med.*55:223.

Winkelstein, J. A.; H. S. Shinn; and W. B. Wood, Jr. 1972. "Heat Labile Opsonins to Pneumococcus: III. The Participation of Immunoglobulin and of the Alternate Pathway of C3 Activation." *J. Immunol.* 108:1681.

CHAPTER 11

Hemophilus influenzae Decomplementation Pattern in Chelated and Nonchelated Serum

D. P. Fine
S. R. Marney, Jr.
D. G. Colley
R. M. DesPrez

Bactericidal activity of various sera against *Hemophilus influenzae* organisms has not uniformly correlated with identification of specific antibody. This suggested to us that possibly *H. influenzae* activated complement directly in the absence of antibody via the recently described C3-shunt mechanism, so that complement would than opsonize the organisms for phagocytosis or lyse them directly. For this reason, we compared the complement activation pattern of *H. influenzae* with known activators of the C3 shunt.

The classic hemolytic complement pathway, which proceeds from C1 through C9, is known to require calcium. Götze and Müller-Eberhard (1971) recently described an alternate complement pathway, the so-called C3 shunt, which activates at the level of C3, proceeding through the later components, but bypassing C1, 4, and 2. They suggested that this pathway might require magnesium rather than calcium; this suggestion was confirmed by Sandberg and Osler (1971).

This work was done at Vanderbilt Medical Center and at Veterans Administration Hospital, Nashville, Tennessee.

This paper was supported by VA Infectious Diseases Training Program, TR-#74, VA Research Part I Funds and grant from U.S.P.H.S., National Institutes of Health, H.E.-08399.

The authors gratefully acknowledge permission by the Williams & Wilkins Company, Baltimore, Maryland, to use Figures 1, 2, and 3, which appeared in D. P. Fine; S. R. Marney, Jr.; D. G. Colley; J. S. Sergent; and R. M. DesPrez, "C_3 Shunt Activation in Human Serum Chelated with EGTA," *Journal of Immunology* 109 (1972): 807-810.

Since the classic C142 pathway requires calcium ion and the C3 shunt requires magnesium ion, we postulated that one might be able to distinguish one pathway from the other by using the chelators ethylene diamine tetra-acetic acid (EDTA) and ethylene glycol tetra-acetic acid (EGTA) which provide differential divalent cation chelation.

Figure 1 shows the basic experimental design of our studies. One ml of undiluted human serum was chelated with either EDTA or EGTA in a final concentration of 10 mM. Control serum received equal volumes of normal saline.

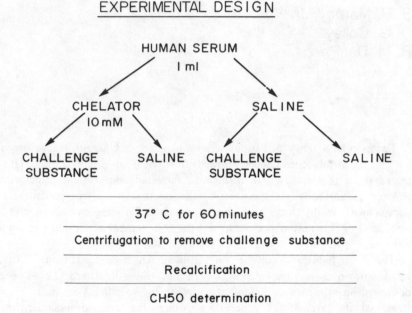

EXPERIMENTAL DESIGN

Fig. 1. Experimental design. (From D. P. Fine, S. R. Marney, Jr., D. G. Colley, J. S. Sergent, and R. M. DesPrez, "C$_3$ Shunt Activation in Human Serum Chelated with EGTA," *Journal of Immunology* 109 (1972): 807-810, with permission of the publishers.)

These sera were challenged with one of a variety of particulate substances (sensitized erythrocytes, zymosan, or whole bacterial organisms) or an equivalent volume of saline, then incubated at 37°C for 60 minutes with frequent mixing. After incubation, the sera were centrifuged to remove the challenge material; the supernatant fluids were withdrawn and those containing chelator were recalcified. Residual hemolytic complement (CH50) was then determined in the supernatant fluids according to the method of Rapp and Borsos (1970).

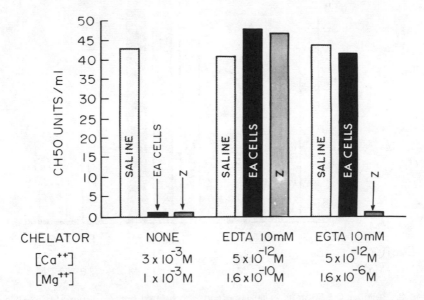

CHELATOR

[Ca^{++}]

[Mg^{++}]

Fig. 2. Residual CH50 units in chelated and nonchelated human serum after challenge with EA cells (2×10^9) and Z(2mg). (From D. P. Fine, S. R. Marney, Jr., D. G. Colley, J. S. Sergent, and R. M. DesPrez, "C_3 Shunt Activation in Human Serum Chelated with EGTA," *Journal of Immunology* 109 (1972): 807:810, with permission of the publishers.)

Figure 2 compares the decomplementation patterns of sensitized erythrocytes (designated EA), known to activate the C142 pathway, and zymosan (designated Z), a yeast cell wall preparation thought to activate the C3 shunt. Residual complement activity in CH50 units per ml is plotted on the vertical axis and the various chelated and nonchelated sera on the horizontal axis. Below each serum is the approximate divalent cation concentration as calculated from the association constants of the cation-chelator interactions. The essential difference between EDTA-treated serum and EGTA-treated serum is the magnesium concentration: while both sera are essentially depleted of calcium ion, EGTA-treated serum has a magnesium ion concentration four logs greater than EDTA-treated serum.

As can be seen, EGTA distinguishes between C142 activation as exemplified by EA cells (which requires calcium and thus does not proceed in EGTA-treated serum) and C3-shunt activation as exemplified by zymosan (which requires magnesium and thus proceeds in EGTA-treated serum.)

Chelated and unchelated sera were then challenged with 4×10^9 *E. coli* organisms, used as a particulate source of endotoxin (Fig. 3). *E. coli* behaved

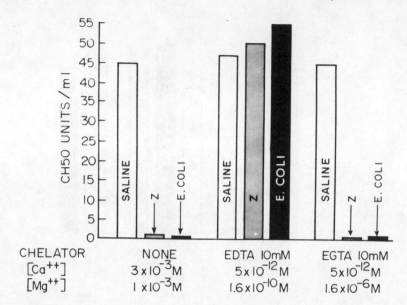

Fig. 3. Residual CH 50 units in chelated and nonchelated human serum after challenge with Z (2mg) or *E. coli* (4 x 10⁹). From D. P. Fine, S. R. Marney, Jr., D. G. Colley, J. S. Sergent, and R. M. DesPrez, "C_3 Shunt Activation in Human Serum Chelated with EGTA," *Journal of Immunology* 109 (1972): 807-810, with permission of the publishers.)

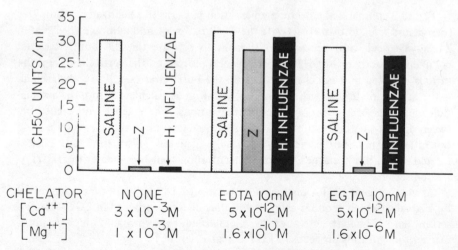

Fig. 4. Residual CH50 units in chelated and nonchelated human serum after challenge with Z (2mg) or *H. influenzae* (4 x 10⁹).

exactly as zymosan, decomplementing unchelated and EGTA-treated sera but not EDTA-treated serum. These data show that complement activation by *E. coli* (and, by inference, endotoxin) requires magnesium but no calcium. This sharply distinguishes it from C142 activation and is consistent with the current premise that endotoxin activates the C3 shunt.

When whole *Hemophilus influenzae,* type b, organisms (supplied by Dr. Sarah Sell) were used in a manner analogous to the *E. coli* organisms, a different pattern obtained (Figure 4). Zymosan (and *E. coli*) decomplemented serum chelated with 10 mM EGTA; *H. influenzae* did not. This demonstrates that *H. influenzae* decomplementation requires calcium and thus proceeds through the C142 pathway only. Interstingly, challenge doses of purified polyribose phosphate ranging from 1 to 40 micrograms produced no decomplementation in this experimental system.

We do not know whether the human serum, which we obtained from healthy adult male donors, contained antibodies to *H. influenzae,* although that is a reasonable assumption. In that case, the most likely interpretation of our results with the whole organisms is that an *H. influenzae*-antibody complex fixes complement through the C142 pathway. *H. influenzae* organisms, at least in their intact state, appear to lack the ability to activate the C3 shunt.

REFERENCES

Götze, O., and H. J. Müller-Eberhard. 1971. "The C3-Activator System: An Alternate Pathway of Complement Activation." *J. Exp. Med.* 134:90.

Rapp, H. J., and T. Borsos. 1970. *Molecular Basis of Complement Action.* New York: Appleton-Century-Crofts.

Sandberg, A. L., and A. G. Osler. 1971. "Dual Pathways of Complement Interaction with Guinea Pig Immunoglobulins." *J. Immun.* 107:1268.

Discussion

David T. Karzon, Presiding

David T. Karzon: We will discuss as a group the preceding four papers concerning various aspects of assessment of antibody. One of the key issues in *Hemophilus influenzae* work is the methodology assay and significance of the various antibody systems.

John B. Robbins: Dr. Anderson, do I assume from the curves that you do not achieve 100% binding of the antigen at any antibody concentration in the reference serum obtained from Stan Klein?

Porter Anderson: No. The effective dilutions simply were not plotted. If you used low antigen concentration and a lesser dilution of Stan Klein's serum, you can bind up to 100% of the antigen.

Robbins: The second question refers to a technical problem that I think is still open. I want to mention it so that others might take it into consideration. Is it possible that C'lq, a protein which binds polyanions and will precipitate with 50% saturated ammononium sulfate, might interact with the type b polysaccharide? C'lq does interact with other precipitate with 50% ammonium sulfate. At high levels of antibody, this nonantibody-induced binding would not produce a sufficient amount of binding to interfere with the assay. The question is, will it interfere at low levels? Now, when I suggested to you that heating the serum to inactive C'lq might be an important facet, you said it looks as if the Igm antibody in its natural state would be affected by heating. When I look back at the literature without doing the experiment, two types of patterns of so-called heat susceptibility of "natural" antibodies emerge. I do not know how clear the differentiation is, because it would appear that, when studying antibodies which behave like polyanions, against endotoxin and gram-negative bacteria which are negatively charged, it can be demonstrated that heating reduces the low level of "natural" antibodies. But when one looks at inactivation of antibodies which react with particles on a one-to-one ratio, as you might observe in virus neutralization, the heating effect upon "natural" antibodies does not seem to be as important. Might there be a possibility of C'lq binding at low levels which would be an important viable? Dr. Schneerson and I have done experiments with Stan Klein's serum in which we isolated the purified antibody by disassocation of the immune precipitate and studied the subclass specifically. We only detected IgG_2 antibody in this preparation.

Richard B. Johnston, Jr.: When Dr. Anderson reacted postvaccination serum with purified PRP, washed the complex, then eluted with hypertonic saline about two thirds of the IgG antibody was IgG_2 and one third was IgG_1. This is perhaps germane to immunity, in that it is very clear that IgG_1 and IgG_3 attached to red cells will bind to phagocytic cells via their Fc piece and form rosettes. IgG_2 will not so bind. I wonder what that means, if the primary IgG antibody response to PRP is IgG_2, as it is to other polysaccharide antigens, and this antibody does not opsonize. Unfortunately, we do not know whether or not IgG_2 anti-PRP antibody will enhance phagocytosis of *H. influenzae,* type b, but we plan to study this.

Robbins: Just one more comment about the bactericidal test. The bactericidal test is an assay for serum antibodies. I would like to point out that there are many bacteria, including the meningococcus, *H. influenzae,* and, of course, *E. coli Easter,* which survive without demonstrable bactericidal effect in the presence of enormous excess of antibody and complement. If you use the bactericidal reaction, antibodies to *E. coli Easter* would not be detected. This is true of Vi antigen of Salmonelli typhi, which is similar to the *H. influenzae* type polysaccharide antigen, in that it is a carbohydrate polymer, negatively charged. I think a bactericidal test is a useful test but the interpretations are limited.

Carl W. Norden: It is exactly what it says: either bactericidal activity is present or not. Either the serum kills the bacteria or it does not. I think that what you are saying is that you are measuring bactericidal activity in the serum and it is only one test of antibody activity. Certainly it does not imply that antibodies are present which might be detected by other techniques. We have tried heating many sera and have not found a difference, at least in bactericidal activity, whether the serum was heated or not.

Robbins: Another question should be directed to Dr. Anderson. What dilution of Stan Klein's serum gives about 20% binding at low antigen concentration? I have calculated roughly, on a graph, the amount of antibody one can detect at the two different serum volumes and at a large serum volume. It seems to be similar in both instances. How much can one dilute Stan Klein's serum and still get binding that enables one to say there is antibody present?

Anderson: In reference to the first point, concerning complete binding of the antigen, the curves as you know, are sigmoid and approach 100% slowly. But if one uses enough Stan Klein serum or any anti-PRP serum, then one binds 100% of this antigen, within clinical limits of precision of the assay. In reference to the heating, immediately after you told me about the possibility, I selected sera from children who had low but detectable serum activity and which had been put into a -70° C freezer within a couple of hours of collection. I then heated some of those sera at 56° C and compared them with the unheated. The results were the same, and this was with a low concentration of antigen. So this remains a difference which we can iron out, perhaps, by exchange of material. Looking at the graph with Stan Klein's serum, 20% binding of the lowest antigen concentration using 100 microliters of serum is at a dilution of 2800; using 20 microliters of serum, it is 940.

Robbins: I was concerned that, since you were measuring very low levels, the binding may be due to nonantibody proteins, such as C'lq. At low levels, where immune responses of very young children might be measured, this might be a problem.

Anderson: Have you evidence that C'lq will bind to native PRP or is this only to the radioactive PRP?

Robbins: No. My caution was provoked by two observations. First, if one uses fresh, unheated potent antiserum with PRP, a double precipitin line in immunodiffusion analysis is obtained. If one then heats the serum, the double-line phenomenon goes away. These authors postulated that this was due to complement proteins adhering independently of antibody. We were concerned that this nonantibody binding might be important at low antibody levels. If you feel confident that it is not, that issue might be closed.

Anderson: I wonder whether *E coli Easter* is resistant to action of complement when anti-O-antibody is used.

Robbins: The anti strain/antibody/Easter 075:H5 contained anti-O-antibody. It precipitates with the O antigen. The Easter strain of *E. coli* is also resistant to the effect of Easter or *H. influenzae,* type b, antiserum in the mouse-protection test. (the LD_{50} of strain Easter is very low: 10^2 organism/mouse). The Vi antigen of Salmonella typhi is also related to the anticomplementary effect and it may very well be that the amount of polysaccharide on this organism is great enough so that the antibody-antigen interaction occurs far enough from the susceptible bacterial site so that the lysis does not occur.

David W. Fraser: Dr. Norden, do young children fail to show a bactericidal response to type b even when their homologous strain of type b is used in the assay?

Norden: In the group from Rochester, five children were tested against their own strain without evidence of any bactericidal activity. We have tried this subsequently with serum from other children and found one or two that have shown bactericidal activity only in the undiluted serum against their own strains, while there was no activity against the two standard strains used in the laboratory. The same observation was reported concerning bactericidal activity of meningococcus. Occasionally against the homologous strain there is activity in very low titres, but not against others. Probably, it would be ideal to test serum from all children against their own strains.

Georges Peter: Dr. Norden, were your hemagglutination assays performed at 37°
or 4°?

Norden: At 37 ° C.

Peter: Dr. Johnston, what is the youngest age at which you have seen opsonization activity in sera from children?

Johnston: It has been found in cord sera, and it has been shown to develop in
many infants in the first year. I am sorry I cannot give you specific figures,
but since we have not finished studying these sera, our data are not yet
collated.

Peter: Does it persist thereafter?

Johnston: Again, my recollection is that it is more often transient than persistent in the first two years of life.

Peter: At least in the one example you showed, activity persisted unchanged for
at least two or three years.

Johnston: Right.

Karzon: What is this age effect due to—is the age effect in those who respond
versus those who do not respond?

Norden: I do not know. However, Dr. Richard Michaels pointed out to me a
very interesting paper published in 1951 by Dr. Rantz, measuring antistreptolysin-O titres, in children with severe streptococcal infection. One can
show almost identical patterns. Up to two years, the children make extremely
poor response in terms of ASLO—either absent or weak. In children aged two
to three years, mean titres are higher; and above three, they are significantly
higher. It may be as Dr. South suggested in her editorial in the *Journal of
Pediatrics,* (1971) that this is simply due to immaturity of the immunologic
system in terms of recognition of *H. influenzae* antigens. This is certainly one
possibility.

Robbins: There are many reasons to consider why young animals do not make as
much antibody as older animals. Some excellent papers written in the thirties
by Leona Baumgartner (1934) and Jules Freund describe this phenomenon
very nicely. I would like to make a suggestion about discrimination of young
from old that might be related to our observations in rabbits. Rabbits fed
cross-reactive *E. coli* antigen respond, when challenged with *Hemophilus influenzae,* type b, with more anticapsular antibodies than those which are not
fed. With polysaccharide antigens, there are a finite number of specificity
sugars that form the antigens of polysaccharide. The age-related phenomenon
may simply represent the length of time required for the population as a
whole to come in contact with these sugars so that a secondary response will
be observed. I think the difference between an infant whose maternal antibodies have disappeared and an adult is that, in an adult, there is a secondary
response and in the infant and child, there is a primary response.

Virgil M. Howie: Dr. Anderson, you tested 28 sera versus homologous strains for bactericidal power. It is my recollection that 17 of them showed a significant rise in individuals with otitis media in two weeks. This is not meningitis, but otitis media. Most of the bacteria were untypable, I think. Two or three were typable strains.

John K. Whisnant: May I ask Dr. Norden if his data suggests differentiating between an "infantile" and an "adult" type of response? Can you tell us how many adults have an infantile response?

Norden: I have seen one adult with *H. influenzae* meningitis and two adults with *H. influenzae* epiglottitis. They have all had a prompt and brisk antibody response.

Whisnant: Of 20 adult volunteers who were immunized with polysaccharide vaccine (Schneerson, et al., 1971) there were some who gave "adult responses" and some who gave "infantile responses." It may be that the level of antibody is not totally age-dependent.

Robbins: The immune response in epiglottitis seems to differ from that in meningitis. This might be age-related because individuals with epiglottitis are older than those with meningitis. However, in epiglottitis, the antibody response is quite high and, in some individuals, rather extraordinarily high. I do not think we have studied a case of epiglottitis for antibodies to type b polysaccharide in which less than two micrograms of antibody were detected in convalescent sera. Some have been quite high. These were two- and three-year-old children.

Johnston: I think Dr. Whisnant's point is a good one. I think that certainly it must be a relationship between polysaccharide versus protein. I think we do not know.

Roger A. Feldman: Dr. Norden's paper earlier commented that he was going to try to immunize people who had no measured immunologic response, and this has come up again. Have you not done this yet?

Karzon: We will come back to this issue when we discuss immunization. Perhaps we can move on at this point.

REFERENCES

Baumgartner, L. 1934. "Relationships of Age to Immunological Reactions." *Yale J. Biol. & Med.* 6:403.

Freund, J. 1936. "Effect of Heterologous Bacterial Products upon Tuberculous Animals." *J. Immunol.* 30:241.

Rantz, L.A.; M. Maroney; J. M. DiCaprio. 1951. "Antistreptolysin O Response Following Hemolytic Streptococcus Infection in Early Childhood." *AMA Arch. Int. Med.* 87:360.

Schneerson, R.; L. P. Rodriques; J. C. Parke, Jr.; and J. B. Robbins. 1971. "Immunity to Disease Caused by *Hemophilus influenzae,* type b. II. Specificity and Some Biological Characteristics of 'Natural,' Infection Acquired, and Immunization Induced Antibodies to the Capsular Polysaccharide of *Hemophilus influenzae,* type b." *J. Immunol.* 107:1081.

South, M. A. 1971. "Enteropathogenic *Escherichia coli* Disease: New Developments and Perspectives." *J. Ped.* 79:1.

SECTION V

CHAPTER 12

Transformation of Human Lymphocytes by a *Hemophilus influenzae* Antigen

Robert H. Alford

Chronic obstructive pulmonary disease is characterized by recurrent and chronic bacterial lower-respiratory infections. The organisms responsible for these exacerbations are not known for certain, but a great deal of indirect evidence implicates the pneumococci and *Hemophilus influenzae* (Burns, 1968; Reichek et al., 1970). Because of the possible role of *H. influenzae* in the pathogenesis of chronic obstructive pulmonary disease, the blastogenic response of human lymphocytes to an extract from *H. influenzae* was evaluated.

The experiments described here were performed using a nontypable (as determined in Dr. Sarah Sell's laboratory) *H. influenzae* strain from an adult with bronchiectasis. An extract from the organism was prepared according to the method outlined in Table 1.

Characterization of this extract is as follows:

1. The dry weight of material was approximately 1.5 mg/ml.

2. Since it was prepared from an unencapsulated strain, it was assumed to contain relatively little polyribose phosphate.

TABLE 1

PREPARATION OF *HEMOPHILUS INFLUENZAE* EXTRACT

48-hr. culture in Levinthal's broth
Wash 3 x in phosphate-buffered saline
Disrupt 2 x in French pressure cell at 16-18 000 lb.
Clarify at 1500 x G
Ultracentrifuge 100,000 x G for 2 hrs.
Dialyze 3 x against saline; 1 x against Hanks BSS.
Millipore filter

3. The ratio of ultraviolet absorption at 280 mu to that at 260 mu was 0.84, indicating the presence of nucleic acid or nucleoprotein.

4. The protein content (Lowry, et al., 1951) was 750 μg per ml, or about 50% of the dry weight.

5. Qualitative acrylamide gel electrophoresis revealed several bands upon staining for protein. Scanning densitometry of such a gel is reproduced in Figure 1 and indicates possibly 16 proteins of differing electrophoretic mobilities.

Utilizing this extract as a stimulant for normal human lymphocytes, the following dose-response curve has been obtained (Fig. 2). Standard methods (Alford, 1970) for lymphocyte culture were used employing 10^6 lymphocytes per culture in a medium containing 20% autologous plasma. Overnight thymidine uptake on the fifth day of culture indicates DNA synthesis which is proportional to the blastogenesis (or transformation) of lymphocytes which has occurred. The maximum uptake (8900 CPM) occurred at a dilution of the extract which introduced 25 μg of protein per culture. This resulted in a ratio of

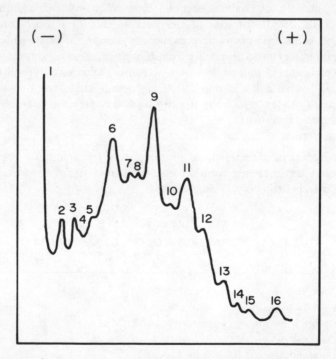

Fig. 1. Densitometric scan of 7.5% acrylamidegel electrophoresis of proteins of *H. influenzae* extract. Buffalo black stain. The anode is on the right. Numbers refer to identifiable protein-containing bands.

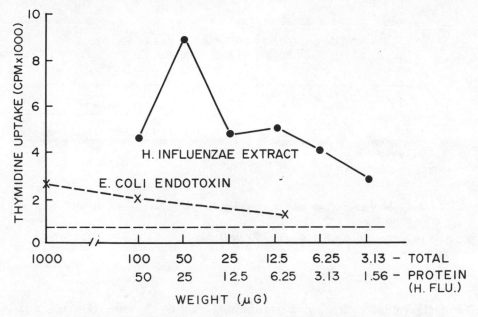

Fig. 2. *H. influenzae* extract and *E. coli* endotoxin-induced transformation of human peripheral blood lymphocytes. The endotoxin is *E. coli* 0127:B8 lipopolysaccharide B, Difco Laboratories. The horizontal dashed line indicates the uptake of unstimulated control cultures.

uptake of stimulated to control cultures of 14. This ratio is called the stimulation index. This concentration, giving optimal blastogenesis, was used in subsequent transformation studies. Note that a dilution of extract containing only 1.56 μg of protein yielded 2800 CPM or a stimulation index of 4.3.

Since endotoxin is a stimulant of human lymphocytes (Oppenheim and Perry, 1965; Heilman, 1970), it is instructive to compare the *H. influenzae* extract dose-response to that of *E. coli* lipopolysaccharide (or endotoxin). The lymphocyte stimulation of 100 μg of this potent endotoxin was less than that caused by a total weight of 6.25 μg of the *H. influenzae* extract. Note also the characteristic, flat dose-response curve of endotoxin. It is reasoned that it is unlikely that much of the blastogenic effect of the *H. influenzae* extract is due to endotoxin-like activity.

Further evidence of freedom of endotoxin-like effect of the *H. influenzae* extract was gained in an experiment in collaboration with Dr. Roger M. Des Prez (Table 2). Endotoxin causes the release of 5-hydroxytryptamine (serotonin) from rabbit platelets (Des Prez, Horowitz, and Hook, 1961). *H. influenzae* ex-

TABLE 2

EFFECTS OF ENDOTOXIN AND *H. INFLUENZAE* EXTRACT
ON PLATELET 5HT RELEASE

	5HT Release* (%)	
	Prior to Ultracentrifugation	After Ultracentrifugation
E. coli endotoxin †	54	3
H. influenzae extract ‡	21	0

*Citrated rabbit platelet-rich plasma incubated for 30 minutes at 37° C, 5HT measured
fluorometrically.

†100 μg lipopolysaccharide B, *E. coli* 0127:B8, Difco

‡200 μg total weight

tract, clarified by low speed centrifugation, will do the same. However, ultra-centrifugation removes this endotoxin effect and the endotoxinlike platelet-perturbing effect of the *H. influenzae* extract without altering its effect upon lymphocyte blastogenesis.

Therefore, the *H. influenzae* extract that has been prepared is low in poly-saccharide, contains nucleic acid, a mixture of proteins, and is virtually free of endotoxin activity. This extract may be termed a complex somatic antigen.

The effect of this complex natural antigen was determined upon the lympho-cytes of ten normal adult subjects as seen in Figure 3. All subjects' lymphocytes responded with at least a threefold increase in thymidine uptake, indicating a considerable degree of blastogenesis. The mean stimulation index of these ten subjects was 12.6, denoting a brisk blastogenic response of lymphocytes of normal adults to *H. influenzae* somatic antigen.

The demonstration of considerable cellular reactivity to *H. influenzae* antigen raises several questions: (1) what is the role of delayed hyper-sensitivity or cell-mediated immunity (as is indicated by lymphocyte transpormation by soma-tic antigen) in resistance to *H. influenzae* infections? (2) Are there cross-reacting bacterial antigens which are responsible for the demonstrated lymphocyte trans-formation? (3) Do those adults who apparently lack antibody to *H. influenzae* have cellular immunity to its antigens? (4) Could *excessive* cell-mediated im-munity—i.e., hypersensitivity to *H. influenzae* antigens—contribute to the *patho-genesis* of an illness? Lymphocytes undergoing blastogenesis release lympho-cytotoxins which nonspecifically cause cellular injury (Pincus, Woods, and Pang,

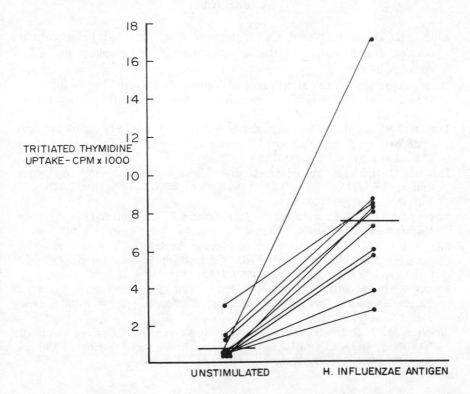

Fig. 3. Lymphocyte transformation of ten normal subjects due to *H. influenzae* somatic antigen. The mean uptake of the unstimulated and *H. infleunzae*-stimulated cultures is indicated by the solid horizontal lines.

1970). Could antigens of *H. influenzae* due to chronic presence (May, 1953) in the respiratory tract stimulate sensitized lymphocytes with the subsequent release of lymphocytotoxins leading to immune injury of bronchial epithelial cells?

These and many more questions about cellular immunity to *H. influenzae* await answers.

REFERENCES

Alford, R. H. 1970. "Metal Cation Requirements for Phytohemagglutinin-induced Transformation of Human Peripheral Blood Lymphocytes." *J. Immunol.* 104:698.

Burns, M. W. 1968. "The Significance of Various Bacteria in Chronic Bronchial Disorders as Determined by Bacterial Antibody Detection." *Australasian Annals of Medicine* 17:289.

Des Prez, R. M.; H. I. Horowitz; and E. W. Hook. 1961. "Effects of Bacterial Endotoxin on Rabbit Platelets: I. Platelet Aggregation and Release of Platelet Factors *in vitro.*" *J. Exp. Med.* 114:857.

Heilman, D. H. 1970. "Mitogenic Activity of Bacterial Fractions in Lymphocyte Cultures. Endotoxins and Other Derivations of Gram-Negative Bacteria." *Int. Arch. Allergy* 39:415.

Lowry, O. H.; N. J. Rosebrough; A. L. Farr; and R. J. Randall. 1951. "Protein Measurement with the Folin Phenol Reagent." *J. Bio. Chem.* 193:265.

May, J. R. 1953. "The Bacteriology of Chronic Bronchitis." *Lancet* 2:534-537.

Oppenheim, J. J., and S. Perry. 1965. "Effects of Endotoxins on Cultured Leukocytes." *Proc. Soc. Exp. Biol. and Med.* 118:1014.

Pincus, W. B.; W. W. Woods; and R. K. Pang. 1970. "Immune-Specific Cytotoxic Factor Formation by Small Lymphocytes." *Journal of the Reticuloendothelial Society,* 7:220.

Reichek, M.; E. B. Lewis; D. L. Rhoden; R. R. Weaver; and J. C. Crutcher. 1970. "Antibody Responses to Bacterial Antigens during Exacerbations of Chronic Bronchitis." *Amer. Rev. Resp. Dis.* 101:238.

CHAPTER **13**

Electron Microscopy Studies of Antibodies to *Hemophilus influenzae,* type b

John P. Robinson
Sarah H. Sell
Shirley S. Schuffman

The negative-staining technique has been a useful method for studying soluble antibody-antigen complexes in the electron microscope (Valentine and Green, 1967; Feinstein and Rowe, 1965; Robinson, 1966; Robinson and Schuffman, 1971). It was found that positively stained preparations were better suited for examining certain precipitated complexes (Robinson and Schuffman, 1971; Robinson, Schuffman and Sell, 1972). The latter technique, when used with thin sectioning, appears to be a useful method for examining complexes of specific antibodies with *Hemophilus influenzae* cells. This is a report of such an examination.

METHODS

Preparation of antigen for immunization. Hemophilus influenzae, type b, (American Type Culture Collection #9795) cells were grown in Levinthal's broth for 18 hours, at which time 0.3 ml was seeded onto Levinthal's agar plates and incubated for six hours (Alexander, Leidy, and MacPherson, 1946). The bacteria, washed from the plate with cold 0.15 M NaCl containing 0.5% formaldehyde at pH 7.2, were suspended in a concentration of 1×10^8/ml. The cultures were grown the day of the animal inoculations and injected immediately after preparation.

Immunization of rabbits. Immunization was accomplished by a modification of the method of Alexander, Leidy, and MacPherson (1946). Animals were

This work was supported, in part, by Grant # AI-06110 from the USPHS National Institute of Allergy and Infectious Diseases, Bethesda, Maryland.

injected with 0.1 ml volume intravenously three times during the first week. The quantity injected was increased by 0.2 ml per week during the following few weeks, until a total volume of 1.0 ml of the formaldehyde-killed suspension was injected. Finally, 1.0 ml of live organisms was injected three times weekly for three weeks. Rabbits were bled by cardiac puncture and their sera were pooled, tested for type specificity, and frozen at -22°C until used.

Preparation of complexes. (a) Cells with capsules intact: Cells to be used for preparation of complexes were grown in Levinthal's broth for six hours. At this time, 2 ml of the broth culture were transferred to conical centrifuge tubes. Type-specific antiserum was added directly to the broth suspension, in 0.1-ml quantities, and the complex was allowed to form and settle for two hours at room temperature. The complex was then fixed by adding an equal volume of 2.5% glutaraldehyde at pH 7.3. Fixation was continued for two hours at room temperature. The aldehyde was then removed and the complex was washed gently with water.

(b) Cells with capsules partially or totally removed: 2-ml volumes of the broth culture were placed in conical centrifuge tubes where the cells were washed in 0.15 M NaCl in 0.005M sodium phosphate buffer at pH 7.0 (PBS) at room temperature. This procedure removes the capsular polyribophosphate (PRP) from the cells (Pittman, 1931). The supernatant from each centrifugation was monitored by the orcinol-sulfuric acid reaction (Bruckner, 1955). Washing continued until no further PRP was detected. After the cells had been suspended in 2.0 ml of PBS, the complex was prepared and fixed as described for cells with intact capsules.

(c) Control preparations: Control preparations consisted of washed and unwashed cells, each incubated with normal serum and with saline. None of the four preparations formed precipitates, but the cells were centrifuged to a pellet and fixed with glutaraldehyde. These pellets were easily dissociated but could be suitably processed for examination in the electron microscope.

Preparation for examination in the electron microscope. After the initial fixation with glutaraldehyde, all preparations were subjected to two hours of fixation at room temperature with 1% osmium tetroxide in 0.1 M phosphate buffer at pH 7.3. They were then dehydrated by graded ethanol solutions and embedded in araldite. Thin sections were prepared and stained by floating on saturated uranium acetate in 50% ethanol followed by lead citrate (Reynolds, 1963).

RESULTS

Figure 1 represents a complex of *H. influenzae*, type b, cells, with intact capsules, and type-specific antibodies. It is readily apparent that material outside

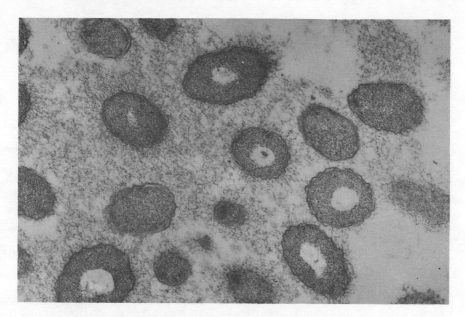

Fig. 1. Positively-stained, flocculated complex of *H. influenzae,* type b, cells, with intact capsules and specific antibodies. (The precipitate was allowed to settle and fixation was started by direct addition of glutaraldehyde to the settled complex. Thin sections of the complex were positively stained as described in methods).

the cell wall is well stained by the methods employed. This stained material does not represent capsular PRP, since control preparations in which unwashed cells were incubated in normal serum or PBS contained none. This is illustrated in Figure 2. The stained extracellular material in Figure 1, then, must be either antibodies or complement. Heat inactivation of serum made no difference in the appearance of these preparations, and it is known that heat-inactivated rabbit sera (56° C for 30 minutes) add no complement nitrogen to complexes (Weigle and Maurer, 1957). This extracellular, stained material, therefore, appears to be antibodies. Figure 3 illustrates, at the arrow, that occasionally individual particles are resolved with the dimensions of IgG molecules. The particle indicated in Figure 3 is about 30 Å by 280 Å, which agrees well with the measurements of antibodies reported by Hall et al. (1959). These probably represent individual antibody molecules bound to the capsule antigen; but since whole serum was used to prepare the complex, it is possible that any given particle examined might be simply a serum protein molecule which is nonspecifically associated in the complex.

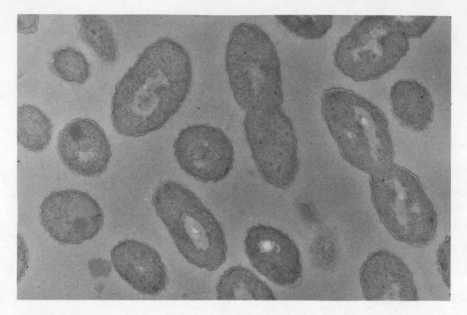

Fig. 2. *H. influenzae,* type b, cells, with capsules intact, which were incubated with normal rabbit serum. It is apparent that the capsular material is not detectably stained by the methods used in these experiments.

When washed cells, with capsules wholly or partially removed, were used in control preparations employing normal serum or 0.15 M NaCl, they appeared no different from those cells illustrated in Figure 2.

Incubation of washed cells with antiserum produced a flocculate of cells trapped in a closely packed mass of dense staining material. This is illustrated in Figure 4. It is apparent that partial or total removal of the capsular antigen produces cells which bind antibodies in a more closely associated manner. The antibodies appear to be associated with each other and the cell walls of *H. influenzae* to form a halo around the cell. Some of the halos extend 1000 Å or more beyond the cell wall.

DISCUSSION

It is apparent that positive staining is a useful method to examine thin sections of precipitated complexes of *H. influenzae,* type b, and its antibodies. Figure 3 illustrates that this method will demonstrate individual antibody molecules in precipated complexes by positive staining; it is simply necessary that the antibodies be sufficiently separated from one another in the complex.

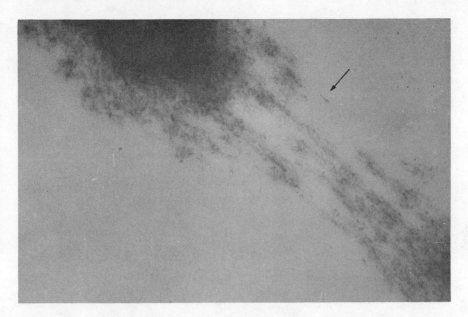

Fig. 3. Higher magnification of a proportion identical to that represented in Figure 1. The arrow indicates a stained particle with the dimensions of gammaglobulin molecules. It is probably an anti-PRP antibody.

In the precipitates which we have examined to date, such separation of antibodies appears to be the exception rather than the rule. This may happen because the components of a precipitate have suffered some denaturation process and, as a result, there are hydrophobic areas on their surface which would associate in an aqueous medium. Due to such aggregation, the reactants in the complex would be expected to associate very closely with one another unless they were bound and held apart. There could be antigen-antigen or antibody-antibody associations through these areas. This would explain some earlier observations of extensive antigen-angiten associations detected in the electron microscope (Robinson, 1966). In the preparations illustrated in Figures 1 and 3, the capsular antigen could serve as a scaffold to hold the attached antibodies in occasional isolated positions. This would not be expected to occur in a complex which contains ferritin molecules as the antigen.

Even though the individual antibodies could be visualized in these experiments, we were not able to distinguish the Fc or Fab portions of the molecule as was reported in the negatively stained soluble complexes of Valentine and Green (1967).

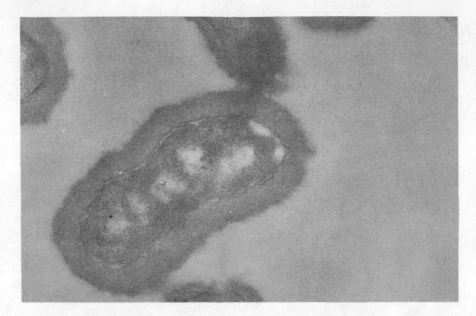

Fig. 4. Precipitated complex of *H. influenzae,* type b cells, with capsules wholly or partially removed and specific antibodies. Tightly packed ring of stained material outside the cell walls often measured more than 1,000 Å in thickness.

When washed cells were used to prepare complexes, there resulted a closely packed, dense-staining layer apparently attached to the cell wall. The thickness of this mass around the cells occasionally reached 1000 Å or more. This distance is too great to be explained by antibody molecules attached at the cell surface with their long axes oriented in a plane perpendicular to the surface of the cell.

The possible explanations that occurred to us were as follows:

(1) The presence of antiglobulins in the sera.
(2) The presence of short fragments of capsular material still attached to the cell wall. Thus an 800-Å long strand of PRP with an antibody attached at the end added an additional 200 Å to its apparent length. This mechanism could explain a layer of stained material of any observed thickness.
(3) The addition of complement.

The use of heat-inactivated antisera to prepare these complexes made no difference in their appearance. This is in agreement with an earlier report (Robinson and Schuffman, 1971). Since such sera add no complement nitrogen to a complex, it is unlikely that complement can explain the thickness of these extracellular layers (Weigle and Maurer, 1957). Further, since the total content of complement in antisera can account for only a small portion of the total mass of a complex, it is unlikely that the addition of complement could add so much material (Kabat and Mayer, 1967).

The presence of antiglobulins in antibody-antigen complexes has been demonstrated in the electron microscope (Robinson, 1966; Robinson and Schuffman, 1971). A layer of any thickness could be explained by the presence of sufficient antiglobulins in the sera. Antiglobulins were demonstrable in these antihemophilus sera by hemagglutination techniques reported earlier (Robinson, 1966), and can, at least in part, account for the results observed here. For such antibodies to be present in these sera, they must either be naturally occurring (Milgrim, 1962) or autoantiglobulins (Robinson and Schuffman, 1971; Gell and Kelus, 1967; Harshman, Robinson, and Najjar, 1963) which were produced during the immunization process.

We feel that either the presence of antiglobulins or the presence of short strands of PRP attached to the cell wall, or both are likely to account for the large layers of dense staining material surrounding the cells. In either case, the authors feel that this report illustrates the usefulness of the positive-staining technique in examing specific immune precipitates.

It is generally accepted that the resistance of virulent *H. influenzae* to host defense is due to the capsular PRP. It has been reported that those antibodies in human sera which are protective for mice against *H. influenzae,* type b, are absorbed and removed by capsular antigen (Alexander, Heidelberger, and Leidy, 1944). Fothergill and Wright (1933) showed that cells without a capsule were more susceptible to the bactericidal activity of antisera than were cells with a capsule. Mpairwe (1971) reported that the bactericidal antibodies could be removed from sera without removing the antibodies against the capsule. Schneerson et al. (1971) indicated that bactericidal and mouse-protective antibodies were removed from sera by adsorption with PRP.

A comparison of Figures 1 and 4 indicates that after partial or total removal of the capsule from type b, *H. influenzae.* Subsequent exposure of these cells to specific antisera results in complexes with increased numbers and more closely associated antibody molecules which attach directly at the cell wall. It follows that removal of PRP would better expose those antigens at the cell wall to the attack by their specific antibodies, which should be present in the antiserum, since whole cells were used to immunize the rabbits. It is, of course, possible that all of these antibodies function co-operatively in host defense and that anticapsular antibodies, in addition to aiding phagocytosis, assist the bactericidal antibodies by better exposing the cell wall antigens after attaching to the PRP.

Additional work is needed to reveal the true mechanism of host immune defense in *H. influenzae,* type b, infections.

REFERENCES

Alexander, H. E.; M. Heidelberger; and G. Leidy. 1944. "The Protective or Curative Element in type b, *H. influenzae,* Rabbit Serum." *Yale J. Biol. Med.* 16:425.

Alexander, H. E.; G. Leidy; and C. MacPherson. 1946. "Production and types a, b, c, d, e and f, *H. influenzae,* Antibody for Diagnostic and Therapeutic Purposes." *J. Immunol.* 54:207.

Bruckner, J. 1955. "Estimation of Monosaccharides by the Orcinol-Sulfuric Acid Reaction." *Biochem J.* 60:200.

Feinstein, A., and A. J. Rowe. 1965. "Molecular Mechanism of Formation of an Antigen-Antibody Complex." *Nature* (Lond.) 205:147.

Fothergill, L. D., and S. Wright. 1933. "Influenzae Meningitis: The Relation of Age Incidence to the Bactericidal Power of Blood against the Causal Organism." *J. Immunol.* 24:273.

Gell, P. G. H., and A. S. Kelus. 1967. "Antiantibodies." In *Advances in Immunology,* vol. VI, edited by F. J. Dixon, Jr., and J. H. Humphrey, p. 461. New York: Academic Press.

Hall, C. E.; A. Nisonoff; and H. S. Slayter. 1959. "Electron Microscopic Observations of Rabbit Antibodies." *J. Biophys. Biochem. Cytol.* 6:407.

Harshman, S.; J. P. Robinson; and V. A. Najjar. 1963. "The Mechanism of Antibody-Antigen Interaction and the Theory of Subcomplementarity between the Reaction Sites of Antibody and Antigen." *Ann. N.Y. Acad. Sci.* 103:688.

Kabat, E. A., and M. D. Mayer, editors. 1967. *Experimental Immunochemistry,* 2nd edition. Springfield, Illinois: Charles C. Thomas.

Milgrim, F. 1962. "Rabbit Sera with Antiantibody." *Vox. Sanguinis.* 7:545.

Mpairwe, Y. 1971. "Immunity to *Hemophilus influenzae,* type b: The Nature of Bactericidal Antibody in Human Blood." *J. Med. Microbiol.* 4:43.

Pittman, M. 1931. "Variation and Type Specificity in the Bacterial Species *Hemophilus influenzae.*" *J. Exp. Med.* 53:471.

Reynolds, E. S. 1963. "The Use of Lead Citrate at High pH as an Electron Opaque Stain in Electron Microscopy." *J. Cell Biol.* 17:208.

Robinson, J. P. 1966. "Electron Microscope Studies of Antigen-Antibody Complexes." *J. Molec. Biol.* 17:456.

Robinson, J. P., and S. S. Schuffman. 1971. "Evidence for Anti-Antibodies in Positively Stained Immune Complexes." *Immunol.* 20:883.

Robinson, J. P.; S. Schuffman; and S. H. W. Sell. 1972. "Electron Microscopic Studies of Complexes of *Hemophilus influenzae,* type b, with specific antibodies." *Immunol.* 23:101.

Schneerson, R.; L. P. Rodrigues; J. C. Parke, Jr.; and J. B. Robbins. 1971. "Immunity to Disease by *Hemophilus influenzae,* type b: II. Specificity and Some Biologic Characteristics of 'Natural' Infection-Acquired, and Immunization-Induced Antibodies to the Capsular Polysaccharide of *Hemophilus influenzae*, type b." *J. Immunol.* 107:1081.

Valentine, R. C., and N. M. Green. 1967. "Electron Microscopy of Antibody-Haptene Complex." *J. Molec. Biol.* 27:615.

Weigle, W. O., and P. H. Maurer. 1957. "The Effect of Chemical and Physical Treatments of Sera on Hemolytic Activities and Fixation of Complement Nitrogen by Antigen-Antibody Precipitates." *J. Immunol.* 79:370.

CHAPTER 14

The Ultrastructure of *Hemophilus influenzae*

Russell P. Sherwin
Jeanette Wilkins

In view of the relative paucity of descriptions of the fine structure of *Hemophilus influenzae,* type b, the organism, isolated from a patient with meningitis, was processed for electron microscopy. Special attention was given to a comparison of the ultrastructure with that described by Reyn, Birch-Anderson, and Lapage (1966), since their report was the only one revealed by our literature search in which electron microscopic details of *Hemophilus influenzae* were presented. The latter report considered *Hemophilus influenzae* as a species possibly related to *Hemophilus vaginalis* (*Corynebacterium vaginale*) and dealt primarily with the ultrastructure of this bacterium rather than with *Hemophilus influenzae.* The present study has also given special attention to the nature of the cell wall, to the appearance of nuclear regions and to the occurrence of mesosomes.

MATERIAL AND METHODS

The organism was originally isolated from the cerebral spinal fluid of a patient with meningitis. Both X and V factors were required for growth, and positive slide agglutination as well as positive Quellung reaction with *H. influenzae,* type b, antiserum were demonstrated. A loop of organisms from a 24-hour chocolate agar supplement B culture was placed in 5 ml of Mueller-Hinton liquid containing 1% supplement B. After 18 hours in a CO_2 incubator at 37° C, the broth suspension of the organisms was centrifuged at 4,000 rpm at

This work was done in the Departments of Pathology and Pediatrics, University of Southern California School of Medicine, Los Angeles, California.

Work supported by grant from NCAPC No. 5 RO1 AP00607, NIAID Contract 72 2056, and the Hastings Foundation.

4° C for 15 minutes. The supernatant was discarded and the organisms resuspended in cold (4° C) 2% glutaraldehyde in cacodylate buffer. The suspension was again centrifuged, as just described, and the pellet secondarily fixed in 1% osmium for ten minutes. The pellet was not embedded in agar, but

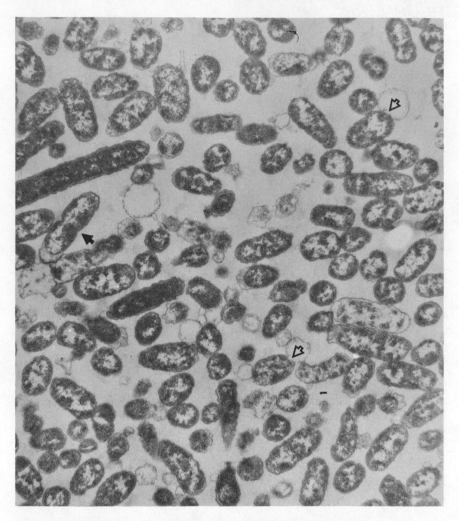

Fig. 1. Low-power view of organisms. A portion of an organism, cut in the longitudinal plane, measures more than 2 micra in length. The width of all of the organisms is relatively uniform, in this section generally averaging 355 nm. There are two examples of "blebbing" (open arrows) and there is one instance (solid arrow) where the bacterium is undergoing central constriction. The bar represents 0.1 micra. (Magnification: 31,050x.)

processed through alcohol dehydration with propylene oxide clearing. Sections were cut with an LKB microtome and mounted on copper grids. Double staining with uranyl acetate and lead citrate followed. The grids were examined with a Hitachi 7 electron microscope.

RESULTS

The organisms varied in size from 355 nm to 530 nm in width and had a maximum observed length of over 3 micra (Figs. 1&2). The wall was typical of

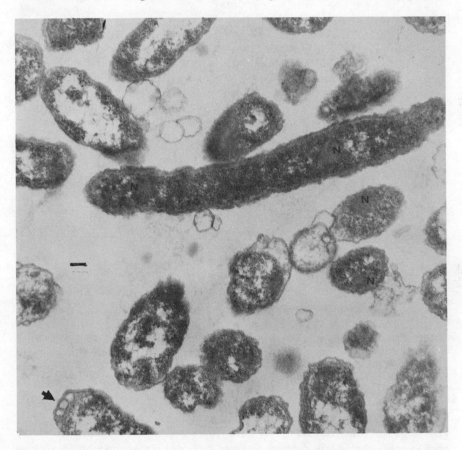

Fig. 2. Nuclear regions. The several nuclear regions (N) shown are in close proximity to or actually abutting cytoplasmic membranes. At the pole of one bacterium, three vesicular structures are noted which appear to represent an early stage of separation of the cell wall from the cytoplasmic membrane (solid arrow). The bar represents one-tenth micron. (Magnification: 68, 310x.)

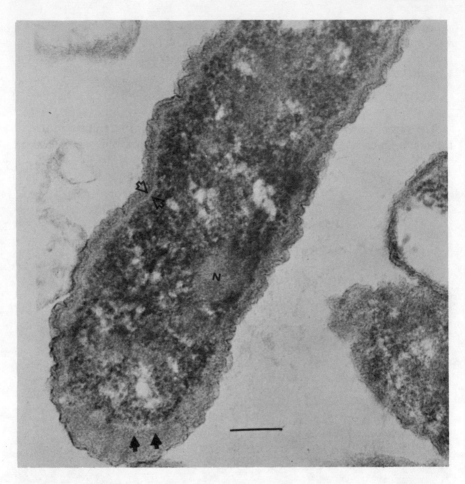

Fig. 3. High-power view of cell wall and cytoplasmic structure. The multimembranous cell wall is separated from the poorly defined cell membrane by an electronluscent space (two solid arrows). A nuclear region (N), in close proximity to the cytoplasmic membrane, is present. Ribosomes are fairly distinct in the region of the two solid arrows. The solid bar represents 0.1 micron. (Magnification: 211,140x.)

gram-negative bacteria, having an ultrastructure composed of multiple wavy membranes and a poorly defined (in these sections) plasma membrane, with an intervening electronluscent space (Fig. 3). In some segments of the outer wall, a triple membrane structure was noted (Figs. 4, 6). The entire wall, including cell membrane, generally averaged 200 Å in thickness. A frequently encountered alteration of the wall was "bleb" or "blister" formation (Fig. 1), a phenomenon

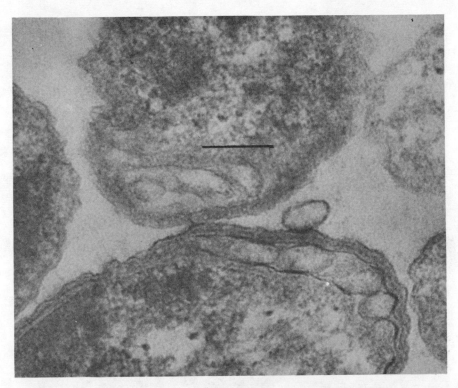

Fig. 4. Cell wall and blebs. Spherical, membranous structures appear to separate the cell wall from the cytoplasmic membrane, but it is not possible from this micrograph to be certain of the location. In addition to the bleblike structures within, there is a single bleb attached to the outer surface of the wall. Note the triple-layer construction of the approximately 200-Å cell wall. The solid bar is 0.1 micron. (Magnification: 209,952x.)

resembling spheroplasting but restricted to a small segment of the outer wall. What appears to be an early stage of "bleb" formation is shown in Figs. 2 and 5 (arrows).

Nuclear regions were often found in the cytoplasm of the bacteria and generally were prominent (Figs. 2 and 4). In Figure 2, a number of the nuclear regions appear to be in close promixity to the cytoplasmic membrane. A specific search was made for mesosomes but, despite the many sections examined, none were identified. Ribosomes (Fig. 3) and irregular, large granules consistent with volutin (Figs. 4 and 5) were commonly noted. Constriction of bacterial organisms was noted fairly often (Fig. 1), implying fairly frequent cell division, and conversely, bacterial degeneration was uncommon. Although a number of "ghost" structures were found (Figs. 4 and 5), they were considered to be more often consistent with tangential cuts of "blebs" than spheroplasts or degenerating organisms.

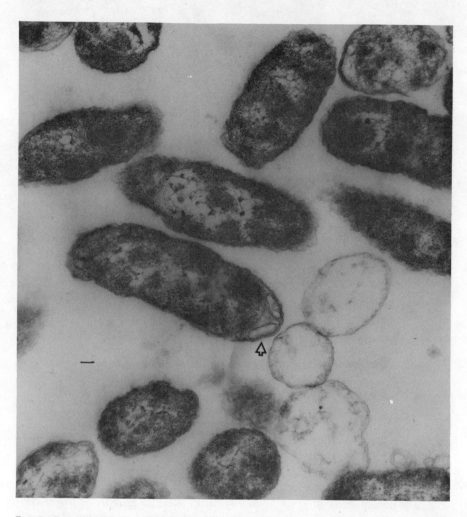

Fig. 5. Early blebbing of cytoplasmic wall. The multiple vesicles appear to be within the confines of the cell wall but are beginning to separate the wall from the underlying and poorly defined cytoplasmic membrane (open arrow). Ghost forms of the cell wall of the organisms are present and presumably are segmental portions of the wall of organisms rather than completely degenerated or spheroplasting bacteria. Irregularly large electron dense granules are present within the matrices of the organisms and are presumably volutin. (Magnification: 52,830x.)

DISCUSSION

The organisms found are similar in many respects to those described by Reyn, Birch-Anderson, and Lapage (1966) in that the organisms have typical gram-negative walls, are very small in size, and fail to demonstrate mesosomes. Not observed in the present study were cytoplasmic loops and, conversely, Reyn's report did not mention blebs. Further, Reyn's report mentions "triple-layered" membranes for the wall; but in the illustrations, Figs. 28 to 30 of her report, the three layers appear to be two dense lines and an intervening electronluscent line. In our study, there appears to be five layers, created by a third electron dense line intermediate between the other two. The latter is consistent with the three-

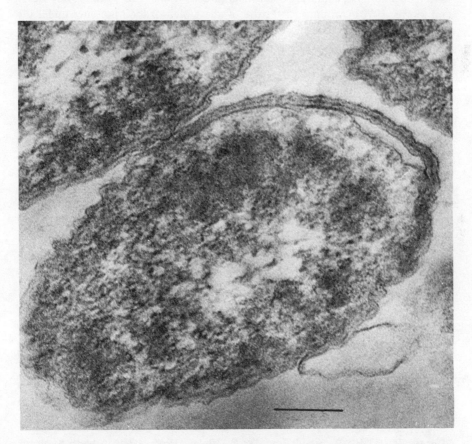

Fig. 6. Cell and ? cytoplasmic membrane. A cytoplasmic membrane has presumably been separated from the cell wall by the formation of a clear space. The solid bar is 0.1 micron. (Magnification: 166, 212x).

layered structure reported by Bayer and Anderson (1965) for gram-negative bacteria other than *Hemophilus influenzae* (Huang and Goodman, 1971; Murray, Steed, and Elson, 1965). The latter point out that fixation at 4° C is necessary to show a three-layered membrane consistently and, since the cell suspensions of Reyn's study were prefixed in osmic acid at room temperature, this may explain the discrepancy. The triple dense-line composition of the wall has the support of a definitive study of the wall of *E. coli* by Bayer and Anderson (1965).

The meaning of the membranous blebs is not clear, but presumably this is not an artifact of fixation, since similar structures have been reported as a phenomenon of nutrient deficiency, that is, bleb formation in the wall of *E. coli* cultured under lysine-limiting conditions (Work, Knox, and Vesk, 1966; Morse and Morse, 1970). An unusual feature of these blebs is their presence under the cell wall as well as on the cell-wall surface (Figs. 4, 5).

The absence of mesosomes in the sections studied of *Hemophilus influenzae* are consistent with their general paucity in gram-negative bacteria, a subject matter recently reviewed by Rogers (1970).

SUMMARY

The ultrastructure of *Hemophilus influenzae* derived from a patient with meningitis has been described. The organism is of a gram-negative type with a triple-track cell wall, underlying electronluscent zone and poorly defined (in these sections) cytoplasmic membrane. Nuclear regions were commonly found in close proximity to cytoplasmic membranes but mesosomes were not identified. Membranous blebs of the cell wall were frequently noted and may be related to a nutrient deficiency.

REFERENCES

Bayer, M. E., and T. F. Anderson. 1965. "The Surface Structure of *Escherichia coli.*" *Proc. Nat. Acad. Sci.* 54:1592.

Huang, P., and R. N. Goodman. 1971. "Ultrastructure of the Cell Wall of *Erwinia amylovora.*" *J. Bacteriol.* 107:361.

Morse, J. H., and S. I. Morse. 1970. "Studies on the Ultrastructure of *Bordetella Pertussis:* I. Morphology, Origin, and Biological Activity of Structures Present in the Extracellular Fluid of Liquid Cultures of *Bordetella pertussis.*" *J. Exp. Med.* 131:1342.

Murray, R. G. E.; P. Steed; and H. E. Elson. 1965. "The Location of the Mucopeptide in Sections of the Cell Wall of *Escherichia coli* and Other Gram-Negative Bacteria." *Canad J. Microbiol.* 11:547.

Reyn, A.; A. Birch-Andersen; and S. P. Lapage. 1966. "An Electron Microscope Study of Thin Sections of *Hemophilus vaginalis* (Gardner and Dukes) and Some Possibly Related Species." *Canad. J. Microbiol.* 12:1125.

Rogers, H. J. 1970. "Bacterial Growth and the Cell Envelope." *Bacteriol. Rev.* 34:194.

Work, E.; K. W. Knox; and M. Vesk. 1966. "The Chemistry and Electron Microscopy of an Extracellular Lipopolysaccharide from *Escherichia coli.*" *Ann. N.Y. Acad. Sci.* 133.

Discussion

Richard L. Myerowitz, Presiding

Richard L. Myerowitz: Have you worked with other capsular types, other than type b, using type-specific antisera? One of the oldest problems in this field is the mechanism of virulence which characterizes the type b organism. By analogy with the pneumococcus, it is thought that perhaps the type b capsule in some way prevents antibody and complement from killing or opsonizing bacteria, while the other capsule types may not. A more definite answer may be obtained using the technique you describe and seeing perhaps a close-knit pattern of antibody on the other capsular types, whereas, in type b, the antibody is far away from the cell wall.

John P. Robinson: I think that might be a worthwhile thing to pursue if we took the strains of greater virulence and compared them to strains with lesser virulence. That might be a good thing to try.

John B. Robbins: I wonder if you have had a chance to try the hybrid antibody technique? You can make an antibody that has dual specificity, one for the capsule and the other for the electron-dense label. That way, you can avoid the complex formation. The other question is, I wonder if you plan to study precipitates composed of antipolysaccharide antibody and bacteria to see how the antibody to the polysaccharide interacts with the bacterial surface.

Robinson: Yes, we hope to do this.

John K. Whisnant: Could nontypable organisms or antibodies to noncapsular antigens in type-specific sera be cemonstrated in this way? We might get an idea to what those particular antigens are related. Are they cell-wall antigens or capsule structures?

Robinson: I think there is certainly potential to that. It is something that has not been studied. We would like to look at it and see what the picture shows.

Jeannette Wilkins: I would like to see you section a phagocytized bacterium inside a leucocyte to see if the cell wall is empty. It may keep its rigidity while the contents spill out of a dead bacterium. An electron microscopic picture might be able to show the details.

Richard B. Johnston, Jr. You may have answered this in a way that I did not understand, but is it possible, on your last picture, that the capsule is seen as strands that come out in fimbria from the cell wall; and that when you wash and manipulate the bacteria, you open up some of the fimbria so that you have antibody to repetitive antigen down the length of the PRP, towards the cell wall?

Robinson: Yes, that is one possibility.

Robbins: I would like to ask Dr. Alford a question. It is a question asked by someone who has spent a long time trying to get the polysaccharide pyrogen-free because, when first isolated from *H. influenzae,* it is very pyrogenic. Your comparison between the endotoxin and *H. influenzae* might be a little more rigorous if you prepared *E. coli* preparations in the same way that you prepare endotoxin. I presume the endotoxin is a typical product which has been phenol-extracted and which tends to form micelles. The phenol extraction alters the endotoxin material so that, in many respects, it does not resemble a material present on the bacterial cell. I wonder if you have been able to do comparable studies with *E. coli* disrupted in the French press.

Robert H. Alford: Yes, *E. coli* extract prepared the same way behaved similarly.

Robbins: Have you prepared the *E. coli* the same way as the *H. influenzae* and do these identically prepared bacterial preparations have different characteristics?

Alford: No. They had the same characteristics. When clarified by low-speed centrifugation, it perturbs the platelet membrane and causes serotonin release. After ultracentrifugation, it is still antigenic but does not cause platelet serotonin release.

David T. Karzon: I am not sure I understood the answer. If you prepare *E. coli* the same way as *Hemophilus,* it acts the same was as *Hemophilus?*

Alford: Yes. We can prepare a number of different bacterial extracts in this way and get an endotoxin-like activity as measured by the platelet assay.

Karzon: How about transformation of that material?

Alford: It transforms lymphocytes also before and after the platelet-injuring activity has been removed by ultracentrafugation.

Robbins: When you studied polyacrylimide gel electrophoresis in your first experiments, how much of the protein remained above the gel? In other words, approximately how much of it enters the gel?

Alford: There is a stainable layer at the interface of the gel that does not enter it. There must be some very high molecular-weight material that does not get into the gel.

Karzon: What do the members of this conference know about cell-mediated immunity in *H. influenzae?*

Robbins: I supply an answer from a literature review. I have not found a case yet with *H. influenzae,* type b, meningitis in infants or children with the so-called primary-cell-mediated deficiency or the combined deficiency. However, cases of x-linked hypogammaglobulinemia and *H. influenzae,* type b, meningitis, including recurrent type b meningitis, are easily found. Now, that is not to say that cell-mediated immunity is not a process that is involved in post-*H. influenzae* host interaction. I have not been able to document clinical evidence to that point. I am curious to see what Dr. Anderson says.

Porter Anderson: I only parrot what Dr. Rosen and Dr. Janeway (1966) say— which is, that, in x-linked aggamaglobulinemia, one of the frequent offenders in recurrent infections is *H. influenzae.* On the other hand, patients with the immune deficiencies that lead to the absence of lymphocytes generally tend to suffer from other chronic problems; for example, fungus infections, and not so much from *H. influenzae* or pneumococcus. But I am saying the same thing, too, that Dr. Robbins does, without having done the literature search.

Johnston: The pathogenicity of *H. influenzae* in normal and immunodeficient patients strongly suggests that it is an extracellular pathogen. These bacteria are rapidly killed once they are ingested but are not ingested efficiently if antibody, C_3, or phagocytic cells are deficient. When cell-mediated immunity is deficient, infections due to obligate intracellular parasites are more threatening. The latter micro-organisms are apparently easily ingested but can survive inside of macrophages unless the macrophages are activated by factors from T-lymphocytes. One might expect on thse grounds (which is no evidence at all) that cell-mediated immunity would not play an essential role in defense against *H. influenzae.* However, it seems to me that Dr. Alford has an experimental system that might get at that question, and I wonder if it is fair to ask him if he has started looking at some of his patients with chronic bronchitis from whom *H. influenzae* has been frequently cultured.

Alford: Yes. The results are very complex, with the patients segregating into at least two groups of differing reactivity. I would not like to comment further on the results at this time, since they are incomplete. I would like to ask a question, though. I am surprised that persisting *H. influenzae* antibodies are not produced until two years of age. Perhaps there exists some T-lymphocyte-mediated immunity before that time as a foundation upon which B-lymphocyte-mediated polysaccharide-induced antibody production is later added. What is the state of children or infants less than two years of age so far as their cellular reactivity to *H. influenzae* antigen?

Sarah H. Sell: We do not know the answer to that question, but it would be helpful indeed. Perhaps a cell-mediated immunity is more important in young infants than is the serum-antibody system.

Karzon: We cannot store cells and we cannot be helped by Dr. Sell's longitudinal serum collection, but it would be interesting to see what newborn and 1-, 2-, and 3-year-old children show in your system.

Johnston: The *in vitro* transformation of cord-blood lymphocytes was studied by Dr. Izzett Berkel and with some of Dr. Anderson's PRP. As i recall, almost all babies responded. Unfortunately, cord lymphocytes will respond *in vitro* to many antigens, and it was hard to know whether the response to PRP was specific or nonspecific. I do not recall, maybe Dr. Anderson does, whether he extended his studies beyond the neonatal period.

Anderson: I remember the general experience was that there was not a clear-cut pattern, but we felt that the capsular antigen had some phytohemagglutinin-like quality; that is, it seemed to be a nonspecific mitogen for lymphocytes, and its effect did not particularly reflect the prior sensitization or the immune experience of the donor.

Whisnant: We attempted to find some cellular differences between normal people and people who have disease. We tested peripheral blood lymphocytes from each group for sensitivity to hyperimmune *H. influenzae,* type b, antibodies. In a very small series of subjects assayed by cyto-toxicity tests by dye exclusion, it seemed that those with disease, particularly epiglottitis, possessed lymphocytes that were more susceptible to the anti-*H. influenzae* antibody than those without disease. We are not yet quite sure what the model means, but it may be a way of establishing some cellular relationship to disease.

REFERENCES

Rosen, F. S., and C. A. Janeway. 1966. "The Gamma Globulin: III. The Antibody-Deficiency Syndromes." *New Eng. J. Med.* 275:709.

SECTION VI

CHAPTER **15**

Natural Infections with *Hemophilus influenzae:* II. Studies of Serum Antibody Activity

Sarah H. Sell
Dorothy J. Turner
Richard B. Johnston, Jr.
Charles F. Federspiel
Roger Vander Zwaag
Linda J. Duke

The exact role of serum antibodies against *H. influenzae* in the immune or protective mechanisms of the human host is not understood. The various methods for serological investigation of influenzal bacillus infections in man are reviewed by Turk and May (1967). The report which originally indicated that antibodies may be protective is the classic study of Fothergill and Wright (1933) which showed that the bactericidal property of whole blood was age-related, with infants from age 6 weeks to 2 years having none, while older children acquired adult levels by age 8 to 10 years. The incidence of meningitis due to *H. influenzae* was highest during ages of lowest bactericidal acticity. This information was complemented by the report of Ward and Wright (1932) that bactericidal activity of serum (+ complement) was comparable to that of whole blood, in man as well as rabbits. In 1939, H. E. Alexander recommended hyperimmune rabbit serum for therapy of meningitis due to *H. influenzae.* However,

Appreciation is expressed to Martha Murtaugh, Shirley Stansell, Linda Arnold, Lucille Hampton, Ana Womack, Sharon Matthews, and Susan Gardner for help in collection and assay of specimens; to Helen Johnson for typing; and to the Pediatric House Staff of Vanderbilt University Hospital for patient care.

This work was supported by U. S. Public Health Service, National Institute of Allergy and Infectious Disease, Grants N. AI-06110 and AI-10286.

since the clinical results of antiserum alone were not always reliable, she also suggested the addition of sulfonamides to the therapeutic regime. In 1944, it was shown by Alexander, Leidy, and Heidelberger that the protective component (for mice) could be removed from the antiserum by absorption with capsular PRP. Turk and Green (1964) reported that hemagglutinating antibodies to capsular antigens developed in a series of patients known to have been carriers of homologous types. However, the significance in terms of protection was unknown.

This report concerns the natural acquisition of serum antibody activity in a group of children who were followed longitudinally for infections with *H. influenzae* during the period 1964-1970.

METHODS

Our longitudinal study, previously described in this symposium, was designed to observe a group of children from birth until age 5 years to try to determine whether antibodies developed following experience with *H. influenzae* in the nasopharynx, with or without associated illness. The subjects were studied monthly until age 6 months and then quarterly thereafter. In addition, studies were conducted during bouts of respiratory illness and one month after each nasopharyngeal culture from which *H. influenzae* was identified. In this way, a blood sample was collected during each episode, and changes in serum antibody activity could be monitored before and after carriage of *H. influenzae,* as well as with advancing age. The serum samples were stored at $-2°$ C immediately after collection and separation.

Since small amounts of serum were contained in many of the samples, micromethods of antibody assay were desirable. We have devised a test for bacterial growth inhibition which is an assay for "bacterial inhibitory substance" (BIS) as an indication of antibody activity. Serum dilutions + bacteria + complement + buffer were mixed in small sterile plastic tubes, shaken for three minutes, after which Levinthal's broth was added and the mixture incubated for five hours. The numbers of bacteria were calculated from dilutions of 1:3 which showed growth. Inhibition was calculated by comparision of the numbers of dilutions of the unknown serum in which the bacteria grew versus dilutions showing growth in a known noninhibitory serum (the complement source).

METHOD OF ASSAY OF BIS

I. *The Test*

1. Into sterile plestic test tube (Falcon Plastics, #2003), using micro-pipettes (H. E. Pederson-Copenhagen), was placed:

    A. For unknown serum:

    0.05 ml test serum & 0.05 ml sucrose veronal buffer (SVB-Rapp and Borsos, '63)

    0.05 ml bacterial inoculum (200 cells in SVB)[1]

    0.1 ml human complement (containing 3-C50 units)

    B. For controls:

    Positive control, which caused complete inhibition of bacterial growth: same procedure as unknown but employing known positive serum.

    Negative control, which caused no inhibition (the complement source)[2]

    0.1 ml SVB

    0.1 ml bacterial inoculum (200 cells in SVB)

    0.1 ml human complement

2. The tubes were shaken at room temperature for three minutes (Thomas Shaking Apparatus # 8927), permitting agglutination as well as some killing.

3. 0.5 ml Levinthal's broth was added before incubation at 37.5° C for five hours (permitting growth well into the logarithmic phase).

II. *Estimate of Bacterial Growth*

1. 1.5 ml Brain-Heart Infusion Broth (BHI) was added to each tube to make 1:3 dilutions and to stop growth.

2. Further 1:3 dilutions of each test tube were then made in quadruplicate, using Cooke Microtitre equipment and plastic trays (Linbro #15MRC96) with flat-bottomed wells which hold 0.3 ml each. They were carried out to 12 places, using 0.05 ml aliquots with 0.1 ml Levinthal's broth as diluent.

---

1. The bacterial inoculum was prepared by diluting a fourteen-to-sixteen-hour Levinthal's broth culture of *H. influenzae*, type b (American Type Culture Collection #9795) in SVB so that 0.05 ml contained 200 to 400 viable bacteria (colony-forming units).

2. The human complement source consisted of serum from an adult female which was shown in thirty tests to be noninhibitory when compared to bacterial growth in series with serum-free Levinthal's broth and buffer in identical dilution and incubation period.

3. After 2% BHI Agar was added to each well, the plates were covered and incubated in a moist chamber at 37.5° C overnight.

4. Growth was estimated by number of dilutions showing colonies when the plate was viewed on a lighted colony counter with a dark background.

III. *Calculation of Inhibition*

1. The numbers of dilutions showing growth were averaged for the quadruplicate determinations of each test.

2. The difference between the averages of the negative control (no inhibition) and the test indicated the degree of inhibition.

3. Percentage of inhibition was determined from the accompanying mathematical (log 3) tables

Mathematics of the assay: A nonparametric statistical test, the Rank Sum Test, was applied to the results of the quadruplicates with significance level of p= .057 or less. The results of 536 serum samples, each in quadruplicate, indicated that 176 had significant inhibition, while 360 did not.

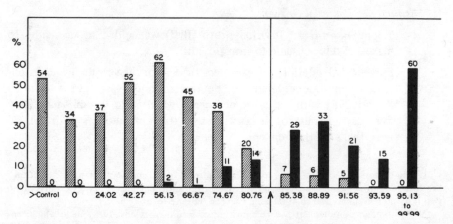

Fig. 1. Chart shows significance by Rank-Sum Test and percentage of inhibition of 536 serum samples.

In addition, the results were calculated in another way. Each well represented a 1:3 dilution of the previous one. The numbers of wells with growth were recorded for each observation of the quadruplicate set. The average for a single serum was calculated. The difference between test and the negative control represented inhibition. From this information, the percent of inhibition could be calculated from the accompanying tables. To determine the amount of inhibition required for significance, separate histograms were prepared showing the distribution of percentage of inhibition in sera with results by the Rank Sum Test, which were judged to be significant or nonsignificant. The two histograms were superimposed. Figure 1 shows that 85.38% was selected as the lower limit of significant inhibition. This represents 1.75 dilutions-difference (each dilution being 1:3 of the previous one) between averages of the tests and noninhibitory control. Table 1 is the mathematical table which was developed for reference.

Passive hemagglutination: Passive hemagglutinating antibodies (HA) were assayed by the method of Anderson, Johnston, and Smith (1972). Fresh human type-O eythrocytes were sensitized with purified polyribophosphate (PRP), kindly furnished by Dr. Anderson.

TABLE 1

MATHEMATICAL REFERENCE FOR ASSAY OF BIS

Inhibition-Difference*	Percentage of Inhibition[†]			
	.00	.25	.50	.75
0	0	24.0164	42.2650	56.1309
1	66.6667	74.6271	80.7550	85.3770
2	88.8889	91.5574	93.5850	95.1257
3	96.2963	97.1858	97.8617	98.3752
4	98.7654	99.0619	99.2872	99.4504
5	99.5885	99.6873	99.7624	99.8195
6	99.8628	99.8958	99.9200	99.9398
7	99.9543	99.9653	99.9736	99.9799
8	99.9848	99.9884	99.9912	99.9933

*Inhibition: Difference between the average of the quadruplicate determinations showing growth in the noninhibitory control minus the average of the quadruplicate showing growth in test serum.

[†]Computed on the basis that each dilution was 1:3 of the previous one and that each determination was performed in quadruplicate.

Opsonizing assay: The ability of serum to promote the phagocytosis of viable *H. influenzae,* type b, ATC strain # 9795, was studied in 274 sera from 25 children, utilizing a slight modification of a previously described spectrophotometric method (Anderson, Johnston and Smith, 1972). Test sera were heated at 56° C for 30 minutes and used in a volume of 0.18 ml per tube, along with 0.10 ml of fresh guinea pig serum (GPS Cordis Laboratories, Miami, Florida) as a complement source. The extent of phagocytosis, measured by the reduction of nitroblue tetrazolium dye, was expressed as Δ OD at 515 nm, which was determined by subtracting the OD with GPS alone from that obtained with GPS and the test serum. The ΔOD achieved with each test preparation was compared to the ΔOD achieved in the same experiment with a heated standard reference serum obtained from an adult immunized with type b capsular polysaccharide. Results were expressed as (ΔOD with test preparation/OD with standard serum) X 100%. In this system, the opsonizing activity of single samples from 17 normal adults averaged 12% of that achieved by the standard high-titred postvaccination serum (range 0 to 46%).

RESULTS

Preliminary studies of BIS: The preliminary studies included determinations of reproducibility. Variability in the serial dilution technique was examined by determining the average dilution showing growth in 10 aliquots of 1:64 rabbit antiserum against type b. All ten aliquots were assayed the same day. In nine of

TABLE 2

RESULTS—PERCENTAGE INHIBITION (BIS)

	Unheated		Heated	
	With Added Complement	Without Added Complement	With Added Complement	Without Added Complement
Rabbit Serum	99.99	99.99	99.99	99.99
Adult	99.99	99.99	99.99	24.02*
Pt. #1 (age 6 months)	88.89	88.89	42.27*	42.27*
Pt. #2 (age 18 months)	91.56	85.38	42.27*	24.02*
Pt. #3 (age 36 months)	88.89	80.76*	88.89	74.63*

*All results below 85.38 were considered to be below the range of significance.

the ten determinations, the average dilution difference was either 1.25 or 1.5, the tenth determination being 2 (see Table 1), indicating very consistent or reproducible results. Variability in the results of the negative control was examined by testing the noninhibitory human serum on 30 consecutive days. The average of the 30 determinations was a dilution of 9, and the sample standard deviation was approximately .75. All but one of the 30 determinations deviated no more than 1.25 from the sample average, and they appeared to be symetrically distributed, 16 being above the sample mean and 14 below.

It was shown that heating at 56° C for 30 minutes did not effect the titre of hyperimmune rabbit serum, but it completely destroyed the activity of a high-titre adult human specimen. Addition of human complement restored the inhibitory effects. However, serum from three young children lost their inhibition by heating and it was not restored in two by addition of the human complement (see Table 2). Recognizing that the patient's own complement might be active in some of the specimens but to an unreliable degree, it was elected to test all sera without heating and to add noninhibitory human serum as complement source.

For determining the effect of the adsorption of sera with PRP, samples with high BIS levels were selected from four subjects, all of whom were between 4 and 5 years of age and had been carriers of type b at one time or another.

Table 3 shows that the inhibitory activity was reduced to insignificant levels in subject A and B but only partially reduced in C and D. It was completely lost after adsorption with whole type b bacterial cells. This was interpreted to mean that somatic antigens in addition to capsular were involved in reactions.

TABLE 3

BIS ASSAYS AFTER ADSORPTION

Subject	Serum Dilution = 1:3		Serum Dilution = 1:2	
	Unadsorbed	Adsorbed with PRP*	Unadsorbed	Absorbed with type b Bacterial Cells[T]
	% Inhibition	% Inhibition	% Inhibition	% Inhibition
A	97.86	24.02	99.89	0
B	97.86	74.62	99.86	0
C	96.30	85.38	99.76	0
D	99.1	85.38	99.92	0

*Adsorbed twice: Total PRP = 10.43 µg/ .05ml serum.

[T]Adsorbed twice: With 1/2 volume packed bacteria (washed once)

(All results below 85.38 were considered to be below the range of significance)

Treatment with 2-Mercaptoethanol did not destroy the inhibition in rabbit or adult human serum. These results were compatible with the interpretation that IgG was involved in the BIS reaction. The reaction in rabbit serum, which was not destroyed by heating, could be due to agglutination which was not complement dependent.

By this assay, 40% (19/40) of the serum samples from healthy adults (blood bank donors) showed significant inhibition of *H. influenzae,* type b. Ten pairs of serum from newborn babies and their mothers were tested. Infants and their mothers had similar inhbition: four pairs were within significant range, while six were not.

Preliminary studies with HA: Fifty-seven (22/40) of the adult (blood bank donors) sera which were also assayed for BIS gave HA titres of 1:2 or greater (up to 512). When this number was enlarged to 103, however, 67% gave such titres.

Of the ten infant-mother pairs, one infant had a titre of 1:2, while eight mothers had 2 or greater (up to 256).

Results from subjects in the study: In the longitudinal study previously described in this volume (Sell et al.) 1,537 samples of serum were collected, and stored at –22° C and were assayed for BIS. Of these same sera, 1,139 were also titred for HA and 274 for opsonizing activity.

Of the cord sera, 27% (27/102) had significant BIS activity, while 8% (6/73) had HA titres of 1:2.

When the results of all assays from each patient were plotted against time, it was apparent that there were antibody rises which were transient, while, in some children, there eventually developed rises which persisted to the end of the study.

Figure 2 shows the patterns of response in one subject with the three assays plotted against age. The arrows at the bottom indicate indentification of *H. influenzae* in nasopharyngeal cultures. There was a significant level of BIS activity in the cord serum and this fell rapidly. There was a transient rise to significant levels lasting between the ages of 28 to 33 months, falling again by 36 months. After age 48 months, the rise was sustained. Type b was identified in the nasopharyngeal cultures multiple times between the ages of 20 and 28 months. The HA titre rose to 1:2 at 54 months of age but was transient. The opsonic activity reached a peak during the first type b carriage and remained elevated.

Figure 3 shows the response patterns of another child. BIS activity, which was noted in the cord serum, was maintained during the first year of life associated with multiple episodes of nasopharyngeal carriage of nontypable and type d strains of *H. influenzae.* There were two later transient rises, one of which followed a second bout of illness associated with type b. When the child was 4

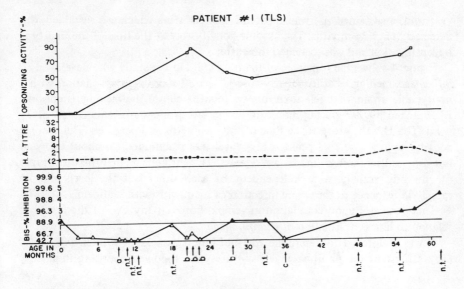

Fig. 2. Patterns of response in one subject with three assays plotted against age.

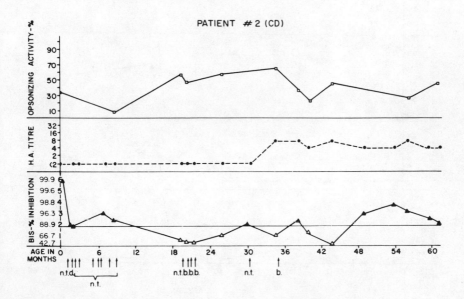

Fig. 3. Patterns of response in second subject with three assays plotted against age.

years old, a sustained rise was apparent. The HA titre, which was sustained, was detected at age 34 months. The opsonic activity rose at the time of the first type b identification and was sustained thereafter.

Figure 4 shows the responses of the only child in the study who developed *H. influenzae* meningitis. BIS activity rose at age 32 months in association with a nontypable strain that fell to zero two months before the meningitis episode. BIS reached 99.99% during the acute illness but dropped off immediately afterward. The HA titre rose at the time of the meningitis and persisted. The opsonic activity rapidly rose to a peak. A high level was maintained for about one year but dropped to the baseline by age 5 years. Thus, it appears that the three types of antibody activity were independent of each other but the levels all rose rapidly in response to the severe infection of meningitis with septicemia.

There was not good correlation in general between any two of the assays in relation to illness or isolation of *H. influenzae*.

It was of interest to determine whether illness associated with *H. influenzae* (any strain) in the nasopharyngeal cultures was followed by rising inhibitory

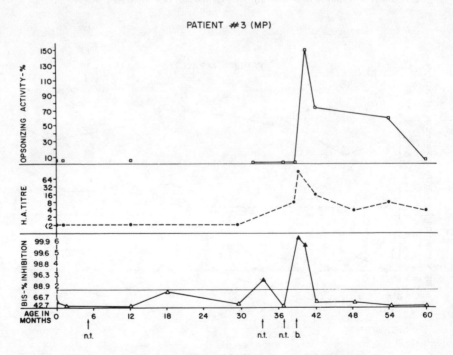

Fig. 4. Patterns of response in third subject with three assays plotted against age.

activity against type b. Table 4 shows results in serum samples collected during the visits immediately preceeding and following defined episodes. It can be seen that after 226 episodes of illness (mild, moderate, or severe) associated with *H. influenzae*, 37% had BIS rises and only 3% occurred in presence of significant BIS. However, after 34% of 498 episodes of no illness and no *H. influenzae*, similar rises were detected. This difference is not statistically significant. Table 5 shows similar results from the passive hemagglutination assays. In fact, 32% of the illness episodes associated with *H. influenzae* occurred while the HA titres were 1:2 or greater.

Table 4 also indicates that there was no difference between the results of BIS after moderate or severe illness episodes associated with *H. influenzae,* type b,

TABLE 4

RESULTS OF BIS ASSAYS OF SERUM SAMPLES COLLECTED BEFORE
AND AFTER OBSERVED EPISODES ALL AGES

Episodes	Totals No.	Low→High No.	Low→High %	High→Low No.	High→Low %	Low→Low No.	Low→Low %	High→High No.	High→High %
H. infl. identified associated with illness (mild, moderate or severe)	226	83	37	7	3	29	57	7	3
No. *H. influenzae* identified No. illness	498	168	34	12	2	311	62	7	1
H. influenzae, type b associated with moderate or severe illness	12	3	25	1	8	7	58	1	8
Pneumococcus (no. *H. influenzae*) assoc. with moderate or severe illness	19	5	26	2	1	12	63	0	0

High: Significant inhibition
Low: No significant inhibition

NOTE: Sera were selected from visit immediately preceding and next visit after index episode. Time interval was at least two months.

than with pneumococcus. About one fourth of each group had rises, but the majority were low before and after the episodes. However, only a rare such episode occurred in presence of significant BIS.

Figure 5 shows the cumulative percentages of children with first rises in BIS and HA activity with age. It is composed of results from the 94 subjects who were followed for three years, including 44 who continued for five years. Transient BIS was noted in 33% by age 1 year, in 61% by age 2 years, and 88% by age 5 years. Persistant BIS, however, was noted in only 3% during the first year, in 14% by age 2 years and 38% by age 5. Persistant HA was noted first at age 16 months. It was present in 14% of the subjects by age 2 years and 52% by 5 years.

TABLE 5

RESULTS OF HA ASSAYS OF SERUM SAMPLES COLLECTED
IMMEDIATELY BEFORE AND AFTER OBSERVED EPISODE ALL AGES

	Totals	Low→High		High→Low		Low→Low		High→High	
Episodes	No.	No.	%	No.	%	No.	%	No.	%
H. influenzae identified associated with illness (mild, moderate or severe)	154	15	10	2	1	87	57	50	32
No. *H. influenzae* identified no illness	410	63	15	17	4	216	53	114	28

High: Titre 1:2 or greater
Low: Less than 1:2

NOTE: Sera were selected from visit immediately preceding and next visit after index episode. Time interval was at least two months.

Twenty-four of the 25 children whose sera were assayed for opsonizing activity had at least a transient elevation to a level of 20% of that achieved by a high titer postvaccination serum. The remaining child had a single elevation to 15%. Opsonizing activity in serum from 17 normal adults averaged 12% of the postvaccination serum. In 15 of the subjects, opsonizing activity remained above 15% for at least the last one or two years during the study. This persistent elevation began as early as 5 months of age, but the average age at its onset was 25 months. Isolation of type b, *H. influenaze,* from NP of asymptomatic child was not regularly associated with concurrent elevation of that child's serum

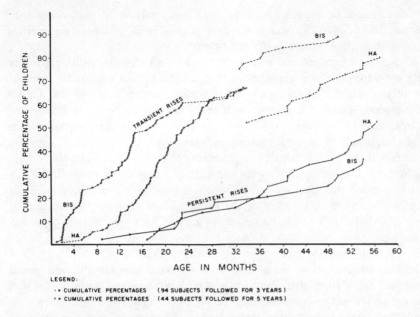

Fig. 5. Cumulative percentages of children with first rises in BIS and HA activity with age.

opsonizing activity. However, in the three children studied who had serious illness associated with type b, there was a definite elevation of opsonizing activity during acute phase of the illness.

DISCUSSION

The results of the serum antibody assays by the three methods in this report emphasize the problems of methodology. The HA test measures only PRP antibodies. The BIS and opsonic activity are more complicated. It was shown by our preliminary studies that while complement was required for human serum BIS activity, it was not needed by rabbit hyperimmune serum. Removal of PRP antibodies by absorption reduced the activity in human serum but whole encapsulated bacterial cells completely removed it. Johnston (in this volume) has shown that opsonization was achieved by serum lacking PRP antibodies and that some opsonizing activity could be achieved by specific antibody in the absence of complement. The results of our assays from infants, when plotted against age of the subject, suggested that the three systems acted independently of each other. Opsonization and BIS, which both involve capsular as well as noncapsular antibodies, might be expected to be more closely related to each other than either to HA. In fact, this was generally true, but levels of these two activites often rose or fell independently of each other.

The peaks of transient activity, as detected by all three methods, especially during the early ages, were intriguing. It is not yet known what these mean in terms of protection. Perhaps they indicate primary immunization so that a more rapid rise occurs after subsequent challenge. They may prove to be important, also, in appraisal of specimens collected over short periods of time during evaluation of antigenicity of immunization procedures.

The fact that we were not able to pinpoint episodes of illness associated with *H. influenzae* in cultures which were specifically followed by rising BIS or HA assays may mean that the time intervals of one month after the illness were not correctly selected in the design of the study. As an example, the subject of Figure 2 carried type b in the nasopharynx at least eight months before the BIS rose to significant levels. Perhaps more sensitive methods might have detected differences which are not apparent in the results reported here.

The over-all patterns of the results from the serial samples collected in this longitudinal study from birth through the first 3 or 5 years of life indicated that persistent serum antibody levels did, indeed, accumulate with age. If *in vitro* activity accurately reflected the status *in vivo*, it appeared that the antibody activity accrued as experience with *H. influenzae* increased, as demonstrated by identification of the strains in nasopharyngeal cultures. It was shown that, while all of the children in the study had documented experience with some strain of *H. influenzae* by age 5 years, only 33% had type b (Sell et al., this volume). Persistent serum BIS activity against type b was identified in 38% and HA titres in 52% by this age. The interpretation must assume that many instances of nasopharyngeal carriage of hemophili did not stimulate detectable levels of BIS antibodies and that HA titres may have been the consequene of missed infections with type b or cross-reacting antigens from other sources (Robbins et al., this volume). It is interesting to note, however, that these proportions with persistent activity compare with the percentages found in the adult sera (blood bank donors) tested during the preliminary studies. If one assumes that all adults must have immunity, then our tests are not very sensitive indicators. On the other hand, the role played by serum antibodies is not yet fathomed. The tests reported here have shown changing patterns with age, however.

The need for standardization of antibody assays is highlighted by this report. There is no way, at present, to translate the serological information gained by this longitudinal study into the terms that can compare our results from BIS with the various bactericidal or radio-immunoassay tests which have been recently reported by others (Anderson, this volume). Due to the numbers of variables, the information collected from this study of natural infections can only be translated directly into units of other tests, if the sera are reassayed for comparison of results from naturally acquired or immunized antibodies.

SUMMARY

A new test was devised for micro-assay of bacterial inhibition of *H. influenzae,* type b (BIS) as an indication of serum antibody activity. By this method, 1,537 sera, collected in a longitudinal study from 104 normal children, followed from birth to age 3 or 5 years, were assayed. For comparison, 1,139 of the same samples were assayed for hemagglutinating antibodies against capsular PRP. Also, 274 sera from 25 of the children were studied for opsonizing activity.

It was shown that there were transient peaks of activity by all assays during the early ages, while persistent levels developed before age 5 years in 38% of the subjects by BIS and 52% by HA. Persistent opsonizing antibodies developed in 60% (15/25) of those studied. These findings indicated that antibody activities accrue with age, apparently from natural infections either with *H. influenzae* or with cross-reacting antigens.

A plea was made for standardization of methodology so that results of studies from various laboratories could be comparable.

REFERENCES

Alexander, H. E. 1939. "Type b Anti-influenzal Rabbit Serum for Therapeutic Purposes." *Proc. Soc. Exptl. Biol.* 40:313.

Alexander, H. E.; M. Heidelberger; and G. Leidy. 1944. "The Protective and Curative Element in type b, *H. influenzae,* Rabbit Serum." *Yale J. Biol. Med.* 16:425.

Anderson, Porter. 1972. "Human Serum Activities against *Hemophilus influenzae,* type b." *J. Clin. Invest.* 51:31.

Anderson, P.; R. B. Johnston, Jr.; D. H. Smith. 1972. "Human Serum Activities against *Hemophilus influenzae,* Type b." *J. Clin. Invest.* 51:31.

Dixon, W. J., and F. J. Massey. 1957. *Introduction to Statistical Analysis.* New York: McGraw-Hill.

Fothergill, L.C., and J. Wright. 1933. "Influenzal Meningitis. The Relation of Age-Incidence to the Bactericidal Power of Blood against the Causal Organism." *J. Immunol.* 24:273.

Harris, A. H., and M. B. Coleman; editors. 1963. *Diagnostic Procedures and Reagents,* p. 140. 4th edition. New York: Am Pub. Health Assn.

Johnston, R. B., Jr.; P. Anderson; and S. L. Newman. 1972. "Opsonization of Phagocytosis of *H. influenzae,* type b." This volume.

Rapp, H. J., and T. Borsos. 1963. "Sucrose Veronal Buffer: Effects of Low Ionic Strength on Immune Hemolysis." *J. Immunol.* 91:826.

Robbins, John; Richard L. Myerowitz; Rachel Schneerson; John Whisnant; Emil Gotschlich; and Liu Darrel. 1972. "Cross-Reacting Antigens of Enteric Bacteria as an Antigenic Source for Natural Antibodies to Bacteria-Causing Meningitis." This volume.

Sell, Sarah H. W.; D. J. Turner, and C. F. Federspiel. 1972. "Natural Infections with *Hemophilus influenzae* in Children: I. Types Identified." This volume.

Turk, D. C., and C. A. Green. 1964. "Measurement of Antibodies Reacting with Capsular Antigens of *Hemophilus influenzae.*" *J. Clin. Path.* 17:294.

Turk, D. C., and J. R. May. 1967. *Hemophilus influenzae: Its Clinical Importance:* London: The English Universities Press.

Ward, H. K., and J. Wright. 1932. "Studies on Influenzal Meningitis: I. The Problems of Specific Therapy." *J. Exp. Med.* 55:223.

CHAPTER 16

Studies on the Prevalence of Antibodies to *Hemophilus Influenzae,* type b

David H. Smith
Suhung Hann
Virgil M. Howie
John H. Ploussard
A. Lynn Harding
Porter Anderson

Hemophilus influenzae, type b, is one of the most frequent causes of systemic infections, including meningitis, in children aged 3 months to 4 years (Haggerty and Ziai, 1960). Such infections are relatively uncommon, however, in older children and are very rare in newborn infants and adults (Fothergill and Wright, 1933; Mathies, Hodgman, and Ivler, 1965; Collier, Conner, and Nyhan, 1967). Seeking an explanation for this age-related susceptibility, Fothergill and Wright in 1933 discovered that whole blood was often bactericidal for an isolate of *H. influenzae* recovered from a patient with meningitis (and later found to be a type b strain)* and that the age-related prevalence of such activity in a population

This work was done in the Infectious Disease Unit, Children's Hospital Medical Center and Beth Israel Hospital, Department of Pediatrics, Harvard Medical School, Boston, Massachusetts.

Work was supported by grants from the Charles H. Hood Foundation, the Massachusetts Cosmetologist Association, Inc., Contract 71-2196 from the National Institute of Allergy and Infectious Diseases, Bethesda, Maryland, and Grant CC 0511 from the National Center for Disease Control, Atlanta, Georgia.

The authors are grateful to Dr. William D. Cochran and the staff of the Boston Hospital for Women, Lying-In Division, for their support and interest; and to Mrs. Hei Sun Lee for assistance. Part of this investigation would not have been possible without the excellent co-operation of Drs. McKeage, Louden, Hagele, D'Souze, and Cutler of Salem, Massachusetts; Dr. Medlinsky of Marblehead, Massachusetts; and the staff, North Shore Children's Hospital, Salem, Massachusetts.

*M. Pittman, 1970: personal communication.

of 133 individuals correlated inversely with that of *H. influenzae* meningitis. They therefore proposed that this bactericidal activity mediated resistance to systemic infection, and that the activity in cord serum was mediated by passively transferrred maternal antibody. The subsequent observations that serotherapy with rabbit anti-*H. influenzae,* type b, serum reduced the mortality of systemic experimental and human infections (Alexander, Heidelberger, and Leidy, 1944; Alexander, Ellis, and Leidy, 1942) and that adsorption with the polyribose-phosphate capsule of *H. influenzae,* type b, eliminated the potency of such sera (Alexander, Ellis, and Leidy, 1942) supported the concept that anti-PRP antibody provides resistance to *H. influenzae*, type b. Furthermore, antibody to PRP, in the presence of complement, is bactericidal and promotes phagocytosis of *H. influenzae,* type b, *in vitro* (Anderson, Johnston, and Smith, 1972).

H. influenzae, type b, has other immunologically distinguishable antigens, some of which are common to untypable and all encapsulated types of *H. influenzae* (Platt, 1939; Tunevall, 1953; May, 1967). These antigens are generally designated as "somatic antigens," although their location within the bacterial cell and their chemical composition have not been well characterized. The role of such antibodies in host resistance has not been well studied, but recent observations have suggested they may also be bactericidal *in vitro* for *H. influenzae,* type b, (Anderson, Johnston, and Smith, 1972).

In order to evaluate the current prevalence of antibodies to *H. influenzae,* type b, we have assayed the sera of certain adults, infants, and children in different regions of the United States. Antibody activity was measured by bactericidal (BC), passive hemagglutination (PHA), and radioimmune-adsorption (RIA) methods.

MATERIALS AND METHODS

The methods used to assay the antibody activities have been described in detail in this symposium (Anderson, Johnston, and Smith, 1973). The source of complement for the BC assays included sera from a boy with x-linked agammaglobulinemia, a healthy adult female with no detectable BC activity against *H. influenzae,* type b, and a precolostral calf. In order to determine the antigen specificity of the BC activity of certain sera, they were absorbed before assay with either PRP or the nontypable *H. influenze,* strain U1 (Anderson, Johnston, and Smith, 1972).

Sera were collected and shipped to the laboratory with varying intervals of exposure to ambient temperature. All were stored at -70° C. A source of complement was added to each specimen before assay for BC activity. Sera indicated as "CHMC" personnel were from adults associated with this institution, most of whom participated in a vaccine study (Anderson et al., 1972). Those from the

"BLI" were collected by Dr. Hann from 150 mothers and their newborn infants at the Lying-In Division of the Boston Hospital for Women. "Huntsville" (Alabama) sera were collected by Dr. Howie and Dr. Ploussard. Sera from children other than newborn infants were from children seeking medical care for acute otitis media. Since the titers in these "acute" sera did not correlate with the bacterial etiology of the otitis media, sera of patients with disease of any etiology, including *H. influenzae,* have been included. The "Salem" sera were the preimmunization sera of children who subsequently received PRP (Peter, Anderson, and Smith, 1973).

RESULTS

Adults. Nearly all the 264 individuals studied had detectable BC activity. Titers of >1.33 (assay mixture contains 75% v/v test serum) were found in all 114 in the CHMC study and in 143 of 150 in the BLI study. The geometric mean titer of those in the CHMC study was 6.8 and that of the parturient mothers was 3.2. There was no significant correlation between the antibody titers and the age of the mothers in the BLI group. Forty-nine randomly selected sera with positive titers were absorbed with PRP, the nonencapsulated *H. influenzae,* strain U-1, or both, prior to assay for BC activity. The BC activity was eliminated from 1 of the sera and reduced in 8 by PRP, and it was reduced in 48 by strain U-1. Thus, detectable BC activity for *H. influenzae,* type b, of healthy adults was generally directed against somatic antigens. The common prevalence of BC "antisomatic" antibodies and the apparent heterogeneity of the somatic antigens of type b strains (Anderson, Johnston, and Smith, 1972) was reflected in differences in assay endpoints when different b strains were used as indicator strains. BC activities of strain b-Eagan and b-Rabinowitz that differed by >4 fold were observed in 11 of the 20 sera tested in the CHMC study and in 13 of 56 in the BLI study. We have found, however, that the susceptibility of each of several other type b strains to randomly selected human sera are essentially identical to that of strain b-Eagan (Table 1).

PHA activity at a titer of 2 or greater was detected in 61% of the CHMC group and in 74% of the BLI group. The geometric mean titer was 3.5 for those in the CHMC study and 4.0 for those in the BLI study. Although BC activity was more common, the PHA and BC activities were weakly correlated (Anderson et al., 1972). The geometric mean titer in the radioimmunoassay of a randomly selected subgroup of 28 of those in the BLI study was 200 ng/ml, with a range of 22 to 5000 ng/ml.

Newborn infants: BLI. The BC activity in cord sera, directed against either PRP or somatic antigens, correlated positively with that in the corresponding

TABLE 1

BACTERICIDAL ACTIVITY OF MATERNAL SERA AGAINST
DIFFERENT STRAINS OF *H. INFLUENZAE*, type b

Mothers	Strains			
	Rab	Eag	Schol	Lup
A.V.	64	32	32	32
D.D.	32	32	32	32
B.G.	16	32	32	32
C.E.	64	32	64	64
G.C.	16	16	16	16
D.G.	4	64	64	64
M.F.	4	64	32	32
D.B.	16	256	256	256
P.M.	16	32	64	32
A.A.	8	128	128	128

maternal serum (Fig. 1) Of 14 premature infants delivered from BLI mothers with BC titers of $\geqslant 2$, all but one had titers that corresponded to that of their mother. The infant delivered after the shortest gestation period in the study, 25 weeks, had no BC activity although his mother's titer was 16 (Fig. 2). None of 56 tested cord sera had PHA activity, although the corresponding maternal serum had a titer of 2 or greater. In RIA, the 28 sera corresponding to the 28 maternal sera described above had a GMT of 60 ng/ml with a range of 6 to 770 ng/ml. Relative to the concentration in the respective maternal serum: 31% were two thirds to equal, 23% were one third to two thirds and 46% were less than one third.

Huntsville: In contrast to the observation that BC activity was widely prevalent among the mothers and their newborn infants in the BLI group, 27% of the newborn infants studied in Huntsville, Alabama, had no BC activity detected at a serum concentration of 1.5 (assay mixture contains 66% v/v serum). Both sets of sera were examined in the same laboratory by the same personnel and under identical test conditions (complement source was pre-colostral calf serum). We therefore conclude that these results indicate significant differences in the prevalence of this antibody activity in the two populations examined.

Children. Table 2 summarizes the prevalence of children with positive PHA and BC activities in the Huntsville group. BC activity was determined at a serum concentration of 50% (reciprocal of dilution = 2) and lower for part of the

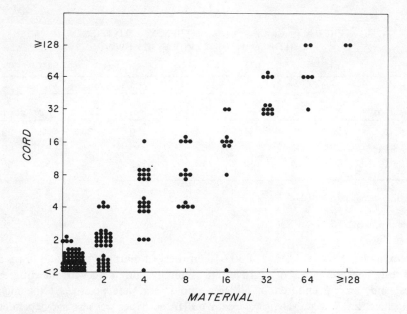

Fig. 1. Comparison of bactericidal activity in maternal and cord sera.

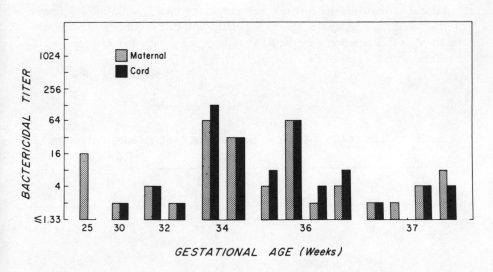

Fig. 2. Comparison of bactericidal activity in the serum of premature infants and their mothers.

TABLE 2

PREVALENCE OF SERUM ANTIBODY ACTIVITIES OF
CHILDREN IN HUNTSVILLE, ALABAMA

Age (mos)	PHA* Activities			BC† Activities					
	$<2^‡$	>2	% positive	<2	>2	% positive	<1.2	>1.2	% positive
<12	267	20	7	184	19	9	34	22	39
13-14	94	34	27	67	7	10	15	10	40
25-48	41	19	32	18	6	25	4	4	50

*Passive hemagglutination
†Bactericidal
‡Reciprocal of serum dilution

group, and at a concentration of 80% (reciprocal of dilution = 1.2) and lower for the rest. The prevalence of positive sera generally correlated with the children's ages, and, among children of all ages, more sera were positive at the higher concentration. The prevalence of positive PHA activities was also age-dependent. The observed differences in the prevalence of PHA and BC activities undoubtedly reflect the sensitivities of the assays and the properties of the immunoglobulins mediating the activity.

Table 3 summarizes the antibody activites in the preimmunization specimens of the Salem, Massachusetts, group. Specific anti-PRP antibody activity was measured in this series only by the RIA method; the geometric mean titers again correlated with the ages of the children.

TABLE 3

SERUM ANTIBODY ACTIVITIES OF CHILDREN IN SALEM, MASSACHUSETTS

Age (mos)	BC Activity		RIA	
	<1.2	>1.2	No. of children	GMT
6-12	6	2	15	8
13-24	15	7	33	34
25-36	10	11	30	66
37-48	23	11	43	120
49-55	4	5	9	330

DISCUSSION

In their study of Boston Children's Hospital that defined an inverse relationship between the prevalence of BC activity against their test strain and that of *H. influenzae,* type b, meningitis, Fothergill and Wright (1933) found BC activity in the blood of all 17 subjects older than 16 years and of 14 of the 16 newborn infants studied. Recently, Norden, Callerame, and Baum (1970) finding no detectable BC activity in the serum of an adult with *H. influenzae,* type b, meningitis at the time of her hospitalization, were led to examine the prevalence of such activity in the serum of 29 other adults in Rochester, New York. Activity at a titer of >2 was detected in 21. These findings raised the possibility that the prevalence of anti-*H. influenzae,* type b, antibody activity now differs from that of 39 years ago, and prompted comment that the prevalence of *H. influenzae,* type b, infections among adults appears to be increasing (Weinstein, 1970). This proposal has been supported by the observations of Graber et al. (1971) in South Carolina that BC activity at a dilution of >4 was detected in only 7 of 64 cord and 4 of 16 maternal sera and those of Feigin et al. (1971) in St. Louis who found no detectable BC activity in the blood of 31 of 101 adults and in 9 of 30 newborn infants.

On the other hand, Schneerson et al. (1971), studying sera of newborn infants in New York City and in Charlotte, North Carolina, found anti-*H influenzae* type b, activity in 1,282 of 1,314 infants tested; and Gump et al. (1971) found bactericidal activity in the serum of 128 of 130 adults. The present results indicate that most adults older than 15 years and newborn infants in Boston have BC activity detectable by our methods. Furthermore, the prevalence of such antibody activity did not relate to a medical occupation, as observed by Feigin et al. (1971). Some of the discrepancies between the results of these serological studies may be more apparent than real. With the exception of Feigin et al. (1971), no recent study has used the methods of Fothergill and Wright, who semiquantitatively assayed the number of colony-forming bacteria in mixtures of whole blood and various concentrations of bacteria after a 24-hour incubation at 37° C. In our experience, assay end-points may be affected by such factors as the amount of PRP (or somatic antigens) in the supernatent fluid of the bacterial culture used in the test, the source of complement, the duration of the incubation of serum, complement and bacteria, the concentration of serum tested, and the degree of bacterial killing used as end-point. (We have not observed, however, that preincubation of human serum at 56° C for 30 minutes adversely affects BC activity). Furthermore, type b strains used as indicators may differ in their susceptibility to a given serum. It will therefore be difficult to determine the relationship of the several recent observations on the prevalence of *H. influenzae,* type b, antibodies to one another and particularly to those of Fothergill and Wright.

Our results indicate further than the prevalence of detectable antibody BC for *H. influenzae*, type b, depends on the population studied. Some of the differences in the several serological surveys cited above are, therefore, real, and undoubtedly reflect differences in exposure to *H. influenzae* or bacteria with antigens common to those of *H. influenzae* to which BC activity can be directed. No attempt was made in our studies to evaluate the epidemiological factors that may correlate with prevalence of BC activity, but it is of interest that most of the newborns studied in Boston and in Huntsville were black and from families of lower socioeconomic status.

Of course, observations regarding the prevalence of antibody are significant only when that concentration of antibody known to prevent disease and the kinetics of the antibody response have been defined. The critical concentration of anti-*H influenzae* antibody b is not known, but we are attempting to resolve this question. The geometric concentration of anti-PRP antibody was approximately 200 ng/ml serum in the "immune" adults and toddler-aged children studied. Since these individuals might generate a higher (protective) concentration of anti-PRP antibody when infected with *H. influenzae*, type b, we have also examined anti-PRP antibody activities in the serum of agammaglobulinemic children prior to their monthly prophylactic dose (0.6 ml/kg) of gamma globulin. This dose has been found emperically to protect these immunodeficient children from systemic *H. influenzae*, type b, disease (Rosen and Janeway, 1966), and thus, we reasoned that their anti-PRP antibody activities should be a better index of a "protective" concentration. The mean concentration in the eight children studied was 230 ng/ml. Further studies are in progress to evaluate the protective efficacy of this concentration of anti-PRP antibody. It is important to note, however, that 200 ng/ml is one-fifth of that detectable in the BC assay, with which the lower limit of sensitivity, in our hands, is 1000 ng/ml (see Anderson, Johnston, and Smith, this volume).

Many of the young children studied had anti-PRP concentrations below 200 ng/ml (see Table 3). This observation does not indicate, however, that they are not protected by this antibody activity. They have had immunogenic contact with PRP or an antigenically related polymer, and thus, as indicated above, they may be able to produce more anti-PRP antibody when infected. The kinetics of such a response have not yet been studied, but "protective" levels of antibody may be produced rapidly enough to prevent systemic disease. Such a proposal is consistent with our serologic findings, the estimated attack rates of systemic *H. influenzae*, type b, diseases, and the considerable clinical experience that indicates that most of these systemic diseases result from the spread of the bacterium from a previous infection of the upper respiratory tract.

We found that BC activity, directed against either somatic antigens or PRP, crossed the placenta and was found in cord serum. PHA activity, however, did not cross the placenta. These *in vivo* data thus support and extend earlier studies that indicated that BC activity directed against PRP in serum is mediated primarily by IgG and PHA actively mainly by IgM immunoglobulins (Anderson, Johnston, and Smith, 1972). The present results further indicate that BC activity directed against somatic antigens is also mediated by IgG globulins. It is evident, therefore, that, if newborn infants are not susceptible to diseases caused by *H. influenzae*, type b, because of passively acquired antibodies, the BC and RIA assays are better *in vitro* tests than the PHA assay for that protective activity.

The BC activity detected in the serum of newborns by Fothergill and Wright was significantly lower than that in the adults they studied. In our investigations, on the other hand, titers of cord serum seldom differed by twofold, or greater, from that of the maternal serum. Since different methods were employed, and Fothergill and Wright did not examine paired sera, the signifiance of this difference between the two studies remains undefined.

All infants of gestational age more than 30 weeks old who were studied had BC titers that were nearly identical to those of their mothers; however, an infant with an estimated gestational age of 25 weeks, who had been delivered from a mother with a BC titer of 16, had no detectable activity. Thus, the placental transfer of these antibodies may start between the twenty-fifth and thirtieth gestational week. If validated by further observations, these results would predict that only very premature infants would be more susceptible to *H. influenzae*, type b, than full-term babies because of deficiency in placental transfer of type-specific antibody.

The results of the present study expand earlier observations made in this laboratory regarding the specificity of the bactericidal activity in *normal serum* (Anderson, Johnston, and Smith, 1972). It is now quite apparent that the BC activity assayed *in vitro* is much more often directed against somatic antigens than against the capsular antigen (PRP). The location, number, and distribution among typable and nontypable strains of *H. influenzae* of the somatic antigens to which bactericidal antibodies are directed remains to be determined. Our results indicate, however, that multiple antigens are involved, that certain of these may be shared by nontypable and type b strains, and that those of b strains may differ. Infection with nontypable *H. influenzae* may therefore provoke an immune response that yields antibody active against type b strains. Such a sequence has been well defined with Group C meningococcus by Goldschneider, Gotschlich, and Artenstein (1969). These results do not detract from earlier observations, however, that purified PRP produces antibodies that are protective *in vivo* and active against all tested b strains *in vitro* (Anderson et al., 1972). Thus, successful immunization with PRP should provoke resistance against *H. influenzae*, type b, infections.

REFERENCES

Alexander, H. E.; C. Ellis; and G. Leidy. 1942. "Treatment of Type-Specific *Hemophilus influenzae* Infections in Infancy and Childhood." *J. Pediat.* 20:673.

Alexander, H. E.; M. Heidelberger; and G. Leidy. 1944. "The Protective and Curative Element in type b, *H. influenzae*, Rabbit Serum." *Yale J. Biol. Med.* 16:425.

Anderson, P.; R. B. Johnston; and D. H. Smith. 1972. "Human Serum Activity against *Hemophilus influenzae*, type b." *J. Clin. Invest.* 51:31.

Anderson, P.; G. Peter; R. B. Johnston; L. H. Wetterlow; and D. H. Smith. 1972. "Immunization of Humans with Polyribophosphate, the Capsular Antigen of *Hemophilus influenzae*, type b." *J. Clin. Invest.* 51:39.

Anderson, P.; R. B. Johnston; and D. H. Smith. 1973. "Methodology in Detection of Human Serum Antibodies to *Hemophilus influenzae*, type b." This volume.

Collier, A.M.; J. D. Conner; and W. L. Nyhan. 1967. "Systemic Infection with *Hemophilus influenzae*." *J. Pediat.* 70:539.

Feigin, R. D.; D. Richmond; M. W. Hosler; and P. G. Shackelford. 1971. "Reassessment of the Role of Bactericidal Antibody in *Hemophilus influenzae* Infection." *Am. J. Med. Sci.* 262:338.

Fothergill, L. C., and J. Wright. 1933. "Influenzal Meningitis: The Relation of Age-Incidence to the Bactericidal Power of Blood against the Causal Organism." *J. Immunol.* 24:273.

Goldschneider, I.; E. C. Gotschlich; and M. S. Artenstein. 1969. "Human Immunity to the Meningococcus: II. Development of Natural Immunity." *J. Exp. Med.* 129:1327.

Graber, C.D.; J. J. Gershanik; A. H. Levkoff; and M. Westphal. 1971. "Changing Pattern of Neonatal Susceptibility to *Hemophilus influenzae*." *J. Ped.* 78:948.

Gump, D. W.; P. Tarr; C. A. Phillips; and B. R. Forsyth. 1971. "Bactericidal Antibodies to *Hemophilus influenzae*." *Proc. Soc. Exp. Bio. Med.* 138:76.

Haggerty, R. J., and M. Ziai. 1960. "Acute Bacterial Meningitis in Children." *Ped.* 25:742.

Mathies, A. W.; J. Hodgman; and D. Ivler. 1965. "*Hemophilus influenzae* Meningitis in a Premature Infant." *Ped.* 35:791.

May, J. R. 1967. "Colonial Morphology, Antigens, and Pathology of *Hemophilus influenzae*." *Sci. Basis Med. Ann. Rev.* 211.

Norden, C. W.; M. L. Callerame; and J. Baum. 1970. "*Hemophilus influenzae* Meningitis in an Adult: Antibody and Immunoglobulins." *N. Eng. J. Med.* 282:190.

Peter, G.; P. Anderson; and D. H. Smith. 1973. "Immunization of Adults and Children with Polyribophosphate, the Capsular Antigen, and *Hemophilus influenzae*, type b." This volume.

Platt, A. E. 1939. "Serological Study of *Hemophilus influenzae*; Two Serological-ly Active Protein Fractions Isolated from Pfeiffer's Bacillus." *Australian J. Exper. Biol. & Med. Sc.* 17:19.

Rosen, F. S., and C. A. Janeway. 1966. "The Gammaglobulins: III. The Anti-body Deficiency Syndromes." *N. Eng. J. Med.* 275:709.

Schneerson, R.; L. P. Rodrigues; J. C. Parke, Jr.; and J. B. Robbins. 1971. "Immunity to Disease Caused by *Hemophilus influenzae,* type b: II. Specificity and Some Biological Characteristics of 'Natural, Infection-Acquired, and Immunization-Induced' Antibodies to the Capsular Poly-saccharide of *Hemophilus influenzae,* type b." *J. Immunol.* 107:1081.

Tunevall, G. 1953. "A Complement Fixation Test for *Hemophilus influenzae.*" *Acta. Pathol. Microbiol. Scand.* 30:203.

Weinstein, L. 1970. "Type b *Hemophilus influenzae* Infections in Adults." *N. Eng. J. Med.* 282:221.

Discussion

David T. Karzon, Presiding

Virgil M. Howie: From patients with otitis media of any cause, presenting in our practice, serum was drawn to determine the hemagglutination (HA) and bactericidal titers against *H. influenzae,* type b. [Otitis media was defined as that condition which causes an accumulation of fluid, rather than air, in the middle ear.] The serum samples were shipped to Dr. David Smith in Boston for the laboratory determinations. The results indicated that, of 28 patients in the 2- to 6-month age group, there was no bactericidal titer greater than one-to-two dilution of serum. There were no other age or titer correlations out of 154 bactericidal titer determinations. Two hundred forty HA titer determinations were performed on 25 patients with otitis media of various causation. As shown in Table 1, the HA titers tended to increase with age. The number of episodes of otitis media as shown in Table 2 tended to be less if the initial episode occurred at 13 months or older. However, there was no relation between HA titer and episodes of otitis media other than that associated with age. The cord serum samples collected in Huntsville, Alabama,

TABLE 1

HEMAGGLUTINATION (HA) TITERS IN OTITIS MEDIA
COMPARED WITH AGE

Age	HA Titers			Totals
	2	2		
1 − 6 mos.	59	6	65	(27.1%)
7 − 12 mos.	60	13	73	(30.4%)
13 + mos.	62	40	102	(42.5%)
Totals	181	59	240	(100%)

$P > .005$

TABLE 2

AGE COMPARED TO EPISODES OF OTITIS MEDIA

Age

Age	Episodes			
	1 − 2	3 or More	Totals	
1 − 12 mos.	67	65	132	(58.7%)
13 + mos.	67	26	93	(41.3%)
Totals	134	91	225	(100%)

P > .01

differed from those in Boston. Of those taken during the summer, July to October, 90% had no bactericidal activity; and during the period from October through January, about 80% had no bactericidal activity. This result was different from the finding by Dr. Smith's group that 90% of the serum samples collected in Boston had bactericidal activity.

Carol W. Norden: We have had comparable experience to Dr. Howie's in terms of cord blood. The bactericidal tests were performed in our laboratory, but we have exchanged some specimens with Dr. Anderson with good correlation of results. We found that only about 20% of the cord bloods had bactericidal activity against *H. influenzae,* type b, strain Eagan.

David T. Karzon: I find these differences in incidence of antibody titer quite extreme. Are they largely explained by technological factors in the laboratory, or are they the resultant of epidemiological phenomona?

Kenneth McIntosh: What about preparation of the serum in terms of immediate refrigeration or freezing?

David H. Smith: We have appreciated no significant changes in antibody activities in sera frozen and thawed several times or that left at room temperature for significant intervals. Furthermore, heating at 56° C for 30 minutes has not affected the bactericidal activity of each of several sera, some of which contain primarily anti-PRP and others which contain only antisomatic antibodies.

Sarah H. Sell: We found that heating serum to 56° C for 30 minutes made a big difference in the results with our BIS test, as shown in Table 2 of our report. Heating destroyed activity which was not restored by human complement in two samples collected from subjects aged 6 months and 18 months. A third sample, which came from a child 36 months old, was not affected by the heating if complement was added. For this reason, we elected not to heat our specimens before testing.

McIntosh: I think if you do not heat sera then it makes an enormous difference in how you get the sera and how they are handled subsequently. Labile factors can be destroyed very easily.

John B. Robbins: I thought I might mention the source of complement in the assay. In the beginning, we found that we could not use normal rabbit serum because it had a demonstrable bactericidal titer. We were obliged to use the serum of a patient with hypogammaglobulinemia which did not by itself alter the ability of the bacteria to survive. We have not done detailed studies on this point, but it has been published that there are important species differences in bactericidal complement. Guinea pig serum, for instance, does not yield a good bactericidal reaction. In some cases, as reported by Fothergill in 1937, guinea pig serum does not give a complement bactericidal reaction with *H. influenzae*, type b. We have utilized precolostral calf serum. This seems to be a satisfactory source of antibody-free complement. Perhaps an alternate substitute, if you do not have the serum of the patient with hypogammaglobulinemia, might be the serum of rabbits taken at 4 to 6 weeks of age assayed to make sure that there are no antibodies in the serum.

Smith: The source of complement is an important consideration for bactericidal assays. We have observed that a nonantibody containing rabbit serum used as a source of complement with a standard source of antibody may give a much higher titer than precolostral calf serum used as a source of complement. Thus, certain antibody-free rabbit sera seem to have a nonimmunological amplification.

Karzon: Is it only an amplification or will it give false positives?

Smith: To date, I think it has given no false positives.

Robbins: We have a little more experience with that. If one defines a false positive as a cidal to bacteria in the absence of another source of antibody, it does not. But the ability of various animals species of complement to elicit the effector reaction—that is, hemolysis of erythrocytes, or lysis of membranes—certainly varies. The size of the holes in the membranes varies from species to species when the source of complement changes and the antibody is the same.

David W. Frazer: Were the titers among children who did not have otitis different from the titers of children who did?

Howie: Other than the reports given here, I do not have information on patients without otitis.

Karzon: Is the chance of a second attack of otitis media due to *H. influenzae* different from the chance of the first attack? In other words, is there any evidence that there is protection against otitis media afforded by prior attacks due to *H. influenzae*?

Howie: It seems to be age-related.

Karzon: Does the second attack occur with a rate which is random for that age, or is the rate diminished after the first attack?

James C. Parke, Jr.: In other words, of all cases of bacterial otitis media—pneumococcal, hemophilus, streptococcal—does the relationship or percentage remain the same, regardless of age?

Howie: Episodes of otitis media seem to be age-related or possibly treatment-related, if antibiotic were used. That is, the better the antibiotic, the more subsequent attacks. The worse the antibiotic used, in terms of being ineffective against hemophilus, the fewer the subsequent attacks.

Karzon: What is the effect of antibiotics on the antibody response?

Howie: I do not know yet.

Karzon: Is the strain of type b important in the serological assays? Are there differences in results if different strains are used in the same test?

Smith: Table 1 in Chapter 16, "Bactericidal Activity of Maternal Sera against Different Strains of *H. influenzae*, Type b," shows the difference in titers by the different strains. That is rather important data, since it illustrates that bactericidal activities may vary by 8-fold to 32-fold, depending on the test strain.

Karzon: The question remains: Can differences in test strains used account, of itself, for all the differences reported?

Smith: It will not make a difference when the bactericidal assays are done with the same strain, but I think it may make a difference if two different laboratories are using two different strains. I also think that the method of preparation of the bacteria is important, and unless there is some standardization of that, one may find big differences in results of studies of prevalence and titers of bactericidal activities.

Howie: Is the difference in the same direction, Dr. Smith?

Smith: No, in the initial experiences, it appeared that b-Rabinowitz was more sensitive than b-Eagan; but in subsequent studies with sera from the Boston Lying-In Hospital, the opposite results were found. We presume that the reasons for this are that the bactericidal activity is directed in many instances against somatic antigens, and that the somatic antigen composition of Rabinowitz and Eagan differs.

Karzon: Did you study strains from the Huntsville area?

Smith: We have done comparative studies. Most type b strains studied, regardless of their origin, reacted similarly to the Strain b-Eagan.

Sell: We have had some experience in testing children's own bacterial isolates against their serum. When the results were compared with tests using our standard strain (American Type Culture Collection Type b-9795), there was greater inhibition of the homologous strains.

Karzon: I think one of the useful things to come out of this conference is standardization of techniques and reagents. I am not fully certain of the implications of this. Is the Rabinowitz a so-called broad or prime strain comparable to similar phenomena in virology? These strains are good indicators because of high activity or whatever term one wishes to apply. Are these strains which contain most of the somatic antigens, or is there marked individual homotypic specificity so that if one wanted to get optimal titers across the board one would have to use a battery? That would be unfortunate.

Robbins: Personally, I would like to see the day when the bactericidal test is not used at all. My reason is that it is a measure of antibody activity as a third-step reaction; that is, one has to measure the interaction of antibody with the bacterial antigen, complement, and an as yet undefined lesion in the bacteria for an end-point. Ideally, I would like to have the antigens in purified form and to measure a direct antigen-antibody interaction. I would think that research efforts should be directed toward working with other antigens. Now that the polysaccharide seems to be prepared and available for a Farr assay, direct antibodies can be measured. I think there are many variables including bacteria themselves which change under laboratory conditions so that research should be directed to having more defined antigens which might be able to distinguish these bacterial antigens and permit more accurate assays of antibody.

Richard H. Michaels: I am afraid that we do not have any idea about what level of which antibody indicates protection from disease. I think there is urgent need for data which will enable us to correlate antibodies with protection.

Karzon: In virology, the neutralization test is considered the "father of all tests" because it is supposed to represent the *in-vivo* protection. If one had to do a single test or assess a new test, one would logically look to the neutralization test, which, through viral binding, prevents cell attachment and penetration. One's instinct is that the cidal test is its counterpart and in fact would represent protection whether or not the operational antigen is PRP or somatic antigens. Is this not so?

Robbins: I would disagree with you, for these reasons: Presuming that in the neutralization test, the antiviral antibody has a very narrow specificity toward that functional portion of the virus that permits attachments to the cells, one can see the subsequent *in-vitro* tissue-culture effect. Now, in this case, there are a whole host of antigen specificities that are measured by the bactericidal assay, the interactions of which are variable. It would be nice if the bacteria did have a single attachment point. My own personal opinion is that we will be able to relate protection to serum antibody directed toward one component, that is the capsule, very soon. If it is related, we will know. If it is not related, our efforts should be directed toward identifying some other active substance from the bacteria.

Karzon: May I provoke further discussion on this point? What is the evidence at this time that the PRP antigen and the antibody directed to it is the functional system in protection? You have said that we will soon know that. How soon will we know it and how?

Robbins: Let us review the evidence that we have and see how faulty it is. I do not know if this is the right time to do it. I am wondering if we could not postpone it until we have had some more papers.

Karzon: Fair enough. We will return to this tomorrow.

Smith: This may be a small point, but one aspect about the *in vitro* test for phagocytosis is that the bacteria are usually dead before phagocytosis by the white cell; that is, the kinetics of the bactericidal reactions are very rapid, and by the time the assay is completed, only dead bacteria are available for phagocytosis. We may be presumptuous to assume that we can translate the *in vitro* reactions to *in vivo* situations.

Karzon: Dr. Johnston, your test is being impuned.

Richard B. Johnston, Jr.: I would prefer to say *scrutinized,* and it should be. I agree 100% with Dr. Smith, and I think that any direct extrapolation from any of these systems to real life must be done with caution. It is difficult to separate, using an *in vitro* system with this particular organism, the bactericidal effect of antibody and complement alone from the bactericidal effect of these two plus the white cells. The same problem, however, is true for enteric bacteria. There is an experiment of nature which may elucidate the role of these two bactericidal systems in defense against enteric organisms, namely, chronic granulomatous disease. In this disorder, patiens have very high levels of antibody and complement, which should permit high levels of bacteriolysis, but they have chronic and lethal infections due to *E. coli, Pseudomonas, Proteus, Klebsiella,* and other organisms, because their phagocytes cannot kill these bacteria, once ingested. That is rather indirect evidence, of course, and I would not say that it settled the issue. However, I think it is purely a matter of cleverness in manipulating the phagocytosis system as to whether we will be able to stretch out the bacteriolytic effect of serum and still get an opsonizing effect, and thereby show a dichotomy, *in vitro.* I still wonder if that will answer the basic question regarding host defense. I do not think it will.

Robbins: We have had some experience with the phagocytic test after reading the very elegant articles by Dr. Johnston. I would like to comment about one thing in those tests. If one adds washed bacteria to washed lymphocytes alone, there is dye reduction; whether or not this is due to phagocytosis, we do not know. If heated complement is added, there is an increment of phagocytosis. Antibody alone will give an increment, also. The final reaction mixture really represents, not phagocytosis *per se,* but increments of phagocytosis which I think make the interpretation difficult.

Johnston: One can see with this particular bacterium some slight reduction of the nitroblue tetrazolium dye in the reaction mixture before the phagocytes are added. However, if the reaction mixture without white cells is tested as a control, the color is not extractable, and, thus, significant dye reduction is not demonstrated in the final result. For example, when white cells are omitted, there might be an OD of about 0.020 to 0.030, in the distinction to a positive reaction of from around 0.300 to 0.400. I think dye is reduced here by oxidative enzymes inside the bacteria; but one can separate this from the dye reduction that occurs secondary to phagocytosis. If serum is replaced with saline, on the other hand, an OD of 0.050 to 0.070 results. Therefore, we routinely subtract the baseline obtained with bacteria, saline in place of serum, and white cells. This leaves the OD, that is, the OD achieved over and above the baseline obtained without serum in the system. There is, indeed, some further enhancement of phagocytosis (dye reduction) on the addition of heated serum, but it is not unexpected, since we and others have shown opsonization by antibody alone.

Porter Anderson: Let me direct a question to Dr. Robbins about antibacterial tertiary or secondary activities. Given an antigenic specificity that may be important, what about the different classes of immunoglobulins in so far as their ability to fix complement and not to fix complement, in reference to the possibility that some classes of antibodies to the given antigen on the bacterial surface may turn out to be a blocking antibody, in some sense, or a lytic reaction. Is a blocking antibody something you have thought about?

Robbins: That is a very good question. One supposes that an antibody with an antigenic specificity might cover it, so that an antibody capable of fixing complement would compete for the antigenic site. The result might be a living antibody-coated bacterium. A possibility is that IgA antibody can serve as that noncomplement-fixing moiety, as we showed in *Salmonella typhimurium.* It is possible that there are subclasses of IgG antibodies to these antigens with noncomplement-fixing properties. I think the possibility is there, although it has not been shown. I do think that this illustrates the complexity of the complement dependent reaction. I advocate working with single isolated systems to measure direct interaction.

Karzon: Dr. Anderson, that idea could be put to the test by adding a noncomplement-activating antibody, such as IgA.

Anderson: One might be able to construct a system to test the possibility. It is difficult to answer. In the host presented with the antigen, what proportion of the antibody might fall into potential blocking types? From my perspective of, say, a year ago, it never occurred to me that there might be vaccination trials before one could, by inferential means, prove that the antibody was protective; but that situation may have changed now. It may be that, rather than having to demonstrate in advance that if the antibody of X-class is raised it would be protective, one might want to go ahead and test the antigen, anyway. A year ago, I would have argued with Dr. Robbins that maybe we should not be too quick to throw out a complicated antigen, antibody, complement, and phagocyte-dependent phenomenon, just because it is hard to work with. But considering the vaccination possibilities now, that may be less important. In reference to the former thinking, we had thought it important to collect as many infecting strains of organisms as possible from children with systemic diseases and try to gather something from the presence or absence of the serum bactericidal or opsonic activity in their acute serum against their own isolates. I think there is still some merit in looking at this, but it is very difficult material to collect. We get about half a dozen such combinations a year.

REFERENCE

Fothergill, L. D. 1937.*"Hemophilus influenzae* (Pfeiffer's Bacillus) Meningitis and Its Specific Treatment." *N. Eng. J. Med.* 216:587.

SECTION VII

Studies on Mechanism of Susceptibility to *Hemophilus influenzae,* type b, Disease: Relationship of Erythrocytes and Histocompatibility Antigens with *Hemophilus influenzae,* type b, Meningitis and Epiglottitis

John K. Whisnant
G. Nicholas Rogentine
John B. Robbins

There is no satisfactory explanation for the pathogenesis of *Hemophilus influenzae,* type b, disease to understand why only a small percentage of non-immune individuals develop disease due to this organism. We are attempting to define susceptibility to *H. influenzae,* type b, disease in terms other than the absence of antibody-mediated immunity and to define host characteristics which may be related to the pathogenesis of disease. Cell-surface leukocyte and erythrocyte antigens were chosen for study because of their previously demonstrated relationship to disease states and because their genetic control is well known (Whisnant et al., 1971).

Experimental animal models have indicated that there may be genetic control of susceptibility to infectious agents. Various inbred strains of mice are either susceptible or resistant to *S. typhimurium* (Cowen, 1960) or to the murine leukemia viruses (Lilly, Boyse, and Old, 1964). This latter heritable trait segregates with the mouse major histocompatibility locus, H-2. Human models for genetic control of susceptibility to infectious disease have also been described. Poliomyelitis and tuberculosis have a high concordant attack rate in identical twins of index cases (Schweitzer, 1961). Recent investigations have attempted to relate disease susceptibility to histocompatibility (HL-A) antigens on lymphocytes. Examples of altered HL-A antigen frequencies in disease include systemic lupus erythematosus in which antigens Al may be decreased and A8 and W15 are increased over normal (Grumet, et al., 1971). Studies of individuals with acute lymphocytic leukemia show an almost twofold increase in HL-A 2 (Rogentine et al., 1972).

The two *H. influenzae,* type b, diseases which we selected for study are meningitis and epiglottitis. These diseases are apparently caused by the same organism. However, except for two incompletely described cases, they are not known to occur in the same individual simultaneously, in spite of bacteremia in both diseases. It can be hypothesized that the marked difference in the nature of these two diseases in different individuals (Berenberg and Kevy, 1958) is related to host factors.

Histocompatibility and erythrocyte antigens have now been determined for 30 epiglottitis patients, 20 meningitis patients, and as many siblings and parents as were available. All individuals studied were Caucasian. The frequencies, as compared to normals, of five of the nine HL-A antigens tested at the first segregational series and four of the eleven antigens in the second series are shown in Table 1. These antigens are the ones in which differences were observed between patient groups and between patients and normals. Antigens A2, A3, and Te59 (W19) are examples of differences in frequency between the two patient

TABLE 1

HISTOCOMPATIBILITY ANTIGEN FREQUENCIES IN PATIENTS
WITH *HEMOPHILUS INFLUENZAE*, type b, DISEASE

		Patients		
Antigen	Normals*	Epiglottitis (29)	Meningitis (20)	P
A2	43.7	52.0	40.0	
A3	22.9	17.0	30.0	
A11	9.8	3.0	25.0	<.01(EvsM)
Lc17	6.2	17.0	15.0	<.02(EvsN)
Te59	11.3	14.0	5.0	
A5	11.3	14.0	5.0	
A13	6.7	14.0	5.0	
Te50	17.4	14.0	5.0	
Te57	3.2	14.0	5.0	<.01(EvsN)

*Average of frequencies in two series of blood bank donors, 200 and 251, respectively.

groups. The difference in All, 25 versus 3% is significant by Chi square analysis with appropriate corrections for alleles. Epiglottitis patients also show an increase over normal frequency for Lc17 (W28) and Te57 (W17) antigens.

The distribution of erythrocyte phenotypes in these patient groups also serves to distinguish between these two disease groups and each from normals. The frequencies of Rh phenotypes show differences which are significant but which are not reflected in individual Rh genes. The MNS antigen system phenotype differences, however, fit a pattern which is explicable in terms of a specific gene, NS (see Table 2). The absence of the first phenotype shown and the increased or normal frequency of the second and third ones in epiglottitis patients is reflected in the increased frequency of the NS gene. Including the double heterozygote NS genes in this figure means that onefourth of all 60 MNS genes in the epiglottitis group are NS. Chi Square for the distribution of MNS genes shown is 24.86, $p < 0.01$.

These lymphocyte and erythrocyte antigens with altered frequencies, that is HL-All and NS, may be either linked to some gene product which is related to disease susceptibility, or the antigens themselves may be involved in the pathogenetic mechanisms of disease (perhaps by being chemically related to the saccharide determinants of capsular antigens). In either case, if susceptibility to

TABLE 2

MNS BLOOD GROUP GENOTYPE FREQUENCIES IN PATIENTS WITH
HEMOPHILUS INFLUENZAE, type b, EPIGLOTTITIS AND MENINGITIS

Genotype	Normals %*	Patients		Siblings	
		Epiglottitis (30)—5†	Meningitis (20)—1	Epiglottitis (19)—5	Meningitis (16)—3
MMss	8.0	0	10.0	5.0	12.0
MNSS	4.0	10.0	0	16.0	6.0
MNSs	23.8	17.0	5.0	26.0	18.0
MS	23.8	27.0	20.0	31.0	25.0
Ms	30.5	20.0	32.0	26.0	28.0
NS	7.0	15.0‡	10.0	10.0	9.0
Ns	38.6	38.0	37.0	38.0	38.0

*From E. R. Giblett, *Genetic Markers in Human Blood* (London: Blackwell Scientific publications, 1969).

†-5 indicates 5 double heterozygotes counted as MS, Ns.

‡Minimum estimate, p=.04; including double heterozygotes as NS, then $p < .01$.

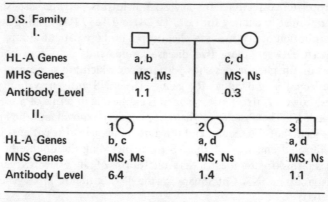

D.S. Family
I.

HL-A Genes	a, b	c, d
MHS Genes	MS, Ms	MS, Ns
Antibody Level	1.1	0.3

II.

	1	2	3
HL-A Genes	b, c	a, d	a, d
MNS Genes	MS, Ms	MS, Ns	MS, Ns
Antibody Level	6.4	1.4	1.1

II.1 Epiglottitis, age 5.   II.2 Meningitis, age 3.
II.3 Clinical Otitis simultaneously.

Fig. 1. Familial pattern of diseases due to *Hemophilus influenzae,* type b.

epiglottitis and/or meningitis is related to these cellular antigens, then genetic analysis of families with both diseases should provide useful information. One such family was made available for us to study by Dr. Richard H. Michaels of the University of Pittsburgh. Two siblings, ages 4 and 5 years, had culture-proven meningitis and clinical otitis respectively. They were HL-A identical and received the same maternal MNS gene (see Fig. 1). A third child, age 6, had acute epiglottitis and was genetically dissimilar from her siblings both by HL-A and MNS genes. We are now aware of five other families in which more than one child has had *H. influenzae,* type b, epiglottitis and/or meningitis. Such studies should establish whether cell surface antigens may be related to a variable disease state (epiglottitis versus meningitis) caused by the same organism.

An alternative hypothesis for the involvement of these genetic markers in pathogenesis or suscpetibility is that they may be linked to basic differences in the immune response of the two groups of patients. Antibody formation against antigens which are simple chemical determinants is known to be under genetic control in mice and in guinea pigs. (Benacerraf and McDevitt, 1972). In each species, the immune-response genes are associated with the major histocompatibility antigen locus. Our preliminary data suggest that such a relationship may be operative in humans with disease caused by *H. influenzae,* type b, in which the capsular antigen determining virulence is a simple chemical structure composed of ribose and/or ribitol phosphate. Analysis of anti-type b capsular antibody

TABLE 3

HEMOPHILUS INFLUENZAE, type b, ANTIBODY LEVELS IN
EPIGLOTTITIS AND MENINGITIS

	µg/ml Antibody		<1µg/ml		1-5µg/ml		5-15µg/ml		>15µg/ml	
	#	mean±S.D.	#	mean±S.D.	#	mean±S.D.	#	mean±S.D.	#	mean±S.D.
Patients *										
Epiglottitis	31	6.01±6.13	4	0.47±.21	13	2.1±1.3	10	7.7±1.1	4	20±0
Meningitis	16	1.93±3.19	12	0.35±.23	2	3.7±.10	2	9.6±1.8	0	
Siblings †										
Epiglottitis	19	2.23±4.35	11	0.40±.31	7	2.5±.92	0		1	20±0
Meningitis	15	4.52±7.06	7	0.53±.19	5	1.7±.45	0		3	18.5±1.8
Parents										
Epiglottitis	52	3.66±5.30	22	0.33±.30	16	2.0±1.3	10	7.4±1.0	4	19.4±1.0
Meningitis	38	5.03±6.32	15	0.45±.50	11	2.7±1.3	7	8.3±1.9	5	19.2±1.6

*Interval since onset of disease to time of Antibody Determination
  Epiglottitis-2.4±2.8, Meningitis-2.1±3.1.

†One nearest age from each family all >2 years of age

levels shows that levels for meningitis patients are lower than for epiglottitis patients (p<.01) (Table 3). The meningitis patients also are distributed differently, according to assigned categories of antibody level (Chi Square =32.43). This over-all mean difference is due to a high percentage of meningitis patients being in a subgroup with low levels of antibody. It is unlikely that division of patients into high, intermediate, and low subgroups is based on differences in ages. The same subgroups are obvious in parents of both groups. In addition, the age distribution within each subgroup of antibody levels is wide, and corrections for age differnces between the two groups fails to nullify the differerences in antibody levels.

We are attempting to relate antibody levels to the cellular antigens studied in these patients. Of the seven patients or siblings having very high antibody levels and on whom we have HL-A typing, five of these seven have the relatively rare HL-A antigen Lc17(W28). One of the seven has an antigen which closely cross-reacts with Lc17, HL-A2. Chi Square for this distribution is 24.2, p<0.01.

In summary, we have shown that individuals who acquire *H. influenzae,* type b, epiglottitis are genetically different from meningitis patients and from normals. Work is in progress to relate these observations to immune responsiveness and to pathogenetic mechanisms in these two diseases.

REFERENCES

Benacerraf, B., and H. O. McDevitt. "Histocompatibility-Linked Immune-Response Genes." *Sci.* 175:273.

Berenberg, W., and S. Kevy. 1958. "Acute Epiglottitis in Childhood." *N. Eng. J. Med.* 258:870.

Gowen, J. W. 1960. "Genetic Effects in Nonspecific Resistance to Infectious Disease." *Bact. Rev.* 24:192.

Grumet, F. C.; B. A. Coukell; J. G. Bodmer; W. F. Bodmer; and H. O. McDevitt. 1971. "Histocompatibility (HL-A) Antigens Associated with Systemic Lupus Erythematosus." *N. Eng. J. Med.* 285:4, 193.

Lilly, F.; E. A. Boyse; and L. J. Old. 1964. "Genetic Basis of Susceptibility to Viral Leukaemogenesis." *Lancet* ii. 1207.

Rogentine, G. N.; R. A. Yankee; J. J. Gart; J. Nam; and R. J. Trapani. 1972. "HL-A Antigens and Disease: Acute Lymphocytic Leukemia." *J. Clin. Invest.* 51:2420.

Schweitzer, M. D. 1961. "Genetic Determinants of Communicable Disease." *Annals, N.Y. Acad. Sci.* 91:730.

Whisnant, J. K.; G. N. Rogentine; D. L. Mann; and J. B. Robbins. 1971. "Human Cell-Surface Structures Related to *Hemophilus influenzae,* type b, Disease." *Lancet* 2:895.

CHAPTER 18

Hemophilus influenzae, type b, Meningitis in Infant Rats

Arnold L. Smith
Damon R. Averill
E. Richard Moxon
Peter F. Weller
Joseph Marino
David H. Smith

Bacterial meningitis continues to be a major health problem of infants and children. Since the introduction of antibiotics, the childhood mortality from this disease has remained at approximately 5% to 10%, while neurological sequelae, such as deafness, seizures, and mental retardation, affect 30% to 50% of the survivors (Sproles et al., 1969; Sell et al., 1972).

The bacteria that most commonly cause childhood meningitis are generally susceptible to available antibiotics. Thus, it seems likely that further reductions in the prevalence, morbidity, and mortality will be realized only through prevention and new modes of management which maintain normal brain metabolism and integrity.

A suitable animal model of bacterial meningitis would allow evaluation of certain aspects of the pathophysiology of this disease, such as the basis of host susceptibility, mode of bacterial invasion, and the biochemical and pathological mechanisms involved in the genesis of neurological sequelae. Furthermore, eventual outcome could be interpreted in terms of these parameters and their relationship to antibiotic therapy.

This work was done in the Infectious Disease Unit, Children's Hospital Medical Center, and Beth Israel Hospital, Department of Pediatrics, Harvard Medical School, Boston, Massachusetts.

Work was supported by grants from the Hood Foundation, Eli Lilly and Company, and the Massachusetts Cosmetologist Association, Inc.

A suitable animal model of bacterial meningitis must meet at least the following three critiera: bacterial invasion of the central nervous system by physiological route; the production of pathological lesions similar to those observed in human disease; and the production of cerebral dysfunction in a significant percentage of survivors.

Several attempts have been made previously to develop a model for the study of meningitis. These models have employed adult animals, and most have introduced the bacteria directly into the central nervous system (CNS), that is, the lumbar subarachnoid space (Flexner, 1907), the cisterna magna (Branham and Lillie, 1932) or the brain (Groff, 1934). These methods do not permit study of the initial stages in the pathogenesis of meningitis; they often produce local, rather than diffuse, inflammation; and they have the unwanted complication of direct trauma to the brain or spinal cord. Weed et al. (1919) produced bacterial meningitis in animals without direct nervous-system inoculation by altering cerebrospinal fluid dynamics in the presence of bacteremia. This model has been employed in most experimental studies, but it requires larger animals which, in turn, limits the size and scope of experiments. It also involves a nonphysiologic manipulation to induce meningitis, namely the withdrawal of cerebrospinal fluid. Neither the neuropathological changes nor the central nervous system function of survivors has been described in these previous models.

We have examined the susceptibility of infant rats to *H. influenzae,* type b, inoculated without trauma to the CNS. Infant rats were chosen because of the known age-related susceptibility of young children to meningitis and because of the large foundation of knowledge of the developmental biology and neurochemistry of rats. Our results indicate that rats also have a marked age-related susceptibility to this bacterium, develop meningitis with classic histologic changes, and, if they survive, demonstrate cerebral dysfunction.

MATERIALS AND METHODS

The bacteria employed were streptomycin-resistant mutants of *H. influenzae,* type b, Eagan (E-1) and the nonencapsular strain U-1 (U-11), which have been described previously (Anderson, Johnston, and Smith, 1972). The methods for culturing the bacteria and performing viable cell counts and bactericidal assays have been described (Anderson, Johnston, and Smith, 1972). Bacteria inoculated into animals were harvested from broth cultures during the exponential growth phase and resuspended in phosphate-buffered saline containing 0.1% gelatin.

All experiments employed Sprague-Dawley rats, derived from strain COBS/CD, which were bred in our animal facilities and maintained as pathogen-free on a defined diet in an environment with controlled temperature, humidity, and light.

The integrity of the cerebral function of animals surviving infection was assessed by the acquisition of, and response in, an operant-conditioning schedule. The test animals were inoculated intraperitoneally at 5 days of age with an LD_{50} dose of type b (E-1), or the same concentration of U-11, organisms. Animals were allowed ad lib access to water from weaning (21 days) to 35 days of age. At that time, access to water was restricted to one hour per day; at 38 days of age, they were placed in an operant-conditioning apparatus for one hour daily and the acquistion observed. Following exposure in the apparatus, the animals were watered for one hour. A force of 5 gms was required to depress the operanda for a reinforcement of 20 microliters of water.

RESULTS AND DISCUSSION

Figure 1 depicts the relation of age to the minimal lethal dose (MLD) of *H. influenzae*, type b, (E-1) inoculated intraperitioneally. As can be seen, there was an 8-log increase in MLD in the first three weeks of life, the time from birth to weaning. Animals inoculated with greater than 10^8 organisms died within two hours following injection; postmortem examination of these animals revealed only diffuse petechiae. Animals inoculated with greater than an LD_{50} but less than an MLD of type b organisms died 18 to 72 hours after inoculation. Inoculation of 10^8 nonencapsulated U-11 organisms was not lethal.

Bacteria were detected in the blood as early as five minutes following the intraperitoneal inoculation of an LD_{50} dose (5×10^3) of type b organisms in 5-day-old animals. The concentration of organisms in blood at 12 hours, 2×10^4/ml, and at 24 hours, 7×10^5/ml, reflected bacterial replication (Fig. 2).

The majority of the animals that succumbed to this infection died by 48 hours postinoculation. Examination of the survivors at that time revealed that 80% have histological evidence of meningitis, as defined by a subarachnoid accumulation of polymorphonuclear cells within a fibrinous exudate and cerebral edema (Figs. 3, 4). The nonencapsulated U-11 strain produced no detectable disease in CNS or in other organ systems.

More recent studies indicate that infant rats also have an age-related susceptibility to the intranasal inoculation of *H. influenzae*, type b, and that infection by this route also produces bacteremia and meningitis. Infection was produced by placing 10μl of a washed bacterial suspension in the anterior nares of non-anesthetized infants rats with a Hamilton syringe. A dose of 10^3 organisms failed to produce detectable bacteremia in any animal, whereas a higher inoculum resulted in a significant incidence of bacteremia and meningitis. (See Table 1.)

The observation that the prevalence of *H. influenzae*, type b, meninigitis in children is related inversely to that of bactericidal antibody has led to the conclusion that deficiency of circulating antibody is the basis of the age-related

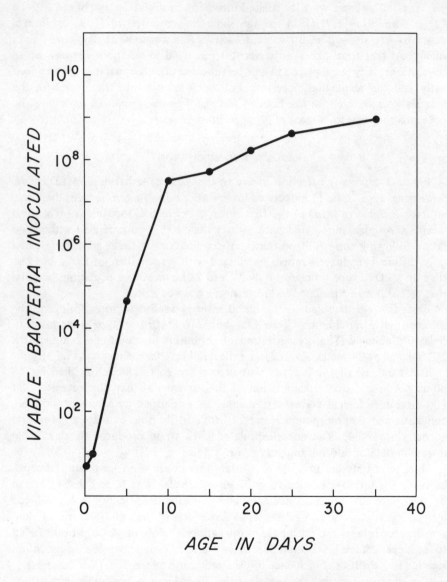

Fig. 1. Relationship between age and minimal number of bacteria which effect death within 96 hours after intraperitoneal inoculation. Data were obtained from experiments involving 390 animals.

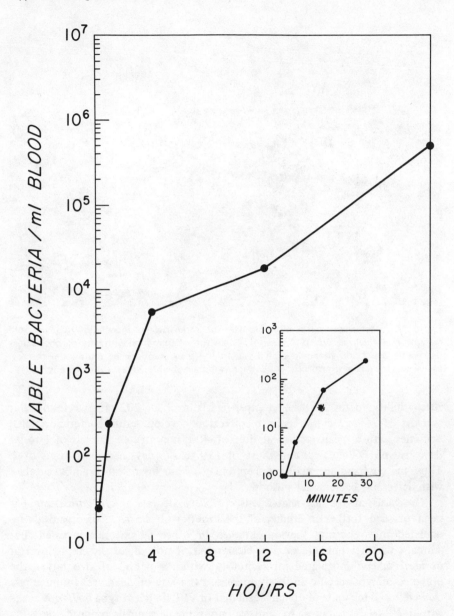

Fig. 2. Temporal course of magnitude of bacteremia following the intraperitoneal inoculation of 10^4 *Hemophilus influenzae,* type b (E_1) into 5-day-old rats.

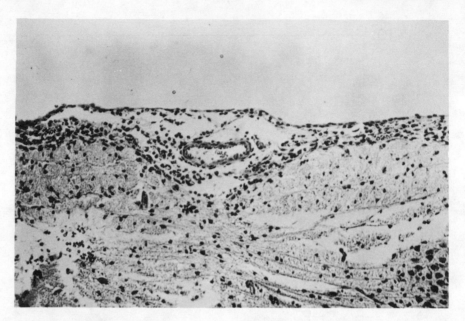

Fig. 3. The subarachnoid space 48 hours after the intraperitoneal inoculation to a 5-day-old rat with *H. influenzae,* type b (Eagan-11). The acute inflammation with polymorphonuclear leukocytes and fibrin strands depicted was in the space surrounding the middle cerebral artery over the left pyriform lobe. The section was stained with hematoxylin and eosin.

susceptibility to this disease. In experiments involving 202 rats, we found that surivors of *H. influenzae,* type b, infection develop serum bactericidal (BC) activities with a mean reciprocal titer of 400; noninfected animals of 1 to 97 days had no BC activity, and those of 119 to 175 days had mean titers of 2. Thus, the observed age-related susceptibility of our infant rats did not correlate with detectable bactericidal antibody.

The basis of the age-related susceptibility of rats to *H. influenzae* has been pursued further in studies of the kinetics of clearance of organisms inoculated intravenously. Previous studies in other laboratories revealed that animals, whether immune or not, clear most, if not all, of the staphylocci or *Escherichia coli* inoculated intravenously within a period of two hours; the presence of type-specific antibody increased the rate of clearance. Immune rats cleared 7 to 8 log-units of nonencapsulated or PRP-deficient type b *H. influenzae* within 10 to 30 minutes. In contrast, nonimmune animals reduced the 8-log inoculum by 1 log unit in 30 minutes to an apparent plateau. The pattern of the response to type b organisms was similar for 1-, 3-, and 8-week-old animals. Thus, the clearance of *H. influenzae*, type b, by rats did not follow the pattern ob-

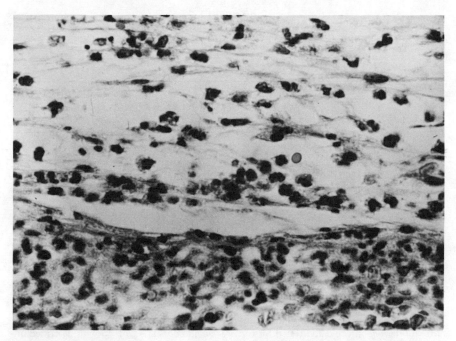

Fig. 4. Subarachnoid space 48 hours after the intraperitoneal inoculation to a 5-day-old rat with *H. influenzae,* type b (Eagan-11). The majority of the animals that succumbed to this infection died by 48 hours postinoculation. Examination of the survivors at that time revealed that 80% have histological evidence of meningitis.

served with other model systems, and the observed age-related susceptibility was not related to the initial clearance of the organisms.

PRP in concentrations up to 1,000 times that amount possessed by 10^8 bacteria did not alter the rapid clearance of 10^8 PRP-deficient organism when added with the bacteria. Finally, if animals possessed anti-PRP antibody, type b organisms were cleared in direct relation to the antibody titers and in a pattern similar to that of nonencapsulated organisms in nonimmune animals.

Survivors of intraperitoneal type b infection had a slower rate of acquisition of the operant schedule than litter mates infected with strain U-11 (Fig. 5). In addition, the final mean response rate per session in survivors inoculated with type b organisms was significantly lower (274 vs. 666) than that of animals inoculated with U-11 (T=4.725; p $\leqslant$ 0.001). This decreased response rate was not dependent upon animal size or force required to depress the operanda. The biochemical basis of this functional cerebral deficiency has not yet been defined,

TABLE 1

RELATIONSHIP OF BACTEREMIA FOLLOWING INTRANASAL INFECTION
WITH *H. INFLUENZAE* b (E-1) TO AGE OF ANIMALS

Inoculum	Age of Animal (Days)	Animals Studied	Animals Bacteremic* (%)
10^7	5	25	19 (76)
10^7	10	20	14 (70)
10^7	15	9	6 (67)
10^7	20	12	9 (75)
10^5	5	25	13 (52)
10^5	10	20	8 (40)
10^5	15	5	0 (0)
10^5	20	–	–
10^3	5	5	0 (0)

*Infant rats were infected and tested for bacteremia 48 hours after infection as described in the text.

but preliminary studies indicated that the total brain DNA concentrations of adult rats surviving *H. influenzae*, type b, infection at 5 days of age was 50% that of control animals.

This model meets criteria required for suitable experimental study of bacterial meningitis, and it provides the unique opportunity to delineate in biochemical and anatomical terms the genesis of cerebral dysfunction caused by this infection. It seems likely that the results of future studies with this model will be applicable to other types of bacterial, and possibly viral, meningitis, and that they may provide insight into the biochemical basis of certain non-infectious causes of cerebral dysfunction. The basis for the susceptibility of young animals to *H. influenzae*, type b, meningitis remains to be defined, but our findings indicate that factors other than bactericidal antibody are operative. It also seems reasonable to suggest that animals have age-related susceptibilities to other bacteria, and that previous failures to achieve meningitis without trauma or local CNS inoculation were due, in part, to the use of adult (and therefore nonsusceptible) animals.

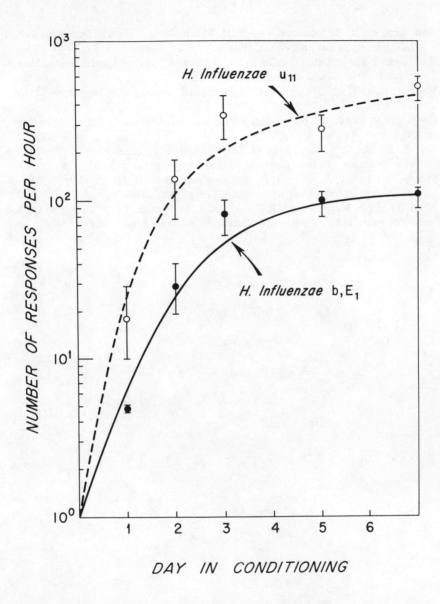

Fig. 5. The acquisition of a continuous reinforcement schedule in 35-day-old rats inoculated intraperitoneally at 5 days of age with *Hemophilus influenzae,* type b (E₁) or *Hemophilus influenzae* U₁₁.

REFERENCES

Anderson, P.; R. B. Johnston; and D. H. Smith. 1972. "Human Serum Activities against *Hemophilus influenzae*, type b." *J. Clin. Invest.* 51:31.

Branham, S. E., and R. D. Lillie. 1932. "Observations on Experimental Meningitis in Rabbits." *Publ. Hlth. Repts.* 47:2137.

Flexner, S. 1907. "Experimental Cerebrospinal Meningitis in Monkeys." *J. Exp. Med.* 9:142.

Groff, R. A. 1934. "Experimental Production of Abscess of the Brain in Cats." *AMA Arch. Neurol.* 31:199.

Sell, S. H. W.; R. E. Merrill; E. O. Doyne; and E. P. Zimsky. Jr. 1972. "Long-Term Sequelae of *Hemophilus influenzae* Meningitis." *Ped.* 49:206.

Sproles, E. T., III; J. Azerrad; C. Williamson; and R. E. Merrill. 1969. "Meningitis due to *Hemophilus influenzae:* Long-Term Sequelae." *J. Ped.* 75:782.

Weed, L. H.; P. Wegeforth; J. B. Ayer; and L. D. Fetton. 1919. "The Production of Meningitis by Release of Cerebrospinal Fluid." *J. Amer. Med. Assn.* 72:190.

Discussion

David T. Karzon, Presiding

Richard L. Myerowitz: Dr. Smith, you showed that neonatal rats are very susceptible to *H. influenzae,* type b, disease. If rats are analogous to rabbits and to man with respect to *H. influenzae,* type b, disease, you would expect the neonates to be resistant because of passively acquired antibody. Is serum antibody transferred transplacentally in rats?

David H. Smith: I do not know the answer to your question. On the other hand, all of the mothers of the babies used in the experiment were tested prior to the experiment for the presence of circulating bactericidal antibodies and they had none. I think the other point is that, in our rat colony, at least, adult rats do not start to develop any detectable bactericidal activity until they are beyond 100 days in age. They are grandparents by then.

Myerowitz: So you deliberately use mothers who lack detectable serum antibody?

Smith: Yes.

John B. Robbins: I would like to suggest another experiment that you may be able to carry out with the serum you have. The antibody from newborn rats is only partly placentally transmitted, but a lot of it is gained by suckling colostrum. Rat colostrum contains IgG globulin with very fast mobility, a so-called T-like globulin which, in some analyses, does not yield a complement-dependent lytic reaction. It may be that the acquisition of antibody at four or five days will not yield a bactericidal reaction but it might be measured by measuring antibodies in an antiglobulin reaction.

Smith: Well, it is possible but we have found no anti-PRP or anti-*H. influenzae,* type b, activity in any of the sera of the mother or infant rats. I do not know whether or not colostrum will contain an antibody which is not in the serum.

Robbins: Yes, for some examples, we had occasion to look at Calvin Kunin's data on the presence of somatic antibodies to *E. coli* 075 in colostrum and in the serum (Kunin, 1962). At least for the one individual colostrol antibodies to the somatic 075 antigen was higher than that of the serum. We have done some experiments (Schneerson and Robbins, 1971) on the resistance of young rabbits to systemic infections and death with *Hemophilus influenzae.*

213

We found that resistance was age-related and that it could be related to the presence of serum antibodies. In rabbits, the placenta is permeable to all immunoglobulin classes and newborn animals are highly resistant. Their susceptibility is demonstrable up to 4 to 6 weeks of age. I would like to mention one aspect of those experiments which might be of interest. Many rabbits developed bacteremia with very low doses of intravenously injected bacteria. The blood cultures were positive for two weeks and there was very little apparent change in the behavior of the rabbits' eating or drinking habits. *H. influenzae,* type b, disease in man may have a prolonged bacteremia phase which might be one important aspect of the pathogenesis.

David T. Karzon: Dr. Robbins, does it not surprise you that rats are not infected with a variety of gram-negative rods or gram-positive organisms that cross-react with *Hemophilus influenzae?* Why should rabbits be so different from rats?

Robbins: We have studied the so-called specific pathogen-free mice of the National Institute of Health that were colonized with streptococcus, Lactobacillus, and another bacterium. We tested all three bacteria and none were cross-reactive. The specific pathogen-free mice, even at 2 years of age, had little detectable type b antibody. The presence of bacteria in the gastrointestinal tract of an animal does not necessarily mean that he has cross-reacting antibodies.

Myerowitz: Another observation in this vein relates to the experience of Dr. Schneerson, when she originally examined rabbits from hutcheries for age-related acquisition of immunity to *H. influenzae,* type b. She found that rabbits, after the age of 4 weeks, uniformly developed natural immunity to *H. influenzae,* type b, and this antibody was protective. NZW rabbits which have been born and raised at NIH all their lives do not develop this natural immuntiy until about 8 to 10 weeks later. We have observed this in two experiments indicating that there are differences in the age of acquisition of natural immunity depending upon the environment. I think that might explain some of the observations.

Smith: I would like to answer that colostrum question again. Not only do the mothers not have the serum antibodies, but the infants, at the time they are infected or killed, also have no detectable anti-*H. influenzae,* type b, antibodies or any other anti-PRP antibodies. There may be some inhibitory globulin in the colostrum, but, if so, the level is below the detection methods of the systems being used so far. Furthermore, it is quite clear from the kinetic studies of the clearance of the organisms that animals that have even a minute amount of anit-PRP clear 6-8 log units of type b organisms in a matter of about 15 minutes. On the other hand, the kinetics of clearance of type b organisms from these animals, when they have no antibody, is just one log drop and a plateau for quite a considerable period of time. So, I think whatever we are observing in terms of this early susceptibility is probably not explicable on the basis of antibody alone. To come back to the question raised in the last discussion group: What evidence is there that anti-PRP has biologic activity? It is evident that a rat with anit-PRP antibody can clear a large number of *H. influenzae,* type b, in a short time.

Karzon: Would the infant rat be a good model in which to feed a cross-reacting bacterium such as *E. coli* Easter to see if there is any protection, by measuring effect on the clearance of bacteremia?

Robbins: It might be a very good model. I think the immunity induced by neonatal feeling of *E. coli* Easter may take five or six weeks to develop.

Karzon: Feed it to the mother?

Robbins: Well, then we will be transmitting anti-*H. influenzae,* type b, antibodies indirectly, by Easter, to the newborn.

Karzon: It might be interesting to see what protection is afforded to the young.

Zeev Handzel: How vigorously are the newborn rats handled?

Smith: I think the question of mortality of noninfected animals depends on the skill of the investigator. When Dr. Arnold Smith is doing the studies, there has been very small mortality. When Dr. Moxum first started, there was a sizable mortality, and none of those data were included: but now the mortality of his noninfected animals is negligible. Furthermore, all of the studies with type b infection are compared to those obtained with animals inoculated with nontypable *H. influenzae.* Intranasal inoculation is obviously done with a lens but we hope to get into a situation where we can have inhalation infection rather than each animal having to be inoculated with 10 lambdas of bacterial suspension.

Karzon: Do they get pneumonia?

Smith: We cannot say, yet. The sections are not back. We looked first at the CNS.

Sarah H. Sell: We have an inhalation system that is capable of delivering large numbers of bacteria to mice. We have been working with 2- to 3- and 4-week-old mice. Those aged 2 weeks cleared the bacteria from their lungs within six to eight hours. From those aged 3 weeks, bacteria could be recovered from all lungs at 24 hours, but at the end of 48 hours, from only about half. By age 4 weeks, the bacteria were cleared between 24 and 48 hours in all.

David W. Fraser: Could you comment on the appropriateness of using blood donors as a control group for children with meningitis or epiglottitis for your histocompatibility testing? Second, are you also strongly suggesting that there was no difference in the age of your meningitis and epiglottitis patients?

John K. Whisnant: What we are essentially saying is, if one plots the number of people that have less than 1, 1 to 5, 5 to 15, and 15 μg/ml of antibody, these antibody divisions have very small standard deviations. We think the data is trimodal, and the proportion of people in each group can be tested by chi-square distinction. For meningitis, the low mode predominates and for epiglottitis, the middle mode is largest. Covariance analysis tells us precisely whether or not there is a relationship to age. There is not. This supports our hypothesis. If you look at antibodies in normal adults, parents of children with the disease, their distribution is trimodal, many low ones, some in the middle, and a few high ones. Vaccine recipients are exactly the same way: some make low levels, some make intermediate levels, and some make high levels of antibody. I understand that it is a statistically difficult problem to say definitely that there are gaps. One proposes arbitrary gaps in the data without being able to prove them, then shows a statistical difference in the distribution.

Frazer: It would be difficult to make that point strongly until you have more epiglottitis patients.

Whisnant: The question of appropriateness of controls is a less difficult one. Normal adults, randomly chosen, and typed in exactly the same way, using the exact same typing serum, show little if any variation in frequency, from race to race, geographic area to geographic area, or by age. We assume that our blood-bank-donor population have the same distribution as the parents of these children. This was confirmed in the genotyping of the families.

Roger A. Feldman: Is your blood-bank-donor population in Pittsburgh genetically the same as the parents of children admitted with meningitis and epiglottitis? I thought these were Dr. Michael's patients.

Whisnant: Only a portion of the epiglottitis patients and families were from Pittsburgh. They were typed in our laboratory with our normal donors. The parents of these other patients are scattered from Florida to Boston. No significant difference was shown in the areas.

Karzon: The question that has been raised and could perhaps be readily clarified may be stated as follows: Is there a socio-economic or any other demographic selectivity in either HLA or red cell antigens that could account for the observed differences?

Whisnant: Basically, no. There are some racial differences in erythrocyte phenotype frequencies. All of these families were white and of European extraction. The normal frequencies which I showed are also for that population.

Robbins: May I ask Dr. Feldman a question? What, in his opinion, is the more acceptable evidence, the parents' genotypes or the genotypes used to match the general population?

Feldman: I was trying to figure what alternative choices of controls would appeal to me. One would choose meningococcal or pneumococcal meningitis cases, since they are children, and I know they are certainly similar in age and perhaps similar in other ways. That is one alternative.

Whisnant: Well, the reason we have not worked on these patients is that Dr. Artenstein will soon have that data prepared.

Fraser: Another choice would be children from the same pediatric hospital who had the same age distribution but different diseases.

Whisnant: That is the reason we divided the study into two disease groups, epiglottitis and meningitis. After all, we evaluated two disease populations. One reason was to find out why the same organism was causing two different diseases, and the other was to include a patient-control group.

Fraser: Have you compared HLA subgroups of affected and nonaffected siblings?

Whisnant: No, it has not been studied.

Feldman: On your slide, you had siblings of the meningitis patients and siblings of the epiglottitis patients. Do you have their HLA subgroups?

Whisnant: They are all type d. The epiglottitis patients were different from their siblings. The most significant study would involve a group of families in which one child had one disease and a sibling the other disease. Each had a one-in-two chance of getting A2 from his parent. One had meningitis, and the other had epiglottitis. I showed one such family. There are several more families in which one had disease and the other did not and the common gene in epiglottitis segregated to the child with epiglottitis.

Feldman: What you are looking for is a group of people who had identical exposure to the infecting agent and did not get ill. The problem is to find people who had identical exposure. You mentioned tuberculosis in twins. An essential part of such a study is to show that both identical twins were infected, that is, they were tuberculin-positive and did or did not get ill. This is why I was interested in age, because some of these siblings are not identically exposed.

James C. Parke, Jr.: Do you ever get the same individuals identically exposed?

Whisnant: We studied siblings. Obviously, I would like to have a whole population of families in which there are twins. The families that I know in which a twin has had meningitis and the co-twin was not infected have turned out to be nonidentical by HLA and by erythrocyte antigens. We know of a family where there are triplets; the two identical ones had meningitis; the third was nonidentical and did not have meningitis.

Sell: What kind?

Whisnant: *H. influenzae,* type b.

Karzon: It is interesting to note, with all this, the low rate of second cases of meningitis due to *H. influenzae,* type b. They all have the same genotype setting.

Whisnant: Until we started looking for it, as a pediatrician, I had never heard of it. It was not taught as part of my training.

Karzon: Are we living with a misconception? Are secondary family cases of *Hemophilus influenzae* meningitis as common as meningococcus?

Smith: We feel that secondary cases occur more with *H. influenzae,* type b, than with meningococcus. We have quite an extensive experience with meningococcal meningitis, and we have had no second meningococcal case in the family. Several people have heard me tell the story of three cases of *H. influenzae,* type b, disease in the same family. A child came in with pneumonia and then, three days later, his one sibling was having a lumbar puncture for meningitis at the same time that his other sibling was having a tracteostomy for epiglottitis. Multiple family attacks of *H. influenzae,* type b, systemic disease have occurred three times in at least five or six years since I have been back at Boston Children's Hospital.

G. John Buddingh: My experience goes over a long period, and I do not have any records, but I do not think that there is any difference between *H. influenzae* and meningococcus.

Robbins: There are 28 cases of meningitis that I personally saw, and three had multiple cases in the same family.

Fraser: One must have denominator information to interpret secondary cases in families because families with *H. influenzae* meningitis cases are larger than those with meningococcus. Among 500 family contacts, there was one secondary case of *H. influenzae* meningitis; and in 200 family contacts, there was one secondary case of meningococcal meningitis.

Whisnant: May I make a plea for information on families in which they have had the two diseases, both meningitis and epiglottitis? We are enlarging our study.

REFERENCES

Kunin, C. M. 1962. "Antibody Distribution against Non-Enteropathogenic *E. coli:* Relation to Age, Sex, Breast Feeding." *Arch. Int. Med.* 110:676.

Schneerson, R., and J. Robbins. 1971. "Age-Related Susceptibility to *Hemophilus influenzae* type b, Disease in Rabbits." *Infect. and Immun.* 4:397.

SECTION VIII

Death Certificates as a Measure of *Hemophilus influenzae* Meningitis Mortality in the United States, 1962-1968

Roger A. Feldman
David W. Fraser
Robert E. Koehler

Death certificates listing as the cause of death *Hemophilus influenzae* meningitis have been compiled by the National Center for Health Statistics since 1949, but the only published information is the annual death rate for the country. *H. influenzae* meningitis is not a nationally reportable disease in the United States, but estimates of the magnitude of this disease problem in the country could be based on the available death data. From a study of *H. influenzae* meningitis deaths, it is also possible to obtain information on the age and race of patients, and geographical and seasonal occurrence of the disease. This report represents an analysis of available death-certificate data on *H. influenzae* meningitis deaths in the United States from 1962 through 1968.

Questions that arise with death-certificate data concern the validity of the recorded diagnosis and the percentage of meningitis deaths that are included in the death listing. Four retrospective studies on the frequency of bacterial meningitis in defined populations have recently been completed (Fraser, 1973). Comparison of the death-certificate data with the retrospective population-based case reviews in the four separate areas in the United States permitted an assessment of the completeness with which fatal cases of *H. influenzae* meningitis are recorded in the National Center for Health Statistics records. This comparison also made possible an assessment of the accuracy with which the identity of the bacterial etiologic agent as determined in the laboratory was recorded on the death certificate.

This work was done at the Center for Disease Control, Health Services and Mental Health Administration, U. S. Department of Health, Education, and Welfare, Atlanta, Georgia.

MATERIALS AND METHODS

Data on deaths attributed to *H. influenzae* meningitis were obtained from the National Center for Health Statistics (NCHS) registry of deaths for the years 1962 through 1968. The NCHS registry receives copies of death certificates from each county and codes and tabulates the diagnoses recorded. With a three-year delay, a detailed but unpublished listing is available for certain infectious disease categories. The information available for each *H. influenzae* meningitis death, with few exceptions, includes: date of death, state and county of residence, age, sex, and race.

The census information used to calculate death rates was drawn from the 1960 state census volumes for general characteristics of the population, including special volume PC(2)-1C, *Nonwhite Population By Race,* from the U. S. Census Bureau, 1960. Information about births in 1965 was obtained from *Vital Statistics,* volume 1, for that year.

Population-based retrospective studies of *H. influenzae* meningitis were available in four separate areas of the country. These areas and the years for which available death-certificate data overlapped these retrospective studies included Charleston County, South Carolina, 1961-1968; Olmsted County, Minnesota, 1960-1968; the State of Vermont, 1967 and 1968; and Bernalillo County, New Mexico, 1964-1968. To measure the validity of death-certificate diagnosis, the etiology on the death certificate was compared with the laboratory results found in reviewing hospital charts. To measure completeness, the deaths from *H. influenzae* meningitis found by record review were compared with those in the NCHS registry.

TABLE 1

H. INFLUENZAE MENINGITIS DEATHS
USA, 1962-1968 BY YEAR

Year	Deaths
1962	388
1963	429
1964	412
1965	390
1966	319
1967	270
1968	251
Annual Average	351

SOURCE: National Center for Health Statistics

In presenting information on death rates by race and state of residence, death rates for blacks were calculated for only the 29 states with more than 50,000 black residents and for Indians in only the eight states with more than 20,000 Indian residents in the 1960 census. Death rates for whites were calculated for all 50 states.

RESULTS

H. influenzae meningitis was listed as the cause of 2,459 deaths in the seven-year period 1962-1968, with 429 the largest number in any single year, reported in 1963 (Table 1).

In the four retrospectively studied populations, there were 14 cases in the NCHS registry for which a chart could be found; each was laboratory-confirmed *H. influenzae* meningitis. Of 24 deaths found to be due to *H. influenzae* meningitis by review of hospital records, only 14 were listed as *H. influenzae* on the NCHS death registry, a completeness of 58%. Of the remaining 10, 9 were listed as due to meningitis, but etiology was recorded as *N. meningitidis* (1), other specified (1), and unspecified (7).

The highest death rates from *H. influenzae* meningitis for any age and ethnic group analyzed were for Indians under the age of 1 year (Table 2). Death rates

TABLE 2

H. INFLUENZAE MENINGITIS: AGE- AND RACE-SPECIFIC
AVERAGE ANNUAL DEATH RATES,
USA, 1962-1968

Age in Years	White	Black	Indian
<1	3.09	7.51	26.71
1-4	0.89	1 32	2.24
5-9	0.10	0 13	0.23
10-19	0.01	0.04	0
20-29	0.00	0 01	0
30-39	0.00	0.00	0
40-49	0.01	0 03	0
50 59	0.02	0 04	0.34
60-69	0.03	0.09	0
70+	0.05	0.06	0
TOTAL	0.16	0.41	1 28

NOTE: Rates are per 100,000 in 1960 census.

TABLE 3

H. INFLUENZAE MENINGITIS

AVERAGE ANNUAL INFANT MORTALITY BY RACE AND AGE IN MONTHS,
USA, 1962-1968

Age in Months	RACE			
	White	Black	Indian	Total
0	2.0	2.1	0	2.0
1	4.1	5.6	0	4.3
2	4.5	7.6	0	4.9
3	4.4	6.0	49.9	4.9
4	4.9	10.1	42.7	5.9
5	4.5	12.6	35.6	6.0
6	3.3	9.1	42.7	4.4
7	3.1	5.6	14.2	3.5
8	3.1	8.3	28.5	4.0
9	3.5	9.1	14.2	4.4
10	2.3	6.2	7.1	3.0
11	1.7	2.3	7.1	1.8
Under 1 year	3.4	7.1	20.4	4.1

NOTE: Rates here show deaths per 100,000 live births per year, 1965 vital statistics.

for blacks were higher than for whites for all age groups. The highest age-specific death rates were for children under 6 months of age in all three races studied (Table 3).

The distribution of death rates by race and state is shown in Figures 1, 2, and 3. Death rates for whites were highest in the Pacific and southwestern states. The death rates for blacks were highest in Oklahoma and Florida, but were generally high in the southeastern states. The death rates for Indians were high in each state for which they were calculated except California.

Although there was a November-through-February peak in the seasonal occurrence of *H. influenzae* meningitis deaths for the nation, the peak was more prominent in 14 southern states than it was in 13 northern states (Figure 4).

DISCUSSION

Two major questions concerning death-certificate data as a measure of *H. influenzae* meningitis deaths in the United States concern the completeness and accuracy with which fatal cases of confirmed *H. influenzae* meningitis are recorded in the NCHS death certificate register.

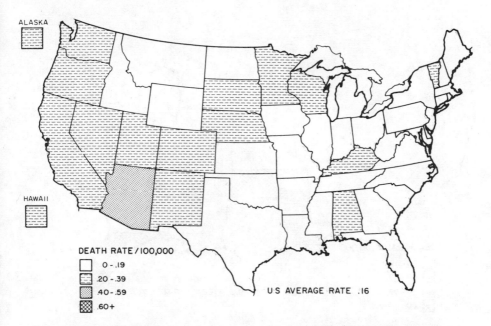

Fig. 1. Average annual *Hemophilus influenzae* meningitis mortality in whites, United States, 1962-1968.

We determined that laboratory data from the medical record were transferred accurately to the death certificate in each of 14 fatal cases in four studied populations. We had no way to measure the correctness of the laboratory identification. Only 58% of the confirmed cases of fatal *H. influenzae* meningitis in the four study areas were listed as *H. influenzae* meningitis on the NCHS registry. Therefore, if one wished to estimate the annual number of deaths from *H. influenzae* meningitis for the country as a whole for 1962-1968, using an admittedly limited evaluation of completeness and validity, the estimated annual number of deaths from diagnosed *H. influenzae* meningitis for the country would be 603, rather than the 351 deaths reported. The use of a single case-fatality ratio for all ages (8.5%), compiled from the data obtained in the four study areas (Fraser, 1972) (Table 4) yielded an estimate of 7,100 cases per year for the period 1962-68.

In computing race-specific death rates, a unique problem arose with respect to the Indian population. Norris and Shipley (1971) noted that, of children in California recorded as Indian on the birth record and dying in the first year of life, approximately one third were recorded as Indian on the death certificate

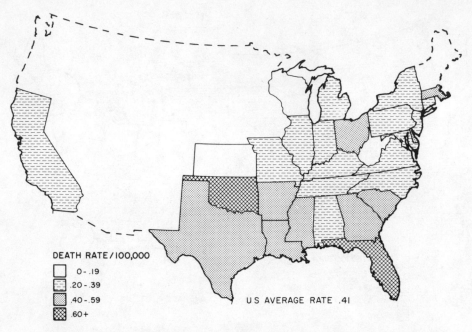

DEATH RATE / 100,000

☐ 0 - .19
▨ .20 - .39
▩ .40 - .59
▩ .60 +

U S AVERAGE RATE .41

Fig. 2. Average annual *Hemophilus influenzae* meningitis mortality in blacks, United States, 1962-1968. (Data is shown here only for states with at least 50,000 blacks in 1960 census.)

(Table 5). Ninety-nine percent of the children recorded as white at birth were recorded as white on the death certificate and 97% of children recorded as black at birth were recorded as black on the death certificates. It appears, at least in California, that death rates for Indians are underestimated.

The highest death rate for each race was for children less than 6 months of age, which is somewhat younger than the age at which the disease was most common in the four populations studied (Fraser, 1973).

The race-specific regional distribution of cases was difficult to interpret because we did not correct for variations in socioeconomic level. Use of race-specific socioeconomic information concerning county populations might lead to a more meaningful analysis. The data available indicated that the highest death rates were for populations which overrepresented the lowest socio-economic group.

A seasonal peak of deaths, as was seen in the 14 southern states, was comparable to published reports concerning *H. influenzae* meningitis in hospital-based studies (Crook, Clanton, and Hodes, 1949). The relative absence of a seasonal peak in the 13 northern states has not been previously mentioned.

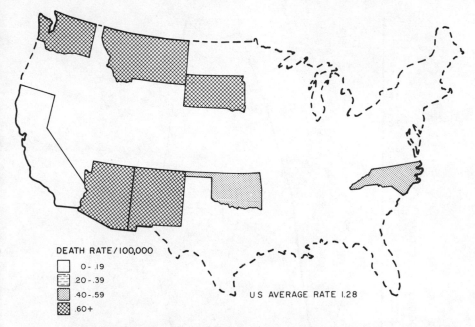

Fig. 3. Average annual *Hemophilus influenzae* meningitis mortality in Indians, United States, 1962-1968. (Data is shown here only for states with at least 20,000 Indians in 1960 census.)

SUMMARY

Death-certificate data on persons in the United States reported as having died of *H. influenzae* meningitis, 1962-1968, were studied. Comparison of the death-certificate data with retrospective population-based chart reviews in four areas of the country showed that transcription of the laboratory data to the death certificate was accurate but incomplete. Only 58% of the fatal cases of *H. influenzae* meningitis found by chart review were recorded in the National Center for Health Statistics death registry. Using the case-fatality ratio of 8.5% found in a study of cases in the four study areas, it was estimated that there were an average of 7,100 cases of *H. influenzae* meningitis diagnosed each year in the United States in the years 1962-1968.

The highest *H. influenzae* meningitis death rates were for children under 6 months of age. At all ages, the death rates were highest for Indians, and the death rates were higher for blacks than for whites.

The distribution of death rates by state showed high rates for Indians in all states with significant Indian populations except California. The highest rates for

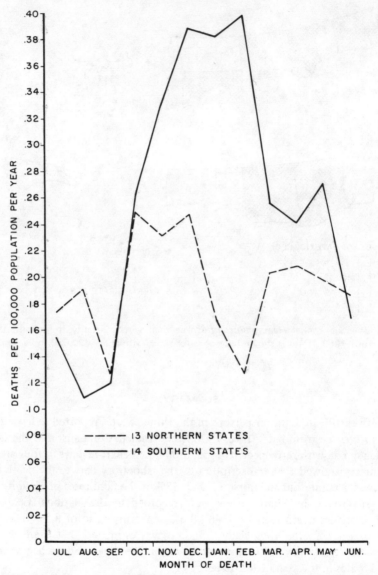

Fig. 4. *Hemophilus influenzae* meningitis: mortality rates by month and region, United States, 1962-1968. NOTE: The thirteen northern states for which data is given are Maine, New Hampshire, Vermont, Massachusetts, Michigan, Wisconsin, Minnesota, North Dakota, South Dakota, Montana, Idaho, Washington, and Oregon. The fourteen southern states are North Carolina, South Carolina, Georgia, Florida, Tennessee, Alabama, Mississippi, Arkansas, Louisiana, Oklahoma, Texas, New Mexico, Arizona, and California.

TABLE 4

DEATH RATE OF *H. INFLUENZAE* MENINGITIS
IN FOUR STUDY AREAS

Study Area	Cases	Deaths	Death Rate %
Bernalillo County, New Mexico (1964–71)	86	7	8.1
Olmsted County, Minnesota (1960–70)	44	2	4.5
Charleston County, S.C. (1960–70)	105	14	13.3
Vermont (whole state) (1967–70)	60	2	3.3
TOTAL	295	25	8.5

NOTE: Data excludes one Charleston County case, missed on chart review but found by review of death certificates.

TABLE 5

COMPARABILITY OF RACE CODED ON LINKED BIRTH AND DEATH
RECORDS FOR INFANTS, CALIFORNIA
1965-67 BIRTH COHORT

Race Coded on Birth Record	Total Number	Race Coded on Death Record Percent of Total Births		
		White	Black	Indian
White	16,801	99.7	0.2	* *
Black	2 885	3.0	96.9	* *
Indian	148	60.8	2.0	36.5

*Less than 0.1 percent.

blacks were observed in Oklahoma and Florida, and the highest rates for whites occurred in the Pacific states and the southwest.

A seasonal peak was evident in deaths in the southeast and in the country as a whole, but not in the northern states.

Further analysis of death certificate records using race-specific socioeconomic data, preferably on a county basis, is needed to interpret the observed differences in death rates by race and region of the country.

REFERENCES

Crook, W. G.; B. R. Clanton; and H. L. Hodes. 1949. *"Hemophilus influenzae* Meningitis: Observations on the Treatment of 110 Cases." *Ped.* 4:643.

Fraser, D. W.; C. P. Darby; R. E. Koehler; C. F. Jacobs; R. A. Feldman. 1973. "The Epidemiology of *Hemophilus influenzae* Meningitis." This volume and unpublished data.

Norris, F. D., and P. W. Shipley. 1971. "A Closer Look at Race Differentials in California's Infant Mortality, 1965-1967." *HSMHA Health Reports* 86:810.

CHAPTER **20**

The Epidemiology of *Hemophilus influenzae* Meningitis

David W. Fraser
Charles P. Darby
Robert E. Koehler
Cecil F. Jacobs
Roger A. Feldman

A retrospective study of the occurrence of *Hemophilus influenzae* meningitis in Charleston County, South Carolina, was undertaken to elucidate associations of meningitis risk with age, race, season, income level, crowding, and sickle-cell disease.

Charleston County has approximately 240,000 residents, of which one-third are black. The county was chosen for this study because its eight hospitals provide the major portion of medical care to residents of southeastern South Carolina (Wickwar, 1968) and each of the hospitals was willing to co-operate with the study.

METHODS

Cases of *H. influenzae* meningitis with onset of symptoms between January 1, 1961, and June 30, 1971, in residents of Charleston County were sought by review of information from four sources:

1. Hospital discharge diagnoses coded under the categories meningitis, meningoencephalitis, and encephalomyelitis
2. Records of bacterial isolates from spinal fluid in the laboratory of Medical University Hospital, which serves five of the eight hospitals in the county

This work was supported by the Center for Disease Control, Health Services and Mental Health Administration, U. S. Department of Health, Education and Welfare, Altanta, Georgia.

3. A series of cases collected by Juan J. Gershanik, M. D., formerly of the Medical University of South Carolina

4. Death certificates citing bacterial meningitis as a cause of death

The following information was abstracted from the hospital record of each case in which *H. influenzae* was isolated from cerebrospinal fluid: age at onset, date of onset, census tract of residence, hemoglobinopathy if present, and outcome.

RESULTS

One hundred and six cases of *H. influenzae* meningitis were found; 15 of these were fatal.

Completeness of case finding. Two of the 15 fatal cases were discovered only because death certificates were used as a case-finding technique. One of these patients died in an emergency ward prior to hospitalization and was never admitted to the hospital; the second patient who had initially been overlooked had been admitted to one of the hospitals in the county. The completeness of the first three (admission-based) methods of finding cases of fatal diagnosed *H. influenzae* meningitis can therefore be estimated at 87% (13/15) for all cases and 93% (13/14) for hospitalized cases.

Age and sex. All but five patients (ages 5, 5, 8, 11, and 26 years) were less than 5 years old. There were no neonatal cases. Incidence was highest for infants 6 to 8 months of age (Table 1). Fifty-four of the 106 cases were in males.

Race and sickle-cell disease. Seventy-three of the cases were in blacks. Using age-adjustment to the age distribution of all Charleston County residents, the rate of *H. influenzae* meningitis was found to be 3.5 times higher for blacks than

TABLE 1

AGE-SPECIFIC INCIDENCE OF *H. INFLUENZAE* MENINGITIS

	Age										
	Months								Years		
	0-2	3-5	6-8	9-11	12-14	15-17	18-20	21-23	2	3	4
Cases	6	20	25	12	7	6	5	4	4	7	4
Incidence*	42	137	171	83	49	42	34	28	7	13	7

*Cases per 100,000 population per year.

for whites: 7.7 cases per 100,000 per year for blacks and 2.2 cases per 100,000 per year for whites. Two of the 73 black patients were known to have sickle-cell disease. This proportion is not significantly higher than expected for black new-borns (.0063) from the known prevalence of sickle-cell trait among black adults in Charleston County (Boyle, Thompson, and Tyroler, 1968).

Season: Forty-four of the cases had onset of symptoms in the months of November, December, and January, compared with nine cases in July, August, and September.

Crowding. The incidence of *H. influenzae* meningitis among whites was highest in the least densely populated census tracts, and it decreased progressively with increasing population density (Table 2). No correlation was found for blacks between population density and the incidence of the disease.

TABLE 2

INCIDENCE OF *H. INFLUENZAE* MENINGITIS
BY RACE AND POPULATION DENSITY OF CENSUS TRACTS

	Total Population Density (thousands of persons per square mile)			
	<.10*	.10-.99*	1.0-9.9*	>10*
White	9.0	2.7	1.0	0 0
Black	5.1	12.1	4.7	8.0

*Incidence of *H. influenzae* meningitis here involves cases per 100,000 per year adjusted to age distribution (<5 years, >5 years) of total Charleston County population.

No association was found for either race between the incidence of *H. influenzae* meningitis and the race-specific proportion of homes in each census tract which were excessively crowded (Table 3).

Income. Among blacks, the incidence of *H. influenzae* meningitis was highest in the poorest areas of the county and fell progressively with rising median black family income. For whites, no association was found, but in Charleston there is little overlap of the ranges of incomes of blacks and whites (Table 4).

DISCUSSION

Bacterial meningitis is a dramatic and serious disease that is readily diagnosed and usually requires hospitalization. As a result, the disease is amenable to a

TABLE 3

INCIDENCE OF *H. INFLUENZAE* MENINGITIS BY RACE AND
RACE-SPECIFIC PREVALENCE OF CROWDED HOUSES BY CENSUS TRACT

	Percent of Houses with ≥1.01 Persons per Room								
	0-4*	5-9*	10-14*	15-19*	20-24*	25-29*	30-34*	35-39*	40-49*
White	2.2	2.7	1.9	2.3	–	–	–	–	–
Black	–	–	–	–	5.7	9.9	5.7	5.7	16.8

*Incidence of *H. influenzae* meningitis here involves cases per 100,000 per year adjusted to age distribution (<5 years, ≥5 years) of total Charleston County population.

TABLE 4

INCIDENCE OF *H. INFLUENZAE* MENINGITIS BY RACE AND
RACE-SPECIFIC MEDIAN FAMILY INCOME IN CENSUS TRACTS

	Median Family Income (thousands of dollars)							
	1.0-1.4*	1.5-1.9*	2.0-2.4*	2.5-2.9*	3.0-3.9*	4.0-4.9*	5.0-5.9*	6.0+*
White	–	–	–	–	3.0	2.7	1.1	2.4
Black	14.0	9.7	7.7	5.4	–	–	–	–

*Incidence of *H. influenzae* meningitis here involves cases per 100,000 population per year adjusted to age distribution (<5 years, ≥5 years) of total Charleston County population.

retrospective hospital-based study. Using cases found only by a search of death certificates, the completeness of finding of fatal cases of *H. influenzae* meningitis in the present study can be estimated at 87%.

In a population-based study, possible associations between various demographic variables and the incidence of a disease can be examined. In the present study, increased risk of *H. influenzae* meningitis was found to be associated with four major variables: age (highest in those 6 to 8 months of age), season (highest from November through January), race and poverty (highest in blacks living in the poorest areas of the county), and population density (for whites only, highest in rural areas).

The age distribution of cases found in Charleston County has been noted in other regions at other times (e. g., Fothergill and Wright, 1933; Smith, 1954).

The predilection for middle infancy is thought to be due to a nadir in circulating antibody against *H. influenzae* during that period (Fothergill and Wright, 1933).

The seasonal peak in late fall and early winter has been noted to be a characteristic of fatal cases of *H. influenzae* meningitis occurring in the southern states in this country (Feldman, Fraser, and Koehler, 1973).

The excess risk of *H. influenzae* meningitis among blacks has been noted previously (Parke, Schneerson, and Robbins, 1972), but the present study suggests that poverty may be more intimately associated with this increased risk than race alone (Table 4). A more complete analysis of the effect of socioeconomic status would require study of a population with larger numbers of poor whites and rich blacks than were available in the present study. If ready access to medical therapy of ear or upper respiratory infections led to prevention of septicemic complications such as meningitis, the high risk of *H. influenzae* meningitis among blacks in poor areas of Charleston might be explained on the basis of an economic barrier to poor blacks obtaining early medical care. If this hypothesis were true, it might explain the relatively high rate of *H. influenzae* meningitis among rural whites (Table 2), who may have a geographic barrier to early medical therapy of "minor" infectious disease.

The hypothesis suggested by this study that risk of *H. influenzae* meningitis is more related to poverty than to race is testable. To this end, we are conducting a similar retrospective study of this disease in Bernalillo County, New Mexico, an area with a white population with a broad spectrum of income levels.

REFERENCES

Boyle, E., Jr.; C. Thompson; and H. A. Tyroler. 1968. "Prevalence of the Sickle-Cell Trait in Adults of Charleston County, South Carolina: An Epidemiologic Study." *Arch. Env. Hlth.* 17:891.

Feldman, R. A.; D. W. Fraser; and R. E. Koehler. 1973. "Death Certificates as a Measure of *Hemophilus influenzae* Meningitis Mortality in the United States, 1962-1968." This volume.

Fothergill, L. D., and J. Wright. 1933. "Influenzal Meningitis: The Relation of Age-Incidence to the Bactericidal Power of the Blood against the Causal Organism." *J. Immun.* 24:273.

Parke, J. C., Jr.; R. Schneerson; and J. B. Robbins. 1972. "The Age and Racial Distribution and Case Fatality Rate of *Hemophilus influenzae*, type b, Meningitis in Mecklenburg County, North Carolina." *J. Ped.* 81:765.

Smith, E. S. 1954. "Purulent Meningitis in Infants and Children: A Review of 409 Cases." *J. Ped.* 45:425.

Wickwar, W. H. 1968. *Health in South Carolina.* Columbia, South Carolina: South Carolina State Board of Health and University of South Carolina Bureau of Governmental Research and Service.

Discussion

John Witte, Presiding

John Witte: I would like to ask Dr. Feldman about his age-specific death data for influenzae meningitis where he showed the highest rates in the under-one-year and the second highest in the 1- to 4-year age groups. That 1-to-4 age group is a very critical one, and I wonder what further breakdown you might have. Are rates higher in 1-year-olds, 2-year-olds, or is there a continuous decline during this period as Dr. Fraser's data on the morbidity showed?

Roger A. Feldman: There was a continuous decline.

Richard H. Michaels: Dr. Fraser, could you explain how you tested for crowding?

David W. Fraser: We used, as our index of crowding, the proportion of houses in a census tract in which there was more than one person per room. This is a crude estimate of the degree of crowding or proportion of crowded people in the population. If we had failed to find a correlation either for crowding or for income, I would say we had failed because of the form of analysis.

John K. Whisnant: Dr. Fraser, I do not understand the curve where you have three or four points in the lower group from the black population, and four in the upper income groups that are white. Since you have totally exclusive, white versus black and low versus high income, how can you draw the conclusiong that the important factor is income instead of race?

Fraser: Without studying blacks and whites of similar economic levels or one race with a spectrum from poverty-to-wealth, I cannot be certain.

Whisnant: The study you propose to undertake in other areas with different racial composition is going to be important.

Fraser: Our proposed study of bacterial meningitis in Bernalillo County, New Mexico, is designed to complement the Charleston study. We should be able to compare rates in poor whites with Spanish surnames to those in wealthier whites with non-Spanish surnames.

Feldman: We are going to use the death-rate data, albeit difficult, to interpret numbers and to analyze by county. We have information by county, by race, on the percentage of the people in the county who are below poverty level, using OEO data. This will bear on the socio-economic data and race. We can determine whether curves for the death rates in poor whites flow together, as you are now suggesting.

Whisnant: I am not saying that they flow together. I am asking obviously because I would be very interested in a strict distribution by race.

Sarah H. Sell: The poor in rural areas, where there are neither physicians nor hospitals with adequate bacteriological laboratories, cannot be compared with poor in the crowded areas of a city who have access to medical facilities, geographically at least.

Witte: That is a good point. There are a number of communities where there is socio-economic data available by census tract that has a large population of whites in the poverty-income group as well as blacks. This would seem a more reasonably approach.

Fraser: Many of the white families in Charleston had $3,000 to $3,500 annual incomes and would be considered impoverished. However, it seems that one must be even poorer than that to increase one's risk of *H. influenzae* meningitis.

David H. Smith: Do you know, in fact, that the individuals involved had given incomes or definite types or crowding, or do you know they lived in areas with certain average income or housing conditions?

Fraser: The latter. It would be extremely interesting to know the family income of the individual cases, but when one is trying to plan a vaccine trial, it is more useful to know that the rates are high in a given region than that children in certain houses are at high risk. It may be that the rich people in the poor areas are the ones getting the meningitis, but that would surprise me.

Smith: When you talked about this, I was not sure whether you "arm-chaired" this or whether you "shoe-leathered" it.

Fraser: I "shoe-leathered" it—the chart reading, at least. I "arm-chaired" the analysis.

Charles F. Federspiel: What was the total morbidity during the 10½-year period?

Fraser: There were 260 definite cases, of which 106 were caused by *H. influenzae*.

Federspiel: Can you calculate a case fatality ratio?

Fraser: For *H. influenzae*, it was 14%.

Feldman: How does that compare to other types of bacterial meningitis?

Fraser: It was 7% for meningicoccal and 36% for pneumoccal.

Georges Peter: What do you estimate the incidence of *H. influenzae* meningitis per 1,000 population to be for those between the ages of 6 months and 4 years or per live births?

Fraser: If one integrated the incidence from birth to the fifth birthday, one would find that 1.8 of every 1,000 children in Charleston developed *H.*

influenzae meningitis before the age of 5 years.

John B. Robbins: We have similar statistics from Mecklenburg County, North Carolina. Before the age of 5 years, one in 400 children born will contract *H. influenzae*, type b, meningitis.

William Schaffner: Dr. Feldman, if I understand you correctly, you do not have any urban-rural breakdown?

Feldman: Correct. Although urban-rural data is on the death certificate, it is the census bureau's definition of urban and rural. We can actually calculate a death rate in rural and urban America.

Whisnant: What is an epidemiological measure of adequate medical care?

Federspiel: There is no adequate answer to that.

Whisnant: I doubt that the University Hospital environment defines better medical care. There are examples of hospital services with academic affiliations where the medical care is awful.

Robbins: One statistic surprised me: the mortality rate of 14%. A survey of the literature of cases seen in hospitals suggests that most centers have a case fatality rate of 3% to 10%. I wonder how you account for your high figure?

Fraser: I cannot speak to it.

Robbins: The reason I ask you is to suggest that people who search for mortality data should also make sure that they are accounting for the children that go directly to the morgue and not to the hospital first.

Fraser: I think this is a real problem. In Charleston, the police brought dead children to the County Hospital and live children to the University Hospital. This may be one explanation. In addition, the case fatality ratio is inflated slightly by the definition of a definite case of bacterial meningitis. Cases that could not be proved premortem but were proved postmortem would be included as definite cases, whereas those that could not be proved while in the hospital and did not die were excluded.

Sell: It think it is fair to point out that Dr. Robert Merrill's group (Sproles et al., 1969) at the University of Virginia, not long ago, reported a 17.5% mortality rate. They had followed up all the *H. influenzae* meningitis cases admitted to University Hospital between 1951 and 1964.

Robbins: As a house officer, in two years, I saw three children brought in dead with culture proven *H. influenzae* epiglottitis. Do you have any information regarding this disease? In looking at death certificates related to *H. influenzae*, you might have come across it.

Fraser: I do not.

Schaffner: I just wanted to make a comment supporting Dr. Fraser's general figures for case mortality for *H. influenzae* meningitis. The case mortality at Vanderbilt Hospital for pneumococcal and meningococcal meningitis are quite consistent with those of the literature.

Peter: I think it does seem high. Dr. Michael's study of the case mortality is significantly lower. Our own data at Boston Children's Hospital in the past 10 years surprised us. Among 271 cases of *H. influenzae* meningitis, we had 4 deaths for a mortality of 1.5%. The figures for meningococcal and pneumococcal meningitis are perhaps slightly higher. That does not take into consideration that perhaps some children died who never reached Children's Hospital, but who might have been transferred to us in the past. Do you have any data about the general incidence in places, such as Minnesota? Your data suggests that the difference in incidence between *H. influenzae* and meningococcal meningitis is related to poverty or race, since there was a threefold difference for blacks compared to whites in the incidence of influenzal versus meningicoccal meningitis. Another interesting point was Dr. Feldman's comment about the lack of seasonal distribution of deaths from *H. influenzae* meningitis in the north.

Certainly our experience in Boston bears out that the pediatricians and house staff recognize the *H. influenzae* season which begins in November and December. There are exceptions, such as the group of cases we saw last June; but by and large, the winter has a much higher incidence.

Fraser: We have studied the incidence of *H. influenzae* meningitis in Olmstead County, Minnesota, from 1935 to 1970 and found that the incidence began rising about 1959. In recent years, the incidence in whites in Olmstead County has been higher than the incidence in whites in Charleston County. It is interesting that the peak of *H. influenzae* meningitis deaths in the record 1952 to 1968 was the year 1963 and has been falling since then. I do not know what to make of the fact that the total number of deaths of all bacterial meningitis peaked in 1963-64 and has been falling since.

REFERENCE

Sproles, E. T., III; J. Azerrad; C. Williamson; R. E. Merrill. 1969. "Meningitis due to *Hemophilus influenzae*: Long-Term Sequelae." *J. Ped.* 75:782.

SECTION IX

SECTION IX

The Frequency of *Hemophilus influenzae* Infections: An Analysis of Racial and Environmental Factors

Richard H. Michaels
William F. Schultz

There is need for accurate information concerning the frequency of infections due to type b, *Hemophilus influenzae*. It is now apparent that the incidence of *Hemophilus* meningitis is not constant; there is considerable variation, with both time and location. A gradual increase in admissions for *Hemophilus* meningitis at the Children's Hospital of Pittsburgh and at other medical centers was the subject of a previous publication (Michaels, 1971). The present report represents a preliminary analysis of racial and environmental factors which might help explain certain recently recognized geographical differences in frequency.

GEOGRAPHICAL DIFFERENCES

Table 1 shows the estimated recent annual incidence of *Hemophilus* meningitis calculated for Pittsburgh and surrounding Allegheny County, Pennsylvania, and also for three other locations: Franklin County, Ohio (Smith and Haynes, 1972); Mecklenburgh County, North Carolina (Parke, 1972); and Madison County, Alabama.* In each instance, the rate was obtained by searching hospital records for cases confirmed by isolating the organism from spinal fluid or blood.

This work was done in the Department of Pediatrics, University of Pittsburgh School of Medicine, and the Department of Epidemiology and Microbiology, University of Pittsburgh Graduate School of Public Health.

Work was supported by a grant (0-18) from the Health Research Services Foundation, Pittsburgh, Pennsylvania.

*V. M. Howie, 1972: personal communication.

TABLE 1

ESTIMATED RECENT ANNUAL INCIDENCE OF *HEMOPHILUS* MENINGITIS

Allegheny County, Pa. (including Pittsburgh)	32
Franklin County, Ohio (including Columbus)	36
Mecklenburg County, N.C. (including Charlotte)	63
Madison County, Ala. (including Huntsville)	71

NOTE: Rate per 100,000 children, age 0 to 4 years.

Each area included an urban center with one or more hospitals which attracted some cases from distant areas; out-of-county cases were excluded in order that the county population (age 0 to 4 years) could be used as the denominator. These estimates are undoubtedly low, since only bacteriologically documented cases were included. The difference in incidence between the northern and the southern counties (approximately twofold) seems too great to be attributable to possible differences in completeness of case finding.

A possible explanation for the higher incidence in the southern localities may reside in their larger black populations. A disproportionately greater number of blacks among *Hemophilus* meningitis patients has been noted by Sproles et al. (1969) from Charlottesville, Virginia, by Nahmias* from Atlanta, Georgia, by Parke (1972) from Charlotte, North Carolina, and by Howie† from Huntsville, Alabama. Preliminary review of recent cases in Pittsburgh, however, revealed no significant excess of blacks among *Hemophilus* meningitis patients when compared to census data for the age group 0 to 4 years for Allegheny County (about 12% black in 1970). It was therefore necessary to consider other factors which might explain the apparent difference between northern and southern blacks in the frequency of this condition. The report of Ounsted (1950) had indicated that patients with *Hemophilus* meningitis tend to come from large families. It thus seemed worthwhile to consider whether factors associated with both race and family size—namely, income and accompanying living conditions—might affect host susceptibility to this infection.

*A. J. Nahmias, 1971: personal communication.
†V. M. Howie, 1972: personal communication.

MEDICAL RECORD STUDY

Medical records from the Children's Hospital of Pittsburgh were inspected for indicators of family economic status. The only two indicators consistently available were whether the patient's family received welfare funds and whether he was cared for by a private physician during hospitalization. Many patients, of course, fell into neither category.

Table 2 summarizes this information for several groups of patients: 286 cases of *Hemophilus* meningitis hospitalized during 1964-1970; 300 consecutive admissions for any reason, age 0 to 4 years, during the fall of 1967—a year selected because it served as the mid-point for the *Hemophilus* meningitis admissions; 100 consecutive admissions for laryngotracheobronchitis during the years 1967-1970 to serve as a comparison group for both the meningitis and the epiglottitis patients; all of the 103 patients discharged with a diagnosis of epiglottitis during the past 17 years (including 86 patients from January 1962 through March 1972); and 35 patients with epiglottitis, considered separately because they had documented bacteremia (all *H. influenzae)* at the time of admission.

Table 2 indicates that the proportion of *Hemophilus* meningitis patients who were black was similar to that of the comparison groups, excepting those with epiglottitis. The proportion of *Hemophilus* meningitis patients receiving welfare funds was similar to that of the "consecutive admissions," but larger than that of the epiglottitis patients. The laryngotracheobronchitis group fell into an intermediate position between meningitis and epiglottitis.

The *Hemophilus* meningitis group appeared to differ from the comparison groups in that only about half had private physicians, as compared to approxi-

TABLE 2.

RACIAL AND ECONOMIC FACTORS IN *HEMOPHILUS* MENINGITIS PATIENTS
AND OTHERS HOSPITALIZED FOR VARIOUS REASONS

Type of Patient	N	Black %	Welfare %	Private %
Hemophilus meningitis	286	15	13	52
Consecutive admissions	300	12	12	66
Laryngotracheobronchitis	100	12	9	60
Acute epiglottitis (total)	103	8	3	74
bacteremic (*H. influenzae*)	35	10	6	67

TABLE 3.

RACIAL AND ECONOMIC FACTORS IN MENINGOCOCCAL,
HEMOPHILUS, and PNEUMOCOCCAL MENINGITIS

Etiology of meningitis*	Black %	Welfare %	Private %
N. meningitidis	6	2	72
H. influenzae	20	12	48
D. pneumoniae	34	28	34

*There were 51 patients of each etiology (all aged 3 months through 4 years).

mately two thirds of the "consecutive admissions." Racial factors were excluded by considering nonblack patients only; 61% of the white *Hemophilus* meningitis patients were cared for by private physicians during their hospitalization, as compared to 74% of the white "consecutive admissions" (146 of 241 versus 195 of 263; x^2=9.96; p <.01).

Table 3 presents an analysis of these same parameters with a comparison of *Hemophilus,* meningococcal, and pneumococcal meningitis; 153 patients are represented, 51 patients matched for age and year from each etiologic category. The *Hemophilus* meningitis group occupied an intermediate position in all three

TABLE 4

NUMBER OF SIBLINGS OF PATIENTS WITH *HEMOPHILUS*
MENINGITIS AND OF PATIENTS HOSPITALIZED WITH OTHER
CONDITIONS

Type of Patient	N	Number of Siblings			Mean Number
		Percentage			
		0	1	≥2	
Hemophilus meningitis	51	4	29	67	2.6
Pneumococcal meningitis	51	22	27	51	2.2
Meningococcal meningitis	51	35	20	45	1.7
Consecutive admissions	298	19	27	54	2.0
Laryngotracheobronchitis	100	21	38	41	1.8
Acute epiglottitis (total)	101	22	36	43	1.5
bacteremic (*H. influenzae*)	33	21	24	55	1.7

respects (percentage black, welfare, or private). No explanation can be offered for this ranking, other than to suggest that the pneumococcal meningitis group might include a disproportionate number of blacks because of patients in the group who also had sickle-cell anemia (5 of the 17 blacks with pneumococcal meningitis also had sickle-cell anemia.)

Table 4 includes information on the number of siblings for each of the previously described groups. It provides clear confirmation of the observation of Ounsted (1950) on family size mentioned earlier. In nearly every case, the *Hemophilus* meningitis patient had one or more siblings, differing in this respect from patients in all other groups (including the epiglottitis patients, who are usually older and for that reason might be expected to have more, rather than fewer, siblings).

CASE-CONTROL STUDY

In order to obtain more precise information on family finances, crowding within the home, and other environmental factors, a case-control study was initiated. This study consisted of interviewing parents of patients and controls of about the same age who were present in the hospital at the same time. A questionnaire was used which would allow comparison of some of the information with the 1970 census data.

Table 5 summarizes preliminary results from the first 40 interviews. For simplicity of presentation, arbitrary divisions were made for family income, education level of father, and degree of crowding. It is planned to interview a total of 100 to 150 families before concluding the study; but even with the small

TABLE 5

SELECTED RACIAL AND ENVIRONMENTAL CHARACTERISTICS OF
FAMILIES OF *HEMOPHILUS* MENINGITIS CASES AND OF HOSPITALIZED CONTROLS

	Cases	Controls
Total families studied	20	20
Nonwhite race	5	3
Families receiving welfare funds	3	3
Family income less than $7,000/year	9	6
Father with less than 12 years' education	7	2
More than one person/room in home	5	2
Upper respiratory infection:		
patient, previous two weeks	10	7
home contact, previous month	8	7

number already interviewed, there is indication of an excess of *Hemophilus* meningitis cases with fathers who have less than high school education, families with less than $7,000 annual income, and households with more than one person per room. It can be seen, however, that the number of families receiving welfare funds are the same in each group.

Another aspect of the study is a test of the assumption—often stated but never documented—that upper respiratory infection is important in the pathogenesis of meningitis. So far, there is little difference between cases and controls in regard to preceding upper respiratory infection. Much larger numbers, of course, will be necessary before these similarities (or differences) can be considered to have much meaning. The use of census data in order to compare the *Hemophilus* meningits families with the general population should be helpful in assessing socio-economic factors, but evaluation of the role of upper respiratory infection in this condition will depend solely on a comparison with simultaneously hospitalized controls.

DISCUSSION

Our studies have shown that the *Hemophilus* meningitis patient in Pittsburgh is apt to have one or more siblings and to come from families of relatively low economic status, but that blacks are not disproportionately affected.

One hypothesis to explain the relativity of large family size is that development of *Hemophilus* meningitis after exposure to the bacterial species may be dose-related and therefore dependent on intimate contact with persons who harbor these organisms, particularly young children. Support for this thesis comes from carriage studies. Turk (1963) and others have demonstrated that families of patients with *Hemophilus* meningitis are very likely to carry type b *H. influenzae* in the nasopharynx. Masters el al. (1958) showed that the carriage rates for adults are usually low, but that higher rates occur in infants and young children. Our preliminary observations concerning income, education, and crowding within the home are consistent with this hypothesis.

Another hypothesis to explain how large family size and these socio-economic factors might contribute to development of *Hemophilus* meningitis is that this environment may favor the occurrence of viral respiratory infection, which in turn may favor the development of *Hemophilus* meningitis. The lack of significant difference in frequency of preceding upper respiratory infection between cases and controls tends to negate this thesis in the preliminary stage, but as the study is extended to involve larger numbers, this possibility will be reevaluated.

The findings concerning welfare patients in Pittsburgh are even more difficult to explain. Data from both the medical record review and the case-control study indicate that disproportionate numbers of *Hemophilus* meningitis patients are not found among families receiving welfare funds. A possible explanation for this paradox is that poverty and associated poor sanitary conditions might favor early colonization with enteric bacteria and other organisms which have cross-reacting antigens for type b, *H. influenzae* (Bradshaw et al., 1971), thus conceivably providing these infants with some degree of protection from *Hemophilus* meningitis.

Another paradox is the epiglottitis patient. There are already clues that the pathogenesis of this infection differs from that of *Hemophilus* meningitis; the affected children are apt to be older, the seasonal distribution tends to be different, and genetic differences have recently been found (Whisnant et al., 1971). It now appears that the epiglottitis patient may come from families with greater financial resources and with fewer children than the *Hemophilus* meningitis patient.

There has been little consideration of a purely racial predisposition to infections due to *H. influenzae* in this report. The main reason is that *Hemophilus* meningitis in Pittsburgh is not significantly more common in blacks than in whites—a situation different from that in the southern locations cited. Perhaps the best place to evaluate a possible black predilection to this disease is in the South. The very fact that blacks are not disproportionately affected in Pittsburgh, however, points to factors other than innately racial ones. Our tentative assumption is that the higher incidence of *Hemophilus* meningitis in certain areas of the South is related to the likelihood that educational and economic deficits may be more widespread among the black population in these areas.

REFERENCES

Bradshaw, M. W.; J. C. Parke, Jr.; R. Schneerson; and J. B. Robbins. 1971. "Bacterial Antigens Cross-Reactive with the Capsular Polysaccharide of *Hemophilus influenzae*, type b." *Lancet* 1:1095.

Masters, P. L.; W. Brumfitt; R. L. Mendez; and M. Likar. 1958. "Bacterial Flora of the Upper Respiratory Tract in Paddington Families, 1952-54." *Brit. Med. J.* 1:1200.

Michaels, R. H. 1971. "Increase in Influenzal Meningitis." *New Eng. J. Med.* 285:666.

Ounsted, C. 1950. "*Hemophilus influenzae* Meningitis: A Possible Ecological Factor." *Lancet* 1:161.

Parke, J. C., Jr.; R. Schneerson; and J. B. Robbins. 1972. "The Age and Racial Distribution and Case Fatality Rate of *Hemophilus influenzae*, type b, Meningitis in Mecklenburg, North Carolina. *J. Ped.* 81:765.

Smith, E. W. P., Jr., and R. E. Haynes. 1972. In press. "Changing Incidence of *Hemophilus influenzae* Meningitis." *Ped.*

Sproles, E. T., III; J. Azerrad; C. Williamson; and R. E. Merrill. 1969. "Meningitis due to *Hemophilus influenzae:* Long-term Sequelae." *J. Ped.* 75:782.

Turk, D. C. 1963. "Naso-Pharyngeal Carriage of *Hemophilus influenzae*, type b." *J. Hyg.* 61:247.

Whisnant, J. K.; G. N. Rogentine; D. L. Mann; and J. B. Robbins. 1971. "Human Cell-Surface Structures Related to *Hemophilus influenzae,* type b, Disease." *Lancet* 2:895.

CHAPTER 22

The Attack Rate, Racial Distribution, Age Incidence, and Case Fatality of *Hemophilus influenzae,* type b, Meningitis in Mecklenburg County, North Carolina

James C. Parke, Jr.
Rachel Schneerson
John B. Robbins

Hemophilus influenzae bacillus, described by Pfeiffer in 1892, induces human disease with the most significant morbidity and mortality in infants and children. The most common serious clinical disease induced by this infectious agent is meningitis, according to Alexander (1965) and Turk (1967). Slawyk reported the first authenticated case of influenzal meningitis in 1899, and in 1922 Rivers emphasized the importance of this organism as a cause of meningitis.

Fothergill and Wright (1933) postulated that the susceptibility to *H. influenzae,* type b, diseases resulted from deficient antibacterial antibodies as demonstrated by the inverse relationship between the bactericidal activity of whole blood and the age-incidence of influenzal meningitis. Norden, Callerome, and Baum (1970) have suggested that the development of immunity toward this organism, based upon an analysis of anti-*H. influenzae,* type b, antibodies, is decreasing in the adult population and that an increase in the incidence of the diseases in the adult could be expected.

H. influenzae infections are not reportable in the United States and there are no good statistics concerning the incidence of any disease caused by these bacteria in a defined population except for the recent report of Parke (1972). The National Center for Health Statistics (1969) reports mortality rates for *H. in-*

This study was supported in part by a contract with the National Institutes of Child Health and Human Development, National Institutes of Health, Bethesda, Maryland, #70-2294.

252   *Hemophilus influenzae*

fluenzae meningitis, and Haggerty and Ziai (1964), Sproles et al. (1969), Crook, Clanton, and Hodes (1949) and Sell (1970) have analyzed mortality and morbidity data from large hospital centers. The need for quantitative information about *H. influenzae,* type b, diseases is emphasized by Michaels's (1971) and Almquist's (1970) reports of an increasing frequency of meningitis and arthritis caused by this organism during the past decade.

This report will present the attack rate, racial distribution, age-incidence and case fatality rate of *H. influenzae,* type b, meningitis in a defined community, Mecklenburg County, North Carolina. The records of all three hospitals in the county coded under the general category of meningitis were reviewed to determine the incidence of *H. influenzae* meningitis, type b, proven by culture, from 1966 through 1971. Deaths were identified by a review of hospital records and confirmed by a search of the death certificates filed at the Vital Statistics Section of the Mecklenburg County Health Department. Population statistics were derived from a study of the census of 1960 and 1970.

DESCRIPTION OF THE COMMUNITY

Since the signing of the Mecklenburg Declaration of Independence on May 20, 1775, the area has become the most populated county in North Carolina. It covers 542 square miles and had a total population of 354,656 in 1970. The black population was 84,254 (24% of the total). Charlotte is the main city of the county with a total population of 241,178 in 1970 and the black population was 72,972 (30% of the total). The urban center of Mecklenburg County is estimated to be 282,461 (80% of the total population).

Three general hospitals in Charlotte provide all of the acute inpatient medical services for the people of the county. Charlotte Memorial Hospital is an 850-bed teaching community hospital and operates the only hospital outpatient clinic facility in the county. There are 67 pediatric beds, including a 14-bed pediatric intensive care unit. Presbyterian Hospital has a total of 504 beds, including 33 pediatric beds. Mercy Hospital has a total of 267 beds, including 22 pediatric beds. Charlotte Memorial and Presbyterian hospitals are private general hospitals for acute care and have an emergency treatment area for private patients.

RESULTS

The etiology of 213 cases of acute meningitis in children admitted to Charlotte Memorial Hospital from 1966 through 1970 is shown in Table 1. The number of deaths are shown on the right of the total cases in each column. The 70 cases of *H. influenzae,* type b, meningitis represent 50% of the total 140 cases of bacterial meningitis diagnosed in that five-year period.

TABLE 1

ACUTE MENINGITIS IN CHILDREN,
CHARLOTTE MEMORIAL HOSPITAL,
1966-1970
Age: Newborn to 15 Years

	1966	1967	1968	1969	1970	Totals
H. influenzae	9/0*	10/0	16/0	20/2	15/0	70/2
Pneumococcal	1/0	8/0	3/3	1/0	5/2	18/5
Meningococcal	7/1	7/0	7/1	2/0	1/1	24/3
Tuberculous	0/0	0/0	1/0	1/1	0/0	2/1
Other Bacterial	10/2	7/2	5/1	1/0	3/0	26/5
Viral	6/0	7/0	8/0	1/0	12/0	34/0
Unknown Etiology	10/1	7/3	9/1	9/1	4/0	39/6

*Incomplete: No statistics available from Presbyterian Hospital for 1966.

TABLE 2

HEMOPHILUS INFLUENZAE MENINGITIS, type b
CHARLOTTE MEMORIAL HOSPITAL,
1960-1971
Ages 0 to 15 Years

Year	No. of Cases	Deaths
1961	3	0
1962	7	0
1963	1	0
1964	7	0
1965	12	2
1966	9	0
1967	10	0
1968	16	0
1969	20	2
1970	15	0
1971	22	0
Totals	122	4

A total of 122 cases of *H. influenzae,* type b, meningitis diagnosed at Charlotte Memorial Hospital since 1961 in children up to 16 years of age is shown in Table 2. Four deaths occurred. There has been an over-all increase in the number of cases diagnosed over this eleven-year period.

A total of 128 cases of *H. influenzae,* type b, meningitis admitted to the three hospitals from 1966 through 1971 is shown by race and residence in Table 3. Mecklenburg County residents accounted for 113 of the cases. Ninety-three of the 128 cases were diagnosed at Charlotte Memorial Hospital.

A total of 113 cases of *H. influenzae,* type b, meningitis occurring in county residents from 1966 through 1971 is shown in Table 4 by year, race and hospital. Eighty-one of the cases were diagnosed at Charlotte Memorial Hospital and 61 (75%) of those cases occurred in black residents. Only one adult patient was diagnosed during the six-year period. Thirty cases were diagnosed at Presbyterian Hospital and four (13%) of those cases occurred in black residents. There were

TABLE 3

HEMOPHILUS INFLUENZAE, type b, MENINGITIS
MECKLENBURG COUNTY,
ALL AGES
1966-1971
128 Cases

	Resident	Nonresident	Total
Charlotte Memorial Hospital			
Total	81	12	93
White	20	4	24
Black	61	8	69
Presbyterian Hospital			
Total	30	2	32
White	26	2	28
Black	4	0	4
Mercy Hospital			
Total	2	1	3
White	2	0	2
Black	0	1	1

TABLE 4

HEMOPHILUS INFLUENZAE, type b, MENINGITIS
MECKLENBURG COUNTY RESIDENTS BY RACE,
ALL AGES
113 Cases

	Charlotte Memorial Hospital			Presbyterian Hospital			Mercy Hospital		
	Total	Wt.	Blck.	Total	Wt.	Blck.	Total	Wt.	Blck.
1966	9	2	7		*SNA		0		
1967	9	3	6	5	5	0	1	1	0
1968	15	2	13	3	3	0	1	1	0
1969	17	5	12	6	4	2	0		
1970	12	3	9	8	7	1	0		
1971	19	5	14	8	7	1	0		
Totals	81	20	61 (75%)	30	26	4(13%)	2	2	0(0%)

*Statistics not available.

no statistics available from Presbyterian Hospital for 1966, and therefore the total number of reported cases represents an incomplete number.

Attack rates. Table 5 compares the 1960 to 1970 population of Mecklenburg County. The total population and the black population less than 5 years of age actually decreased slightly during the 10-year period.

The lowest attack rate of *H. influenzae,* type b, meningitis was 2.6 cases per 100,000 population in 1966. Nine recorded cases of meningitis occurred in county residents, but there was incomplete reporting from one hospital.

The attack rate in 1969 was 6.5 cases per 100,000 population. Twenty-three cases of meningitis occurred in county residents.

The highest attack rate occurred in 1971 and was 7 cases per 100,000 residents, based upon an estimated population of 370,000 and 27 cases of meningitis diagnosed in county residents.

It is of interest to examine the attack rate in the susceptible age group of less than 5 years. The lowest attack rate of *H. influenzae,* type b, meningitis in this age group during the six-year period was 39 cases per 100,000 children in 1967. There were 13 resident children in that age group who had proven *H. influenzae,* type b, meningitis.

The lowest attack rate for the less-than-5-year-old black residents was 53 cases per 100,000 black children in 1967.

The highest attack rate for the less-than-5-year-olds occurred in 1971 and was 80 cases per 100,000 children. For the less-than-5-year-old black child, the highest attack rate also occurred in 1971 and was 165 cases per 100,000 resident black children.

Table 6 shows the most susceptible age group to be between 3 months and 3 years, accounting for 89% of the cases. Three cases of *H. influenzae,* type b,

TABLE 5

MECKLENBURG COUNTY POPULATION

	All Ages			Up to Age 5 Years		
	Total	White	Black	Total	White	Black
			(25%)			(30%)
1960	272,111	205,410	66,701	33,944	23,917	10,027
			(24%)			(28%)
1970	354,656	270,402	84,254	32,219	23,049	9,170

TABLE 6

HEMOPHILUS INFLUENZAE, type b, MENINGITIS:
AGE DISTRIBUTION AND AGE INCIDENCE,
MECKLENBURG COUNTY RESIDENTS,
1966-1971

Age Group	Number of Cases			Age of Incidence
	Total	White	Black	(#Cases/ #Months in each age group)
0-2 months	3	2	1	1.5
3-6 months	24	10	14	6
7-12 months	34	14	20	5.7
1-2 years	33	18	15	2.8
2-3 years	10	2	8	0.8
3-6 years	6	1	5	0.2
More than 6 years	3	1	2	
Totals	113	48	65	

meningitis were diagnosed in infants less than 3 months of age and three cases (aged 9 years, 13 years, and 45 years) were diagnosed in individuals beyond age 6 years. The age-incidence was determined by dividing the number of cases in each age group by the number of months for that group. The highest age incidence occurred in the 3-to-6-months group.

Deaths due to acute bacterial meningitis in Mecklenburg County residents from 1966 through 1970 are shown in Table 7. Four deaths occurred in 86 cases of *H. influenzae*, type b, meningitis from 1966 through 1970 and all in black individuals. The over-all mortality rate was 4.6% and for black patients, 8.0%. One of these was a 45-year-old black female who had previously been in good health. A 1-year-old black infant died at home and a diagnosis of *H. influenzae*, type b, meningitis was made by isolation of the organism from cerebrospinal fluid obtained by lumbar puncture and a postmortem examination.

H. influenzae, type b, meningitis accounted for four of the 49 deaths due to bacterial meningitis in Mecklenburg County from 1966 through 1970. Excluding the neonatal and geriatric age groups, *H. influenzae*, type b, meningitis accounted for three out of 19 deaths that occurred in infants, children, and young adults with acute bacterial meningitis.

One death occurred in 27 cases of *H. influenzae*, type b, meningitis during 1971. The over-all mortality for type b meningitis from 1966 through 1971 is 4.4%.

DISCUSSION

The estimate of the incidence and case fatality rate of *H. influenzae*, type b, meningitis in Mecklenburg County may be minimal for several reasons: (a) Some individuals with acute meningitis of unspecified etiology may have had *H. influenzae*, type b, disease; (b) one of the hospitals had no available statistics for 1966; (c) Mecklenburg County residents may have been treated for *H. influenzae*, type b, disease outside the county. However, if the over-all incidence of *H. influenzae*, type b, meningitis in Mecklenburg County (4.8 per 100,000 population per year) is representative, an estimate is derived of approximately 10,000 cases annually in the United States.

The relative frequency of *H. influenzae*, type b, meningitis in infants and children in Mecklenburg County is consistent with data reported by Wehrle, Mathies, and Leedoin (1968), Smith (1954), Seriki (1970), Dodge and Swartz (1965) and Michaels (1971).

The over-all case fatality rate of 4.4% for *H. influenzae*, type b, meningitis in Mecklenburg County is slightly lower than in other series reported by Sell (1970), Smith (1954) and Michaels (1971).

TABLE 7
DEATHS DUE TO ACUTE BACTERIAL MENINGITIS,
MECKLENBURG COUNTY, NORTH CAROLINA,
1966-1970

Year	H. Influenzae	Pneumococcus	Meningococcus	Tuberculous	Other Etiology	
					Specified	Unspecified
1966	0	1 (58 yrs)*	2 (4, 44 yrs)	0	2 (21 days, alpha strep; 7 days, *E. coli*)	5 (80, 65, 47, 17 yrs; 1 mo)
1967	0	3 (80, 76, 63 yrs)	1 (16 yrs)	0	1 (61 yrs, Listeria monocytogenes)	6 (46, 18, 13 yrs; 6 mos.; 2 newborns)
1968	2 (45, 1 yr)	3 (6, 4, 1 mo.)	4 (8, 2, 1 yr; 6 mos)	0	1 (58 yrs., *E. coli*)	2 (17 yrs; 2 mos.)
1969	2 (2 yrs; 5 mos)	6 (78, 66, 57, 52, 43, 28 yrs)	1 (49 yrs)	1 (2 yrs)	0	2 (15 mos: newborn)
1970	0	2 (14, 1 mo)	2 (17; 3 yrs)	0	0	0

NOTE: Deaths due to acute bacterial meningitis, Mecklenburg County, North Carolina, 1966-1970, include all admissions to the hospitals.
*Age at death.

The age distribution of individuals with *H. influenzae,* type b, meningitis in Mecklenburg County is similar to that reported by Fothergill and Wright (1933), Alexander (1965), Turk and May (1967) and Schneerson et al. (1971).

SUMMARY

The attack rate, racial distribution, age incidence, and case fatality rate of *H. influenzae,* type b, meningitis in a defined community has been presented.

A total of 113 cases (65 black) of *H. influenzae,* type b, meningitis occurred in Mecklenburg County residents from 1966 through 1971 and the case fatality rate was 4.4%. Five deaths occurred: four children and one adult; four black and one white.

The highest age incidence was 3 months through 3 years.

The average attack rate was 4.8 cases per 100,000 county residents per year with a high of 7 cases per 100,000 in 1971.

The attack rate for children less than 5 years of age varied from a low of 39 in 1967 to a high of 80 cases per 100,000 children of that age group in 1971.

The attack rate for black children less than 5 years of age was approximately four times that of whites.

REFERENCES

Alexander, H. E. 1965. "The Hemophilus Group." In *Bacterial and Mycotic Infections of Man,* edited by R. B. Dubos and J. G. Hirsch. Philadelphia: J. B. Lippincott.

Almquist, E. E. 1970. "The Changing Epidemiology of Septic Arthritis in Children." *Clin. Orth. and Related Res.* 68:96.

Crook, W. G.; B. R. Clanton; and H. L. Hodes. 1949. *"Hemophilus influenzae* Meningitis: Observations on the Treatment of 110 Cases." *Ped.* 4:643.

Dodge, P. R., and M. N. Swartz. 1965. "Bacterial Meningitis: A Review of Selected Aspects: H. Special Neurologic Problems, Postmeningitic Complications, and Clinicopathological Correlations." *New Eng. J. Med.* 272:954, 1003.

Fothergill, L. D., and J. Wright. 1933. "Influenzal Meningitis: The Relation of Age-Incidence to the Bactericidal Power of Blood against the Causal Organism." *J. Immunol.* 24:273.

Haggerty, R. J., and M. Ziai. 1964. "Acute Bacterial Meningitis." *Adv. Ped.* 13:129.

Michaels, R. M. 1971. "An Increase in Influenzal Meningitis." *New Eng. J. Med.* 285:666.

Norden, C. W.; M. L. Callerome; and J. Baum. 1970. *"Hemophilus influenzae* Meningitis in an Adult: A Study of Bactericidal Antibodies and Immunoglobulins." *New Eng. J. Med.* 282:190.

Parke, J. C., Jr.; R. Schneerson; and J. B. Robbins. 1972. "The Attack Rate, Age Incidence, Racial Distribution and Case Fatality Rate of *Hemophilus influenzae,* type b, Meningitis in Mecklenburg County, North Carolina." *J. Ped.* 81:765.

Rivers, T. M. 1922. "Influenzal Meningitis." *Amer. J. Dis. Child.* 24:102.

Schneerson, R.; L. P. Rodrigues; J. C. Parke; and J. B. Robbins. 1971. "Immunity to Disease Caused by *Hemophilus influenzae,* type b: II. Specificity and Some Biologic Characteristics of Natural, Infections-Acquired, and Immunization-Induced Antibodies to the Capsular Polysaccharide of *Hemophilus influenzae,* type b." *J. Immunol.* 107:1081.

Sell, S. H. 1970. "The Clinical Importance of *Hemophilus influenzae* Infections in Children." *Ped. Clin. N. Amer.* 17:415.

Seriki, O. 1970. "Pyogenic Meningitis in Infancy and Childhood." *Clin. Ped.* 9:17.

Slawyk, E. 1899. "Ein fall von allgeneininfection mit influenzabacillenx." *Ztschr. F. Hyg. U. Infektkr.* 32:443.

Smith, E. S. 1954. "Purulent Meningitis in Infants and Children: Review of 409 Cases." *J. Ped.* 45:425.

Sproles, E. T.; J. Azerrad; C. Williamson; and R. E. Merrill. 1969. "Meningitis due to *Hemophilus influenzae:* Long-Term Sequelae." *J. Ped.* 75:782.

Turk, D. C., and R. L. May. 1967. *Hemophilus influenzae: Its Clinical Importance.* London: English Universities Press.

U. S. Department of Health, Education, and Welfare. National Center for Health Statistics. *Vital Statistics of the United States,* vol. II, pt. A. Washington, D. C.: Government Printing Office.

Wehrle, P. F.; A. W. Mathies; and J. H. Leedoin. 1968. "The Critically Ill Child: Management of Acute Bacterial Meningitis." *Ped.* 44:991.

Discussion

John Witte, Presiding

John Witte: Before opening the general discussion, I would like to make a few comments and refer back to some of the analogies with viral diseases that we have heard several times in the last two days. Obviously, one of the big differences in *Hemophilus* infections, compared to those diseases for which we have had vaccines licensed recently, is the absence of good national morbidity data on which to evaluate the efficacy of the vaccine. Almost everything that has been presented this morning has been related to *H. influenzae* meningitis. Very little has been said about some of the other illnesses that are caused by the bacterial species. I wonder if, as we get into the discussion, we can think of some ways by which we can get more comprehensive data that will give a better understanding of the epidemiology of the various ways in which this infection expresses itself.

David W. Fraser: I wonder if Dr. Michaels and Dr. Parke have any estimates of the completeness of their case findings. I am concerned that differences in completeness of studies may explain apparent geographic differences in incidence of the disease. Where do people in Mecklenburg and Allegheny Counties go for medical care?

Richard H. Michaels: Case finding in Pittsburgh has been carried out primarily by searching laboratory records for infections documented by isolation of *H. influenzae* from the blood or spinal fluid. Survey of autopsy records at the Children's Hospital revealed no cases of *Hemophilus* meningitis that had not already been identified through the bacteriology laboratory—not surprising, perhaps, since we were concerned only with meningitis proven to be caused by this organism. In regard to the question about where residents of Allegheny County get their medical care, migration outward is unlikely but migration inward is a common occurrence. Approximately 25% of the patients with *Hemophilus* meningitis at Children's Hospital come from outside the county. Ours is the only hospital for children in Pennsylvania west of Philadelphia. Patients therefore come to us from all over western Pennsylvania and parts of adjacent states. It is hard to imagine the circumstances under which a resident of Allegheny County might be treated for meningitis outside of the county, unless he became ill while on a family trip.

261

Fraser: How about using death certificates as an independent cross-check? The diagnosis on the death certificate may not be correct, but by reviewing hospital records of each patient who is cited on his death certificate as having died of *H. influenzae* meningitis, you could estimate the completeness of your other methods of case finding.

Michaels: We have not surveyed death certificates in Pittsburgh or Allegheny County.

James C. Parke, Jr.: We ran several checks on this. The first place we started was hospital records signed out as *H. influenzae,* type b, meningitis and then having those deaths recognized, we reviewed the records. Secondly, we went back to the hospital records looking for meningo-encephalitis, encephalitis, or brain abscesses et cetera, and made another check for *H. influenzae* infection and deaths. Thirdly, we went independently to the Vital Statistics Section of the County Health Department and looked at the death certificates and identified all deaths. The hospital records were searched again to insure that those deaths were confirmed. I do not think we overlooked any deaths.

Fraser: What percentage did you pick up by using death certificates that you would not have found through other means?

Parke: There were more deaths reported on death certificates as *H. influenzae* meningitis than actual cases when we searched the records.

Fraser: Agreed. You had to discard a considerable number; but when you did this, how many more had you found by using death certificates?

Parke: There were three additional deaths that were not due to *H. influenzae,* type b.

Fraser: Out of a total of how many deaths?

Parke: Out of four, there were three additional ones that were rejected.

Witte: How can similar data be collected for epiglottitis? What is the morbidity due to otitis media associated with *H. influenzae?* We need to have some idea what the expected background infection is for these diseases and their various parameters.

Parke: From our review of records, there were approximately two cases of epiglottitis per year. This seems to be a rather standard number over a period of years, but in most of those instances, we were not able to document the diagnosis, since there was not a positive blood culture for *Hemophilus.* This was more often a clinical rather than a culture-proven diagnosis. *Hemophilus* otitis media was recognized in our clinic population but not among hospital admissions. Review of hospital records for this diagnosis was found to be an impossible task.

Michaels: I am pessimistic about obtaining reliable incidence data for epiglottitis for another reason. It can masquerade as severe laryngotracheo-bronchitis or croup. An anecdote will illustrate my concern. When a former colleague moved from Babies Hospital in Manhatten to a Department of Pediatrics in Brooklyn about 15 years ago, he was told that epiglottitis did not occur there. There was surprise that there was so much epiglottitis recognized in upper Manhatten. He discovered about 10 cases, however, during his first year in Brooklyn. I suspect that there is more epiglottitis in some areas than in others. It certainly appears to be more common in the northeastern part of this country than in the south, for example, but hard data are going to be difficult to get.

Witte: I wonder if the Boston delegation has any comments on this?

Smith: Epiglottitis is a dramatic disease and generally, by the clinical picture, one has a fairly good idea whether or not the diagnosis is epiglottitis. It is very uncommon and it would be difficult to collect data over a long period of time in a reasonably large population. On the other hand, I would submit that the accuracy, if people are looking for it, can be reasonable. As far as the otitis media is concerned, it is going to be difficult, but possible, to determine the prevalence of *H. influenzae* in this clinical syndrome. I would submit that it is going to be almost impossible to get any kind of attack rate based on nasopharyngeal culture data. Culture of middle-ear exudates is necessary. Dr. Howie has done this for the last several years and can tell us how many children come into his office in each age group. If you give him enough money and people to search his records, he can tell you how many children in Alabama he sees in relation to the total population. I think that the prevalence of *H. influenzae* otitis at Huntsville can be calculated.

John K. Whisnant: May I make some comments about the rarity of epiglottits? At least in several centers there are ample cases for study. At Yale, in New Haven, there were 17 cases in 13 months. In Pittsburgh and surrounding areas, there were 31 cases of blood-culture-proven epiglottitis in the last ten years, with four occurring in the last few weeks. Dr. Michaels also has data to show that the syndrome is probably four times this common, but positive blood cultures were not always obtained. If a careful search is done, including examination of postmortem records, epiglottitis may be a cause of sudden infant-death syndrome. Those children who are found dead in their cribs may have had *H. influenzae,* type b, identified in the blood culture. Just from anecdotal impression, I know of five cases where positive culture was obtained.

Smith: I think you may be right, and there is more epiglottitis than is usually appreciated. On the other hand, I think the number of cases is still small. I would not like the group to gain the impression that *H. influenzae* is a common cause of the acute-sudden-death syndrome in infants.

Whisnant: I did not say meningitis. I said epiglottitis. I am only raising the possibility.

Smith: There have been some fairly extensive bacteriological studies in surveys of the acute-sudden-death syndrome in several cities. I do not think that *H. influenzae,* type b, epiglottitis diagnosed either pathologically or microbiologically has been a common cause.

Witte: I would like to ask Dr. Michaels about the negative data to which he alluded with regard to either antecedent or concurrent viral infections in association with meningitis or epiglottitis.

Michaels: Among the first 28 families interviewed for our case-control study, 8 of 14 patients with *Hemophilus* meningitis had a history of upper respiratory infection during the two weeks prior to admission. The proportion for simultaneously hospitalized controls was 7 of 14. With additional interviews, there is still little difference. We will have much larger numbers for analysis before the study is concluded.

John B. Robbins: Dr. Thomas Shope at Yale University tried to isolate viruses and study the antiviral antibody in sera of nine consecutive cases of epiglottitis, in New Haven. Perhaps because of the nature of the disease, or limitation of the screening for viruses and antibody, he was unable to find a consistent pattern between viral upper respiratory infection and *H. influenzae,* type b, epiglottitis.

Georges Peter: I am interested in the age distribution of Dr. Parke's cases. I think the highest incidence occurred in the 3-to-6-months-old group. We went back and looked at our age incidence in Boston in recent years and compared the data to Fothergill and Wright's original data which came from the same hospital. Table 1, here, on bacterial meningitis at CHMC in Boston shows that the figures are very nearly identical in each age group, both now and in the 1930s. The mode is in the 6-to-12-month-old group now as well as in 1930.

David T. Karzon: Information regarding the secular trend of the incidence and age distribution of *H. influenzae* meningitis would be rewarding. Data from several sources would indicate that cases of *H. influenzae* meningitis are increasing. Over the years, the increased incidence of paralytic poliomyelitis which occurred with improved hygeine was accompanied by a shift from infants to an older age group. In the case of *H. influenzae* meningitis, if there were a decrease in the number of adults with antibody as determined by Norden (this volume) one might expect an increase in cases by early infancy and also in young adults. It is also legitimate to question whether the relatively low rate of disease in the early months of life is due to transplacental antibody or the limited epidemiological contact of small infants.

Michaels: We have published data on some of these questions (*New Eng. J. Med.* [1971] 285:666), and also have some recent information. Review of more than 650 cases of *H. influenzae,* type b, meningitis at the Children's Hospital of Pittsburgh showed a rise of more than 400% during the period 1941-1970.

TABLE 1

BACTERIAL MENINGITIS AT CHMC, BOSTON

Age	1961–1969		Fothergill and Wright (1920–1932)
	Number	% of Total	% of Total
0-3 mos.	8	2.9	2.7
3-6 mos.	27	9.9	10.7
6-12 mos.	70	25.6	30.7
1-1½ yr.	49	18.0	17.3
1½-2 yr.	40	14.7	13.3
2-3 yr	35	12.8	14.7
3-4 yr.	23	8.4	1.3
4-5 yr.	8	2.9	0
>5 yr.	13	4.8	9.3
Total	273	100.0	100.0

The proportion of patients who were less than 3 months of age, however, remained about the same (3% for the 1940s, 3% for the 1950s and 4% for the 1960s.) On the other hand, about 10% (6 out of 62) of the patients admitted since December 1970 were less than 3 months old. The difference is not statistically significant but is certainly something to watch. The situation for older children is more reassuring. A secular trend might be expected to show up at both ends of the pediatric age scale but we have found no evidence of a shift toward older children and adolescents. About 2% (1 out of 62) of the *Hemophilus influenzae* meningitis admissions to Children's Hospital since December 1970 were 6 to 15 years of age and this proportion is actually lower than that observed in the past (3% for the 1940s, 5% for the 1950s, and 4% for the 1960s.)

Robbins: We have searched every article we can find in the world's literature regarding age distribution—about 70 articles. There does not seem to have been a change in the age distribution which would give some clue to any change in the acquisiton of immunity; that is, in adult life or immediately after birth. I would like to point out two deficiencies in such an analysis, however. The first is that many of the reviews were written by pediatricians who studied their own cases; thus we do not have good data for adult life (after the age of 50 or 60) to determine whether this disease seems to be more prevalent during the age group 50 or older as it appears to be for pneumococcal meningitis. The second point is that, in trying to make a table from this literature review data, one is unable to evaluate the most critical variable, that is, the prevalence of *H. influenzae,* type b, at 0 to 3 months of age. Thus the impression exactly parallels the one you have shown from Boston Children's Hospital records. Perhaps investigators should stay alert for the two areas that would reveal changes in immunity, that is, in the very young and in people over 40 to 50.

Smith: I think Dr. Karzon's statement is still valid and I would emphasize that we consider our experience with a bit of tongue in cheek. I think there are still a number of epidemiological questions about *H. influenzae* in general and meningitis in particular. I think, perhaps, just a word on a historical note is in order. Certain of the observations which we are making with great wisdom today have, in fact, been made previously. We should not terminate our discussion of the epidemiology of *H. influenzae* without giving credit to the fact that certain of the guidelines under which we are operating were made by our predecessors ten to twenty years ago. Recent information has made us a lot wiser but I think everyone should recognize the fact that there were others who were also wise.

SECTION X

Cross-Reacting Antigens of Enteric Bacteria as an Antigenic Source for "Natural" Antibodies to Bacteria Causing Meningitis

John B. Robbins
Richard L. Myerowitz
Rachel Schneerson
John K. Whisnant
Emil Gotschlich
Darrel T. Liu

"Natural antibodies with activity against pathogenic bacteria such as meningococci, *Salmonella typhi, Shigella, Vibrio cholera,* and pneumococci and many nonpathogenic bacteria such as *E. coli* and *Pseudomonas* have been demonstrated in most adult domesticated and laboratory animals, as well as in adult human beings (Burg, 1907; Lovell, R., 1932, 1934, 1939; Silverthorne, 1936; Gibson, 1930, 1932; Mackie and Finkelstein, 1928, 1930, 1932a; Mackie, Finkelstein, and Van Rooyan, 1932; Schwentker, Janney, and Gordon, 1943; Ikari, 1964; Svehag, 1964; Bull and McKee, 1921; Abdoosh, 1936; and Swanson and Goldschneider, 1969). Most investigators now accept the concept that the antigenic stimulus for these "natural" antibodies are not necessarily the homologous organism, but may be cross-reacting substances frequently found in enteric, nonpathogenic bacteria (Michael, Whitby, and Landy, 1962; Michael and Rosen, 1963).

A convincing demonstration of the immunogenicity of cross-reacting antigens was reported by Springer, Horton, and Forbes (1959), who observed that antibody to human B erythrocytes, detectable in 2-month-old chicks, were absent in

This work was done in the National Institute of Child Health and Human Development, NIH, Bethesda, Maryland; the Rockefeller University, New York City; and the Brookhaven Laboratories, Upton, Long Island.

chicks raised in a germ-free environment. Monocontamination of germ-free chicks with an *E. coli* 086, an organism with the specificity sugar of the B blood group substance (D-fucose), resulted in the formation of antibodies against blood group B. Subsequently, Springer, Williamson, and Brandes (1961) demonstrated that D-fucose and B. blood group substance reactivity were found in many Enterobacteriacae, including *Salmonellae* and *E. coli.*

Following the demonstration of the cross-reactions between enteric and nasopharyngeal bacteria and the capsular polysaccharide of *Hemophilus influenzae*, type b (Bradshaw et al., 1971), "natural" immunity to other pyogenic organisms that cause meningitis were re-examined. In particular, we were intrigued by the observations that most children and young army recruits have serum antibodies against meningococcal Group A polysaccharide despite the rarity of this organism in this country for the last twenty years (Goldschneider, Gotschlich, and Artenstein, 1969; Feldman, 1965; Evans, Artenstein, and Hunter, 1968; Gotschlich et al., 1972).

In this report, serologic reactions were sought amongst collection of *E. coli* and other enteric bacteria for cross-reacting antigens to *Neisseria meningitidis*, Group A, and three other pyogenic bacteria, *N. meningitidis*, Group C, and *Diplococcus pneumoniae*, types I and III.

METHODS AND MATERIALS

Representative serotypes were chosen of *E. coli, Citrobacter, Klebsiella, Salmonella*, and *Arizona* from the World Health Organization and the Center for Disease Control, urinary tract organisms from the collection of Drs. Edward Kass and Marvin Turck, and organisms from human and animal feces. Representative strains of Group D streptococci and the bacilli groups were supplied by Dr. Viola Young, Baltimore Public Health Laboratory, Baltimore, Maryland.

Rabbit meningococcal Groups A and C antisera and horse pneumococcal types I and III antisera were used to identify the cross-reactions. Pneumococcal types I and III capsular polysaccharides were kindly donated by Dr. Benjamin Prescott, National Institute of Allergy and Infectious Diseases. Group A and C meningococcal, types I and III pneumococcal polysaccharides were available in highly purified form (Gotschlich, Liu, and Artenstein, 1969). The method of identification of the cross-reacting bacteria was simple. Overnight growth on broth or individual colonies from tryptic soy agar, taken as thick saline suspensions, were reacted with the various antisera in agarose gel (Marine Colloids, Maine), for 48 hours at 4° C and the gels observed for precipitin lines. The cross-reacting antigens were prepared from cultures in tryptic soy broth grown to stationary phase, precipitated sequentially with cetavlon, alcohol, and then extracted with phenol.

TABLE 1

ENTERIC BACTERIA WITH CROSS-REACTIVE ANTIGENS

Strain Designation	Species	Serotype	Cross Reaction	Specificity Capsular	Specificity Other
Sh 17	B. pumilis		N. meningitidis grp. A	+	
C 32	E. coli	010:H4	N. meningitidis grp. A&C		+
WHO*290	E. coli	010:H4	N. meningitidis grp. A&C		+
12975 FED	E. coli	0 undet‡:H42	N. meningitidis grp. C		+
BOS 12	E. coli	016:NM	N. meningitidis grp. C.	+	
MT 97	E. coli	undetermined	N. meningitidis grp. C.	+	
WHO 11	E. coli	048:NM	D. pneumoniae type I	+	
WHO 42	E. coli	0113:H21:K75	D. pneumoniae type I		+
WHO 30	E. coli	07:H4:K7	D. pneumoniae type III	+	
WHO 252	E. coli	014‡:NM	D. pneumoniae type III	+	
WHO 165	E. coli	050:H7:K56	D. pneumoniae type III	+	
BOS Y2	E. coli	0150:NM	D. pneumoniae type III	+	
ISB 1353	E. coli	050:H1	D. pneumoniae type III	+	
LH	E. coli	014‡:NM	D. pneumoniae type III	+	

*Organisms designated "WHO" were kindly provided by Dr. F. Orskov from the reference collection of the Escherischia Center, World Health Organization.

†O group undetermined due to roughness.

‡Rough variant also contains cross-reactive antigen.

RESULTS

Table 1 shows the results obtained from a collection of 1,406 bacteria studied for cross-reactions to four pyogenic bacteria (Schneerson et al., 1972).

Neisseria meningitidis, Group A. Three strains of bacteria were initially shown to react with meningococcal Group A antisera; one *Bacillus pumilus* designated strain Sh 17 and two *E. coli* strains: C32 and WHO 290. The Sh 17 antigen cross-reacted with Group A polysaccharide antigens (Fig. 1). Absorption with the Group A polysaccharide removed the reactivity of the Group A antiserum with Sh 17 but not with the two *E. coli* strains. N-acetyl-D-mannosamine, closely related to the specificity sugar of the Group A polysaccharide line, dissolved the precipitin line between the Sh 17 antigen and considerably reduced the intensity of the Group A precipitin reaction, but did not affect the reaction between the Group A antiserum and the *E. coli* noncapsular antigens. Antiserum produced by immunization with whole Sh 17 organisms reacted with a complete identity reaction with the meningococcal Group A polysaccharide and the Sh 17 antigen. This precipitin reaction was almost completely dissolved by N-acetyl-D-mannosamine phosphate. Chemical analysis of the purified Sh 17 antigen revealed D-mannosamine phosphate and a teichoic acid component, polyglycerol phosphate (Robbins et al., unpublished).

Examination of 20 *Bacillus pumilus* strains from the reference collection of Dr. Ruth Gordon, Rutgers University, New Brunswick, New Jersey, yielded six *B. pumilus* with meningococcal Group A polysaccharide cross-relativity.

Neisseria meningitidis, Group C. Two *E. coli*, designated BOS 12 and MT 97, cross-reacted with the meningococcal Group C polysaccharide. Absorption of the Group C antiserum with the purified Group C polysaccharide removed the reactivity to the BOS 12 and MT 97 but did not detectably alter the reaction toward three other *E. coli* preparations, indicating that their cross-relativity was due to noncapsular antigens. It was of interest that the Group C noncapsular cross-reactions yielded identity precipitating reactions with the noncapsular cross-reacting organisms to the meningococcal Group A antiserum. This finding suggests that there is a noncapsular antigen of meningococci, Groups A and C, that is antigenically related to these *E. coli* strains.

Immunization of several rabbits and burros with *E. coli* BOS 12 and MT 97 yielded potent meningococcal Group C polysaccharide antisera, thus providing additional proof of their cross-reactivity. Chemical analyses have identified the *E. coli* cross-reacting antigen as polyneuraminic acid, indicating chemical as well as serologic similarity to the meningococcal Group C polysaccharide (Liu et al., 1971).

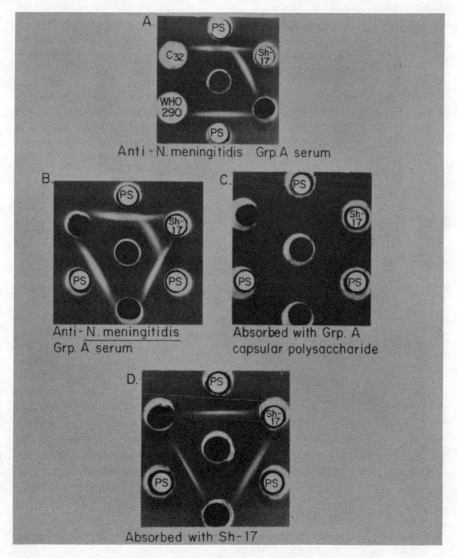

Fig. 1. Cross-reactions of *Escherichia coli* and *Bacillus pumilus* (Sh-17) with meningococcal Group A antigens. Immunodiffusion analysis using rabbit meningococcal Group A serum in the center well.

A. Reaction of C 32 and WHO 290 (*E. coli*) with noncapsular antibodies and reaction of Sh-17 (*B. pumilus*) with a cross-reaction to the Group A polysaccharide.

B. Unabsorbed serum reacting with purified Group A meningococcal polysaccharide and Sh-17 extract.

C. Antiserum absorbed with Group A polysaccharide showing loss of reactivity with Sh-17 extract.

D. Absorbed antiserum with Sh-17 extract show loss of reactivity with the homologous antigen, the Group A polysaccharide.

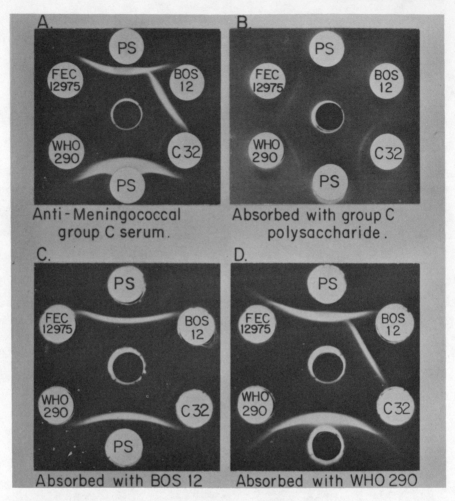

Fig. 2. Cross-reactions of *Escherichia coli* with meningococcal Group C antigens. Immuno-diffusion analysis with Group C meningococcal antiserum with *E. coli* showing capsular and noncapsular cross-reactions.

- A. Unabsorbed serum with BOS 12 cross-reacting with the purified Group C poly-saccharide (PS) and the nonidentity reactions that are noncapsular with FEC 12975, WHO 290, and C 32.
- B. Antiserum absorbed with purified Group C polysaccharide showing lack of reaction with BOS 12 and the persistent reaction with the noncapsular cross-reacting *E. coli*.
- C. Antiserum absorbed with BOS 12 showing persistent reactions with noncapsular cross-reacting *E. coli* and diminished reaction with Group C polysaccharide.
- D. Antiserum absorbed with noncapsular cross-reacting *E. coli* showing lack of reaction with other noncapsular cross-reacting *E. coli* and intact reactions with BOS 12 and Group C polysaccharide.

Diplococcus pneumoniae, types I and III. Two *E. coli*, WHO 11 and WHO 42, yielded precipitin reactions with pneumococcal type I antiserum. WHO 11 cross-reacted with the type I polysaccharide as adjudged by the loss of precipitin reactivity between WHO 11 with pneumococcal type I antiserum previously absorbed with the type I polysaccharide. The absorbed antiserum still reacted with WHO 42, indicating its noncapsular reactivity. In our initial study (Fig. 3), six *E. coli* strains reacted with pneumococcus, type III, antiserum. Many more have since been identified. The *E. coli* cross-reactive antigen yielded a line of partial identity reaction which was removed by absorption of the pneumococcal type III antiserum with the purified type III polysaccharide. All *E. coli* preparations had a serologically identical cross-reactive moiety as a common line of precipitation was observed with all preparations using pneumococcal type III antiserum. Further, absorption of the antiserum against type III with any of these *E. coli* preparations removed reactivity with the other five.

D-glucuronic partially dissolved the precipitin line of the type III polysaccharide and the cross-reacting *E. coli* antigens and the pneumococcal type III antiserum (Fig. 4). Antiserum raised by intravenous injection of one of the cross-reacting *E. coli* organisms, WHO 252, precipitated with the type III polysaccharide.

DISCUSSION

In this study, enteric bacteria were found to possess cross-reacting antigens to the capsular and noncapsular antigens of meningococci and pneumococci. Previously reported cross-reactions between enteric bacteria and virulence factors of pyogenic bacteria include *E. coli* K antigens and pneumococcal polysaccharides and a recently reported serologic relation between *E. coli* K and meningococcal Group B polysaccharide (Grados and Ewing, 1970; Heidelberger et al., 1968). Thus, it appears that structural analogs of many pyogenic bacterial antigens may be found in the "normal" flora of human beings and animals.

Antibodies to *H. influenzae*, type b, and to meningococci have been demonstrated in the sera of adult human beings and several laboratory animals (Bull and McKee, 1921; Abdoosh, 1936). The development of these "natural" antibodies is age related. It has been proposed that "natural" antibodies may confer protective immunity to these two forms of purulent meningitis. The low nasopharyngeal carriage rate of *H. influenzae*, type b, and the recent report of bacteria from the normal flora of human beings and animals that cross-react with the *H. influenzae*, type b, capsular polysaccharide suggest that "natural" antibodies to this organism may arise by stimulation with cross-reactive structures. In the case of meningococcus, it has been shown that "natural" antibodies may arise as a result of the asymptomatic carriage of the homologous bacterium (Gotschlich, Liu, and Artenstein, 1969). However, it is unlikely that this

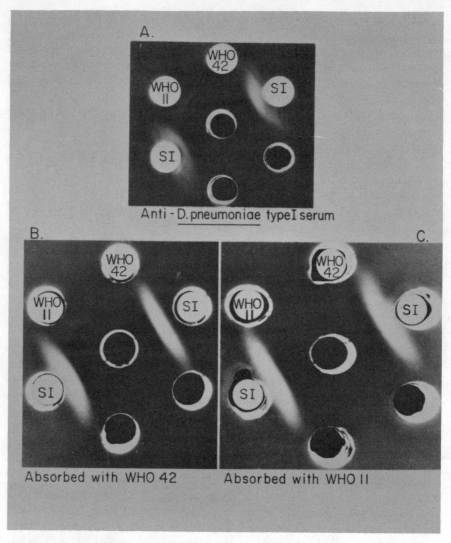

Fig. 3. Cross-reaction of *E. coli* with capsular and noncapsular antigens of *D. pneumoniae,*
Type I. Immunodiffusion analysis using rabbit anti-*Diplococcus pneumoniae*, Type I,
antiserum in the center well and *E. coli* extracts in the outer wells.
  A. Unabsorbed serum showing cross-reaction between S I polysaccharide and WHO 11
     and the noncapsular reaction with WHO 42.
  B. Serum absorbed with the *E. coli* with a noncapsular cross-reaction with WHO 11.
  C. Serum absorbed with WHO 11 (capsular cross-reaction) showing persistent reaction
     with WHO 42. The cross-reaction is too slight to detect a decrease in the reactivity
     with S I with this technique.

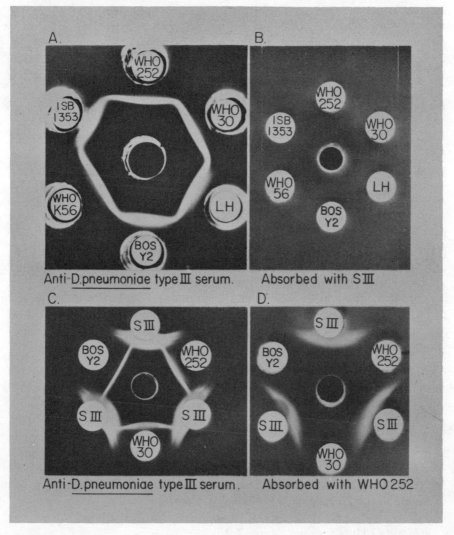

Fig. 4. Cross-reaction of *E. coli* with *D. pneumoniae,* Type III, capsular polysaccharide. Immunodiffusion analysis of *E. coli* supernatants using rabbit anti-*Diplococcus pneumoniae,* Type III, antiserum in the center well.

A. Unabsorbed serum showing the identity reaction of the various *E. coli* extracts.
B. Serum absorbed with S III polysaccharide.
C. Unabsorbed serum showing cross-reactions with the *E. coli* extracts and the purified S III polysaccharide.
D. Serum absorbed with a purified *E. coli* polysaccharide (WHO 252) showing lack of reactivity with other *E. coli* extracts and the diminished reactivity with S III.

stimulus is the only mechanism for the synthesis of antibodies. The evidence is strong for antigenic stimulation by cross-reactive antigens in the case of Group A meningococcal polysaccharide. Epidemiological surveys have demonstraed the almost complete absence of Group A meningococci in the United States since 1953. Thus, the identification of an antigen in *Bacillus pumilus* cross-reacting with the meningococcal Group A polysaccharide may provide an explanation for the prevalence of antibodies to Group A polysaccharide in children and young adults.

One intriguing finding has been the recent identification of a *Bacillus* strain that is cross-reactive with meningococcal Group A, *H. influenzae,* type b, and pneumococcal type III polysaccharides. The possibility exists, then, that bacteria with multiple cross-reactions to pyogenic bacteria will be found. Since the immunogenicity of multiple reactor organisms has not been tested, it is premature to speculate about their values in immunoprophylaxis against meningitis caused by these organisms. However, the number of specificity sugars for the capsular polysaccharides of invasive bacteria such as *Hemophilus influenzae*, type b, meningococcal Groups A, B, and C, and the types of pneumococci frequently associated with diseases, is finite. Thus, a more sensitive search and/or genetic manipulation may provide a bacterium or a group of bacteria with all appropriate capsular antigens. Such a bacterial strain or combination might be fed to newborns and thus accelerate the process of "natural" immunity to diseases caused by these species.

REFERENCES

Abdoosh, Y. B. 1936. "Natural and Immune Bactericidins for Gonococcus." *J. Hyg.* 36:355.

Bradshaw, M. W.; R. Schneerson; J. C. Parke, Jr.; and J. B. Robbins. 1971. "Bacterial Antigens Cross-Reactive with the Capsular Polysaccharide of *Hemophilus influenzae,* type b." *Lancet* 1:1095.

Bull, C. G., and C. M. McKee. 1921. "Antipneumococcus Protective Substances in Normal Chicken Serum." *Amer. J. Hyg.* 1:284.

Burg, E. 1907. *Arch. Hyg.* 62:239.

Evans, J. R.; M. Artenstein; and D. H. Hunter. 1968. "Prevalence of Meningococcal Serogroups and Description of Three New Groups." *Amer. J. Epidemiol.* 87:643.

Feldman, H. A. 1965. "Meningococcal Disease." *J.A.M.A.* 196:105.

Gibson, H. J. 1930. "Observations on the Occurrence, Characteristics, and Specificity of Natural Agglutinins." *J. Hyg. Camb.* 30:337.

Gibson, H. J. 1932. "Natural Agglutinins and Their Relationship to Somatic and Flagellar Antigens of Bacteria." *J. Immunol.* 22:211.

Goldschneider, I.; E. C. Gotschlich; and M. Artenstein. 1969. "Human Immunity to the Meningococcus: II. Development of Natural Immunity." *J. Exp. Med.* 129:1327.

Gotschlich, E. C.; M. Ray; R. Trian; and K. J. Sparks. 1972. "Quantitative Determination of the Human Immune Response to Immunization with Meningococcal Vaccines." *J. Clin. Invest.* 51:89.

Gotschlich, E. C.; T. Y. Liu; and M. Artenstein. 1969. "Human Immunity to the Meningococcus: III. Preparation and Immunological Properties of the Group A, Group B, and Group C Meningococcal Polysaccharides." *J. Exp. Med.* 129:1349.

Grados, O., and W. H. Ewing. 1970. "Antigenic Relationships between *Escherichia coli* and *Neisseria meningitidis.*" *J. Inf. Dis.* 122:100.

Heidelberger, M.; K. Jann; B. Jann; F. Orskov; and O. Westphal. 1968. "Relations between Structures of Three K Polysaccharides of *Escherichia coli* and Cross-Reactivity in Antipneumococcal Sera." *J. Bact.* 95:2415.

Ikari, N. S. 1964. "Bactericidal Antibody to *Escherichia coli* in Germ-Free Mice." *Nature* 202:879.

Liu, T. Y.; E. C. Gotschlich; F. T. Dunne; and E. K. Jonssen. 1971. "Studies on the Meningococcal Polysaccharide: II. Composition and Chemical Properties of the Group B and C Polysaccharide." *J. Biol. Chem.* 246:4703.

Lovell, R. 1932. "Presence of Agglutinins of Bacteria of Salmonella Group in Sera of Normal Animals: Preliminary Report. *J. Comp. Path.* 45:27.

Lovell, R. 1934. "The Presence and Significance of Agglutinins for Some Members of the Salmonella Group Occurring in the Sera of Normal Animals." *J. Comp. Path.* 47:107.

Lovell, R. 1939. "Corynebacterium syogenes Antitoxin Content of Animal Sera." *J. Path. and Bact.* 49:329.

Mackie, T. J., and M. H. Finkelstein. 1928. "A Study of Nonspecific Complement Fixation of Normal Serum and Certain Nonantigenic Substances." *J. Hyg. Camb.* 28:172.

Mackie, T. J., and M. H. Finkelstein. 1930. "Complement Fixation by the Interaction of Normal Bacterial Suspensions: A Contribution to the Study of Natural Immunity." *J. Hyg. 30:1.*

Mackie, T. J., and M. H. Finkelstein. 1932. "The Bactericidins of Normal Serum: Their Characters, Occurrence in Various Animals, and the Susceptibility of Different Bacteria to their Action." *J. Hyg.* 32:1.

Mackie, T. J.; M. H. Finkelstein; and C. E. Van Rooyen. 1932. "The Comparative Bactericidal Action of Normal Serum, 'Whole' Blood, and Serum-Leucocyte Mixtures; with Further Observations on the Bactericidal Mechanisms of Normal Serum." *J. Hyg. 32:494.*

Michael, J. G.; J. L. Whitby; and M. Landy. 1962. "Studies on Natural Antibodies to Gram-Negative Bacteria." *J. Exp. Med.* 115:131.

Michael, J. G., and F. S. Rosen. 1963. "Association of 'Natural' Antibodies to Gram-Negative Bacteria with the γ_1—macroglobulins." *J. Exp. Med.* 118:619.

Robbins, J. B.; R. L. Myerowitz; M. Argaman; D. Liu; and E. C. Gotschlich. Manuscript in preparation. "Serologic and Chemical Analysis of the Cross-Reactions between Meningococcal Group A and C Polysaccharides and Enteris Bacterial Antigens."

Schneerson, R.; M. Bradshaw; J. K. Whisnant; R. L. Myerowitz; J. C. Parke, Jr.; and J. B. Robbins. 1972. "An *Escherichia coli* Antigen Cross-Reactive with the Capsular of *Hemophilus influenzae,* type b: Occurrence among Known Serotypes, and Immunochemical and Biologic Properties of *E. coli* Antisera to *H. influenzae,* type b." *J. of Immunol.* June.

Schwentker, F. F.; J. H. Janney; and J. E. Gordon. 1943. "Relation between Scarlet Fever Morbidity and Streptococcus Carrier Rates." *Amer. J. Hyg.* 38:27.

Silverthorne, N. 1936. "Presence of Meningococcus in Nasopharynx of Normal Individuals and Bactericidal Property of Blood Against Meningococcus." *J. Ped.* 9:328.

Springer, G. F.; R. E. Horton; and M. Forbes. 1959. "Origin of Antihuman Blood Group B Agglutinins in White Leghorn Chicks." *J. Exp. Med.* 110:221.

Springer, G.; P. Williamson; and W. C. Brandes. 1961. "Blood Group Activity of Gram-Negative Bacteria." *J. Exp. Med.* 113:1077.

Svehag, S. E. 1964. "The Formation and Properties of Poliovirus Neutralizing Antibody: IV. Normal Antibody and Early Immunity." *J. Exp. Med.* 119:517.

Swanson, J., and I. Goldschneider. 1969. "The Serum Bactericidal System: Ultrastructural Changes in Neisseria Meningitidis Exposed to Normal Rat Serum." *J. Exp. Med.* 129:131.

CHAPTER 24

Immunization of Adults and Children with Polyribophosphate, the Capsular Antigen of *Hemophilus influenzae,* type b

Georges Peter
Porter Anderson
David H. Smith

The increase in prevalence of serious infections caused by *Hemophilus influenzae,* type b, and the high rates of mortality and morbidity from meningitis, which have remained relatively unchanged during the antibiotic era, have prompted consideration of active immunization for *H. influenzae,* type b. That antibody can provide resistance against such infections has been documented by the efficacy of passive immunization in experimental and clinical infections (Alexander, 1944) and of gamma globulin prophylaxis in individuals with X-linked agammaglobulinemia (Rosen and Janeway, 1966). Considerable evidence indicates that the capsular polysaccharide, polyribophosphate (PRP) of *H. influenzae,* type b, is critical for the pathogenicity of the organism. Furthermore, PRP absorption removed the protective activity of rabbit anti-*H. influenzae,* type b, sera (Alexander, Heidelberger, and Leidy, 1944). Thus, PRP has been considered the candidate immunogen for *H. influenzae,* type b.

This work was done in the Infectious Disease Unit of Children's Hospital Medical Center and Beth Israel Hospital Department of Pediatrics, Harvard Medical School, Boston, Massachusetts.

Work was supported by grants from the Milton Fund, the Medical Foundation, Inc., the Hood Foundation, and the Maternal and Child Health and Crippled Children's Services Program of the Massachusetts Department of Public Health and by contract 71-2196 from the National Institute of Allergy and Infectious Diseases, Bethesda, Maryland.

The authors are grateful to Hei Sun Lee and A. Lynn Harding for technical assistance and to our colleagues for fruitful discussions. Part of this investigation would not have been possible without the excellent co-operation of Drs. McKeage, Louden, Hagele, D'Souza, and Cutler of Salem, Massachusetts; Dr. Medlinsky of Marblehead, Massachusetts; and the staff, North Shore Children's Hospital, Salem, Massachusetts.

Previous investigation (Schneerson et al., 1971; Anderson et al., 1972) has indicated that PRP can be prepared in a form that is nontoxic and immunogenic for adults. This manuscript reviews certain of our observations with PRP immunization of adults (Anderson et al., 1972) and the available data from studies designed to determine the toxicity and immunogenicity of PRP for children.

MATERIALS AND METHODS

The vaccine (Anderson et al., 1972), methods of storing serum, and measuring antibody by bactericidal (BO), passive hemagglutination (PHA), and opsonic methods (Anderson, Johnston, and Smith, 1972) have been described previously. The method of measuring anti-PRP antibody by a radio-immunoprecipitation method has been described at this symposium (Anderson, Johnston, and Smith, 1973).

The adults immunized with PRP have been described (Anderson et al., 1972). The children immunized were referred by six pediatricians in private practice in Salem, Massachusetts. The purpose of the study and the description of the vaccine was explained to the parents of the children by their pediatrician and by members of our staff before immunization. This method of selection resulted in a group of children considered in good health, who were primarily from middle-income families and who were all Caucasian. The studies were performed in the offices of the referring pediatricians and their local hospital. HEW and institutional guidelines regarding clinical investigations were observed.

Reactions for the first three days postimmunization were recorded on post-cards by the child's parents, who were instructed to inspect the injection site for erythema, induration, and pain; to record the recipient's rectal temperature on each of the three evenings following the immunization; and to notify their pediatricians of fever exceeding 101° and other noteworthy symptoms. Blood was obtained by venipuncture in each child before and at three and six weeks after immunization. In the later stage of the trial, a 12-week blood was obtained in place of the six-week specimen.

RESULTS

Studies with adults. Initial studies were performed in 62 adult volunteers who received PRP in doses of 0.01 to 100 μg intramuscularly or intradermally. Figure 1 depicts the kinetics of the antibody responses of three adults immunized with 10, 50, and 55 μg PRP. In all three recipients, PHA and BC activity increased sharply at about one week, ceased rising by two weeks, and remained stable for at least sixteen weeks. A slight increase in opsonic activity was detected at four days but the kinetics of this activity were otherwise similar to that of the BC and

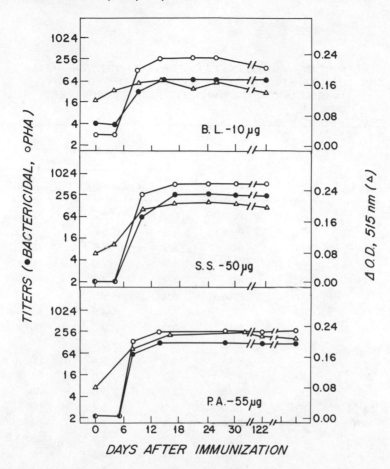

Fig. 1. Antibody responses of three adults immunized with PRP. (From P. Anderson, G. Peter, R. B. Johnston, Jr., L. H. Wetterlow, and D. H. Smith, "Immunization of Humans with Polyribophosphate, the Capsular Antigen of *Hemophilus influenzae,* type b," *J. Clin. Invest.* 51 (1972):39, with permission of the publishers.)

PHA activities. The results depicted in Figure 1 also illustrate that the antibody activities of P. A., as well as those of four other volunteers (not shown) who responded to 3 to 50 μg PRP, did not change following a booster dose of 1 μg PRP given six months after the primary immunization.

PRP doses of 0.01 μg in two subjects did not raise anti-PRP activity but 0.1 μg produced significant rises in roughly half and 1 μg or greater stimulated antibody in essentially all recipients (Table 1). The intradermal and intra-

TABLE 1

THE EFFECT OF VARIOUS DOSES OF PRP GIVEN INTRADERMALLY
OR SUBCUTANEOUSLY ON THE BACTERICIDAL AND PASSIVE
HEMAGGLUTINATION ACTIVITIES OF ADULT VOLUNTEERS

| | | | | Geometric mean of reciprocal titers[†] | |
Dose (μg)	Route	Activity	Fraction with increase*	Preimmun.	Postimmun.
0.01	ID	BC	0/2	22	22
		PHA	0/2	5.6	8.0
.1	ID	BC	3/7	6.6	13
		PHA	3/7	3.6	11
.1	SC	BC	4/7	7.3	16
		PHA	6/7	3.0	22
1	ID	BC	8/10	4.0	53
		PHA	9/10	2.0	56
1	SC	BC	5/6	2.5	14
		PHA	5/6	2.8	25
3	ID	BC	3/3	5.0	81
		PHA	3/3	2.5	200
10	ID	BC	8/9	5.4	50
		PHA	9/9	1.4	69
	SC	BC	7/7	4.9	35
		PHA	7/7	3.3	58
50 or 55	ID	BC	3/4	2.4	91
		PHA	4/4	1.2	180
100	SC	BC	5/7	7.2	64
		PHA	6/7	2.0	58

NOTE: ID, intradermal; SC, subcutaneous; BC, bactericidal activity against strain b-Eagan;
PHA, passive hemagglutination.
*The number of individuals with an increase greater than one twofold dilution/the number
injected.
[†]The antilog of the mean of the logs of the reciprocal titers. For this calculation titers of <2
were assumed to be 1 and titers of ≥256 were assumed to be 256.

muscular administration of PRP produced significant rises in Ab titers. Not evident in the table is the observation that, in general, individuals who received 1 μg or more PRP and who did not have an increase in antibody activity had relatively high preimmunization titers.

The vaccine was generally innocuous. Approximately three fifths of the adults receiving the vaccine intradermally had erythema at the injection site which developed after one day and disappeared by two days and which was accompanied in a few instances by induration. No visible reactions resulted from the intramuscular injection. Slight tenderness at the injection site was noted by four of seven recipients of 100μg. Two individuals who received 10 μg intradermally reported headache, one of whom also had malaise and fatigue, for which other causative factors than the vaccine could not be excluded. One individual manifested an immediate wheal and flare reaction. This response occurred during a booster immunization with 1 μg PRP given at the time the individual's serum contained 60 μg of precipitable anti-PRP antibody in 1 ml of serum (PHA titer of 320).

Studies with children. Children were immunized with single doses of 1, 5, 25, or 100 μg PRP given intramuscularly. The immunizations were generally well tolerated. A few children developed coincidental illnesses, including one with otitis media and another with pharyngitis, for which they were seen by their pediatrician. These children are excluded from the data presented in Tables 2 and 3.

The local reactions are summarized in Table 2. Reactions were more frequent among recipients of the 100-μg dose, occurring in 12 children. Most local reac-

TABLE 2

REPORTED LOCAL REACTIONS DURING 3 DAYS SUBSEQUENT TO PRP
IMMUNIZATION OF CHILDREN

Reaction	PRP Dose (μg) and Volume (ml)			
	1 (0.1)	5 (0.4)	25 (0.1)	100 (0.4)
Erythema	1	0	0	3
Pain	0	0	1	7
Erythema & Induration	0	0	1	1
Erythema & Pain	0	0	0	1
Erythema & Induration & Pain	0	1	0	0
Total Reactions	1	1	2	12
No. of Children	34	35	36	35

tions consisted of pain which was mild, was elicited only by palpation, and disappeared in most by the second day and in all by the third day. Similarly, erythema and induration usually were noted only on the evening after immunization and was one inch or less in diameter. In no case did the parents consider these local reactions marked enough to notify their pediatrician.

Table 3 summarizes the systemic reactions. Fever was most commonly observed among the recipients of 100 μg. Eighteen of 25 of these children had fevers up to 101°. The significance of this is not clear, since young children

TABLE 3

REPORTED SYSTEMIC REACTIONS DURING 3 DAYS SUBSEQUENT
TO PRP IMMUNIZATION OF CHILDREN

Reaction	PRP Dose (μg) and Volume (ml)			
	1 (0.1)	5 (0.4)	25 (0.1)	100 (0.4)
Fever $<101°$F	2	5	3	8
Fever $\geqslant 101°$F	1	3	0	3
Fever $\geqslant 101°$F & Local Reaction	0	0	0	1
Rash	0	2	1	0
Vomiting, Anorexia	0	0	0	1
No. of Children	34	35	36	35

occasionally have evening temperatures in this range without obvious explanation. If one accepts only temperatures of 101° or greater as abnormal, only 6 of 140 vaccine recipients had a febrile response. The highest temperature reported was 101.8°. Fever usually occurred on the first or second day and in two thirds of cases was observed only on the first day. Of the 24 children with any fever, only three children had systemic symptoms. Two siblings had mild rashes of the face and arms, and a third child vomited the night after immunization with subsequent anorexia. Causes for these symptoms not related to immunization could not be ruled out. Of 24 children with fever, only three had local reactions.

In all cases, these local and systemic reactions were mild, and in most cases, they would have been unnoticed had the parents not been instructed to make specific observations.

Serological data is available from 125 of the 140 vaccine recipients (Table 4). Significant antibody response has been defined as a rise in antibody concentra-

TABLE 4

RESPONSE TO PRP OF CHILDREN

	Dose (μg)			
	1	5	2 5	1 0 0
No. of Recipients	32	33	34	26
No. with Response				
at 3 weeks	18	28	29	13
Geometric Mean Titer (ng/ml)				
Pre-PRP	130	42	100	28
	(n = 32)	(n = 33)	(n = 36)	(n = 26)
Post-PRP				
3 wk	470	910	1110	110
	(n = 32)	(n = 33)	(n = 34)	(N = 26)
6 wk	530	950	830	210
	(n = 29)	(n = 31)	(n = 30)	(n = 10)
12 wk	—	–	–	50
				(n = 16)

tion greater than two standard deviations of the pre-immunization concentration. This definition thus gives a 95% confidence limit. In nearly all cases, these rises were 50% or greater. By this definition, 1 μg of PRP produced antibody rises in 18 of 32 children, or 56%. In contrast, 5 and 25 μg produced rises in nearly 90% of recipients. With 100 μg, only half of the recipients demonstrated rises. Geometric mean titers were distinctly higher in the 5- and 25-μg groups than in the 1- and 100-μg recipients.

The geometric mean titers of children in each group of vaccine recipients were similar at six weeks to those at three weeks. The number of children with significant responses to these doses at six weeks was similar to that at three weeks; thus, the rise in antibody activity generally occurred in the first three weeks after immunization. The geometric mean titer of the 12-week sera of the recipients of 100 μg was distinctly lower than that of their counterparts bled at six weeks.

The relationship of age to immunological response to all doses of PRP is depicted in Table 5. Among infants 6 to 12 months of age, only 1 of 13 or 7.7% responded to any dose of PRP; in contrast, 78% of 112 children over 1 year of age responded. Older children also had the greatest increase in postimmunization titers: 24 of 32 of the children older than 3 years who received 5 or 25 μg had 10-fold or greater antibody rises, compared to 14 of 31 between 1 and 3 years.

TABLE 5

RELATION OF AGE AND DOSE TO PRP IMMUNIZATION

Age (mos.)	Dose (μg)				Total (%)
	1	5	25	100	
6-12	0/3*	0/1	1/3	0/6	1/13 (7.7)
13-24	3/6	6/7	11/12	4/8	24/33 (73)
25-36	5/9	7/8	4/4	8/8	24/29 (83)
37.48	9/12	13/14	11/13	1/4	34/43 (79)
> 48	1/2	2/3	2/2	–	5/7 (71)
Total	18/32	28/33	29/34	13/30	88/125 (70)

*Number responding/Total

DISCUSSION

PRP administered to adults at doses as little as 0.1 μg elicited antibody activity, measured by PHA and BC methods in certain individuals. Higher doses were more often effective and generated greater increases. The kinetics of the response were similar to those observed in adults immunized with other polysaccharide vaccines (Heidelberger et al., 1946; Artenstein et al., 1970). Antibody levels of individuals with preimmunization activity increased over a period of 10 to 14 days to maximal values. These were maintained for at least 16 months and were not boosted by re-immunization. This persistence of antibody activity following a single dose of antigen is consistent with the previous proposal that polysaccharide vaccines may persist in the immune system (Heidelberger et al., 1946). The basis for the lack of response to booster doses of PRP remains undefined, but certain possible explanations have been discussed previously (Anderson et al., 1972).

Adults immunized intradermally often manifested a tuberculinlike response. This response was not observed in adults and children immunized intramuscularly. The basis of this reaction has not been defined, but its characteristics differ from those of vaccines containing endotoxin. The possibility that this reaction is cell-mediated is under evaluation in our laboratory. Immediate wheal and flare reactions have been observed following the intradermal inoculation of PRP in some patients following the intravenous administration of therapeutic doses of rabbit-anti-*H. influenzae,* type b, serum (Dingle and Seidman, 1941). This type of reaction was observed only in one individual in the present series; an adult with very high concentrations of anti-PRP antibody who received a booster dose of PRP.

Studies with children indicate that PRP is well tolerated and immunogenic. However, several major questions remain to be answered. Does the poor response of infants to PRP (see Table 5) indicate an inability of PRP to stimulate a primary response? Most of the children immunized in this series and responding to PRP were older than 18 months and may have been having a secondary exposure to the antigen. On the other hand, the lack of response of infants immunized may have been dose- as well as age-related: only four of the 13 infants of 6 to 12 months received the optimal doses of 5 or 25 μg. What will be the response to multiple PRP injections during early infancy, as is the current practice with most existing bacterial vaccines? Will the administration of PRP in conjunction with DPT affect the response to PRP? Clearly, infants of 3 to 12 months are at highest risk to *H. influenzae*, type b, meningitis, the primary target of an active immunization program. Thus, studies on dosages and vaccine schedules in young infants should have the highest priority.

Why do children seemingly respond poorly to 100 μg of PRP? Is this really a poor response or only the result of circulating PRP binding anti-PRP antibody which then cannot be detected by present assays? Calculations based upon the assumption that PRP is not degraded and circulates freely in the total body extracellular water and upon the observation that PRP can precipitate 50 times its weight of anti-PRP Ab* indicate that a 10-kg infant given 100 μg of PRP would have 40 nanograms of PRP per ml of extracellular water. This circulating PRP would be the equivalent of 2000 nanograms of anti-PRP Ab/ml and thus could mask a substantial antibody response. This possibility is currently under investigation in our laboratory.

Anti-PRP antibody has been shown to protect animals from experimental *H. influenzae*, type b, infection (Alexander, Heidelberger, and Leidy, 1944; Anderson et al., 1972), and indirect evidence indicates that it provides human beings with type-specific resistance. However, the concentration of circulating anti-PRP antibody that will protect man against invasive *Hemophilus influenzae*, type b, diseases remains to be defined. To gain some insight into this question, the concentration of circulating anti-PRP has been measured in six agammaglobulinemic children prior to their monthly gamma globulin injections. These injections empirically protect these children from invasive *H. influenzae*, type b, infections to which they are so susceptible before therapy is initiated. Levels in these six agammaglobulinemic patients ranged from 210 to 350 nanograms of anti-PRP antibody and the geometric mean titer was 270. In addition, the geometric mean titer by RIA of a randomly selected group of

*R. B. Johnston, Jr.: unpublished data.

healthy young adult and, presumably, immune women was 200 µg/ml. The postimmunization geometric mean titer for the 5- and 25-µg vaccine recipients greatly exceeds these figures. Further insight into this problem will be provided by analysis of the sera of patients convalescent from systemic *H. influenzae*, type b, diseases.

The observation that a single dose of PRP can elicit antibody activities in adults and children that exceed those of certain individuals considered to be "immune" without serious side effects and that the antibodies are bactericidal and opsonic *in vitro* and protective in laboratory animals supports the thesis that immunization of humans with PRP might confer active immunity to *H. influenzae*, type b. Further studies with this vaccine, particularly in infants, appear to be indicated.

SUMMARY

Single doses of 1 to 100 µg PRP are immunogenic and well tolerated by adults and children. The kinetics of the response in adults is similar to that observed following immunization with other polysaccharide vaccines. A single intramuscular dose of 5 and 25µg produces antibody rises in approximately 90% of children to levels that exceed those found in presumably immune individuals. Further studies of PRP vaccine, particularly in infants, are needed.

REFERENCES

Alexander, H. E. 1944. "Treatment of type b *Hemophilus influenzae* Meningitis." *J. Ped.* 25:517.

Alexander, H. E.; M. Heidelberger; and G. Leidy. 1944. "The Protective or Curative Element in type b, *H. influenzae* Rabbit Serum." *Yale J. Biol. Med.* 16:425.

Anderson, P.; G. Peter; R. B. Johnston, Jr.; L. H. Wetterlow; and D. H. Smith. 1972. "Immunization of Humans with Polyribophosphate, the Capsular Antigen of *Hemophilus influenzae*, type b." *J. Clin. Invest.* 51:39.

Anderson, P.; R. B. Johnston, Jr.; and D. H. Smith. 1972. "Human Serum Activities against *Hemophilus influenzae*, type b." *J. Clin. Invest.* 51:31.

Anderson, P.; R. B. Johnston, Jr.; and D. H. Smith. 1973. "Methodology in Detection of Human Serum Antibodies to *Hemophilus influenzae*, type b." This volume.

Artenstein, M. S.; R. Gold; J. G. Zimmerly; F. A. Wyle; W. C. Branche, Jr.; and C. Harkins. 1970. "Cutaneous Reactions and Antibody Response to Meningococcal Group C Polysaccharide Vaccines in Man." *J. Infect. Dis.* 121:372.

Dingle, J. H., and L. R. Seidman. 1941. "Specific Polysaccharide as Cutaneous Test for Evaluation of Serum Therapy in Influenza Bacillus Meningitis." *Proc. Soc. Exp. Biol. Med.* 46:34.

Heidelberger, M.; C. M. MacLeod; S. J. Kaiser; and B. Robinson. 1946. "Antibody Formation in Volunteers Following Injection of Pneumococci or Their Type-Specific Polysaccharides." *J. Exp. Med.* 82:303.

Rosen, F. S., and C. A. Janeway. 1966. "The Gamma Globulins: III. The Antibody Deficiency Syndromes." *N. Eng. J. Med.* 275:709.

Schneerson, R.; L. P. Rodrigues; J. C. Parke; and J. B. Robbins. 1971. "Immunity to Disease Caused by *Hemophilus influenzae*, type b." *J. Immunol.* 107:1081.

CHAPTER 25

Quantitative Measurement of "Natural" and Immunization-Induced *Hemophilus influenzae,* type b, Capsular Polysaccharide Antibodies

John B. Robbins
J. C. Parke, Jr.
Rachel Schneerson
John K. Whisnant

INTRODUCTION

Most invasive diseases caused by *Hemophilus influenzae* are due to type b organisms and occur during infancy and early childhood (Pittman, 1931; Alexander, 1965; Fothergill and Wright, 1933; Turk and May, 1967; Dawson and Zinnemann, 1952; Sinclair, 1941; and Nelson, 1972). Our decision to study the induction of type b serum antibodies in infants was based upon evidence suggesting that the capsular antigen is important in the acquisition of immunity to this organism. The evidence for the protective nature of anticapsular antibodies may be summarized:

1. Of the six *H. influenzae* capsular types, type b causes almost all invasive diseases (meningitis, epiglottitis, osteomyelitis, etc.) (Pittman, 1931; Alexander, 1965; Fothergill and Wright, 1933; Turk and May, 1967; Dawson and Zinneman, 1952; Sinclair, 1941; and Nelson, 1972).

2. The protective effect of hyperimmune animal serum is type-specific, as shown by the loss of its activity following absorption with the type b capsular polysaccharide (Pittman, 1933; Alexander, Heidelberger, and Leidy, 1944; Schneerson, et al., 1971).

This study was supported in part by the National Institute of Child Health and Human Development on Research Contract No. 70-2294.

3. The inverse relationship between the age incidence of *H. influenzae,* type b, meningitis and the prevalence of serum antibacterial antibodies parallels the age-related development of anti-type b antibodies as measured by passive hemagglutination (Fothergill and Wright, 1933; Schneerson, et al., 1971).

4. Individuals with X-linked hypogammaglobulinemia are susceptible to severe and repeated attacks of *H. influenzae,* type b, meningitis (Rosen and Janaway, 1966). Passive immunization of these individuals with pooled immunoglobulin shown to contain anti-type b antibodies confers a high degree of protection against invasive diseases caused by this organism (Schneerson et al., 1971).

5. "Acute" serum samples from patients with *H. influenzae,* type b, diseases showed no detectable serum anti-type b antibodies (Schneerson et al., 1971). Following convalescence, most individuals developed serum antibodies (Schneerson et al., 1971; Peter et al., 1971; Norden et al., 1972).

Normal adults, with pre-existing serum anti-type b antibodies, injected with the purified *H. influenzae,* type b, polysaccharide responded with a prompt and sustained serum antibody response (Schneerson et al., 1971; Anderson et al., 1972). These volunteers showed no untoward reactions. Our preliminary studies of the serum antibody response of infants and children showed lower antibody levels than those observed in adults. Previous studies utilized passive hemagglutination to assay anticapsular antibodies (Schneerson et al., 1971) which was capable of detecting approximately 0.2 to 0.5 μg/ml of antibody as estimated by comparing the endpoint titration of a human serum and a rabbit serum with their concentration of precipitating antibody. Approximately the same amount of serum antibody was detected by the complement-dependent bactericidal reaction. These methods have two serious limitations at low levels of antibody. The first is that the antibody concentration is expressed as an endpoint titration of a series of doubling dilutions. Second, the complement-dependent bactericidal reaction may be induced by noncapsular *H. influenzae* antibodies (Peter et al., 1971; Norden, 1972).

In this study, a newly developed radioimmunoassay has provided a quantitative method to characterize the adult and infant human serum antibody response to injection of the *H. influenzae,* type b, capsular polysaccharide.

MATERIALS AND METHODS

Radioimmunoassay. An I^{125} derivative of the *H. influenzae,* type b, capsular polysaccharide (Rodrigues, Schneerson, and Robbins, 1972) was prepared by a modification of the method proposed by Gotschlich (Anderson et al., 1972). Two ml of *H. influenzae,* type b (strain "Rab") polysaccharide (5.0 mg/ml) (Gotschlich et al., 1972) were brought to pH 10.0 with constant stirring. Cyanogen bromide (50 mg/ml H_2O Eastman Chemicals) was added (0.1 mg CNBr/mg polysaccharide) and the pH maintained at 10.0 for one hour at room temperature by addition of 0.1 N NaOH. C^{14} labelled tyramine (specificity activity 1 microcurie/mg, New England Nuclear) in 0.5 M $NaHCO_3$ was added and the reaction continued for one hour at room temperature and for 15 hours at 4° C. The reaction mixture was centrifuged at 65,000 xg, 4° C, for two hours and the supernatant passed through a 2.5 x 30 cm Sephadex G-25 column equilibrated with phosphate buffered saline, pH 7.4. The molar ratio of tyramine to polysaccharide in the tyrosylated derivative as determined by C^{14} to pentose was approximately 8/1. This product was radiolabeled with 2 millicuries I^{125} by the iodine monochloride method (McFarlane, 1958). The specific activity of several iodinated derivatives varied from 70,000 to 90,000 CPM/μg.

An adult serum (S.K. immunized with 50 μg. of the purified polysaccharide) was used as a reference standard. The antibody concentration of this serum was determined by quantitative precipitation analysis. The reaction mixture consisted of 2.0 ml of S.K. serum previously heated to 56°C for 30 minutes and dilutions of the type b polysaccharide. Following incubation at 37° C for 30 minutes and for 48 hours at 4° C, the precipitates were collected by centrifugation, washed twice with phosphate-buffered saline pH 7.2, and then dissolved in 0.8% sodium lauryl sulfate. Assuming an extinction coefficient (280 nm) for human immunoglobulin of 14.0, the antibody content of the reference serum was found to be 40 μg Ab/ml.

Fetal calf serum (Grand Island Biological Co.), assayed for the absence of gamma globulin by cellulose acetate electrophoresis, was used to dilute the reference standard (S.K.) and other serum samples with high antibody levels. A 50 μl serum sample and 10 μl of the I^{125} antigen were delivered to a microfuge tube (Beckman Instruments). The tubes were capped and mixed, incubated at 37° C for 30 minutes and overnight at 4° C. Sixty μl of the supernatant were removed and counted for two minutes in an auto gamma counter (Nuclear Chicago). The maximum I^{125} antigen binding capacity of the undiluted reference serum for the I^{125} polysaccharide was 90% to 95% and this value was adjusted to 100% in the standard curves (Fig. 1). Curves were constructed for these concentrations of antigen and dilutions of the reference serum. The antigen concentration of 0.1 μg/ml was chosen because most adult preimmune sera bound 30% to 90% of the antigen. Serum samples that had less than 30% binding were assumed to contain less than 0.04 μg Ab/ml. The coefficient of variation for the assay was 10% at 7.0 μg Ab/ml and 7% at 0.8 μg/ml. The antibody concentrations are expressed as μg Ab/ml but were converted to logarithms to normalize

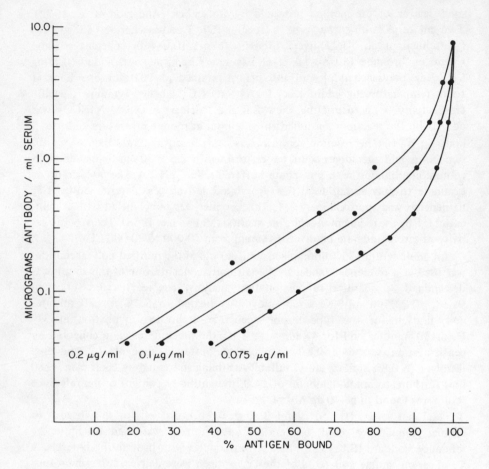

Fig. 1. Curves showing relationship between the concentration of precipitating antibody of a reference serum standard (SK) and the binding of various concentrations of an I125 derivative of the *Hemophilus influenzae,* type b, polysaccharide.

the data for statistical analysis. Postimmunization antibody levels were compared to preimmune levels by paired t-tests.

Antigen for immunization. H. influenzae, type b, capsular polysaccharide, prepared by a modification of a previously published method (Rodrigues, Schneerson, and Robbins, 1972), was dissolved in phosphate-buffed saline or precipitated from 0.05 M sodium acetate on 2 mg aluminum hydroxide.

Bacteriologic. H. influenzae, type b, and bacteria possessing antigens cross-reacting with the type b capsular polysaccharide were sought in nasopharyngeal and rectal cultures using the antiserum-agar technique (Bradshaw et al., 1971; McFarlane, 1958). *E. coli* possessing the cross-reacting antigen were typed by Dr. George Hermann, Enterobacteriology Unit, Center for Disease Control, Atlanta, Georgia.

RESULTS

Anti-type b antibodies of pooled human immunoglobulin (Cohn Fraction II). To estimate the minimal protective level of serum anti-type b antibody, the serum concentration of passively administered antibodies in patients with X-linked hypogammaglobulinemia was determined. Published values for the catabolic rate (tl/2=20 days) and extracellular equilibration (40%) of immunoglobulin were used to predict the serum antibody concentration three weeks following injection (Waldman and Strober, 1969; Gitlin and Janeway, 1960). Analysis of 86 commercially available human immunoglobulin preparations, including hyperimmune tetanus antitoxin and pertussis globulin, showed an average level of 39 μg type b antibody/ml of immunoglobulin (range 20-73). Assuming an immunoglobulin dose of 0.05 to 0.1 ml/kg injected every three weeks, the average serum anti-type b antibody level prior to the next injection of immunoglobulin was calculated to be 0.12 to 0.24 μg Ab/ml. Patients receiving 0.05 ml/kg (low dose) of immunoglobulin containing 20 μg Ab/ml (lowest concentration) would have about 0.06 μg Ab/ml. Based upon these calculations, we have estimated the minimal protective level of anti-type b antibodies to be 0.06 to 0.1 μg Ab/ml.

"Natural" anti-type b antibodies in normal adults. The mean anti-type b antibody concentration in sera of 422 normal blood bank donors of the Clinical Center of the NIH and from 100 pregnant women at term at the Jacoby Hospital at the Albert Einstein College of Medicine, Bronx, New York, and the 20 adult volunteers prior to immunization was 1.39 μg Ab/ml (S.D. = 3.02, range 0.04 - 26.0). Ninety-five percent of the adults had anti-type b antibody levels greater than 0.04 μg Ab/ml. Since most adults are protected against *H. influenzae,* type b, disease and since the mechanism of protection is presumed to be serum antibody, then the protective level may be estimated to be 0.04 to 0.1 μg Ab/ml.

Serum antibody response of adult volunteers immunized with type b polysaccharide. As previously reported, immunization of 20 adult volunteers with 50 μg of *H. influenzae,* type b, polysaccharide resulted in increase of the pre-existing serum antibodies within three weeks (Schneerson et al., 1971). Sera from these adults were re-examined by the radioimmunoassay with additional

TABLE 1

SERUM ANTIBODY RESPONSE OF ADULT VOLUNTEERS
INJECTED WITH 50 μg OF *H. INFLUENZAE*,
type b, CAPSULAR POLYSACCHARIDE

Subject*		Micrograms Anti-type b Antibody/ml Serum		
	Preimmune	3 weeks	3 months	3 years
1	0.04	1.4	2.0	6.0
2	0.07	1.7	1.5	2.8
3	0.08	3.2	2.8	3.2
4	0.10	0.4	1.1	1.1
5	0.11	1.2	1.2	1.2
6	0.12	22.0	20.0	20.0
7	0.15	1.7	1.8	2.2
8	0.15	30.0	30.0	18.0
9	0.20	1.8	1.8	0.9
10	0.25	40.0	41.8	39.2
11	0.40	0.7	0.8	2.3
12	0.58	18.0	32.0	5.4
13	0.58	9.3	21.8	39.0
14	0.68	0.8	0.8	1.3
15	0.80	15.0	15.0	5.4
16	0.80	50.0	50.0	51.8
17	0.90	1.5	4.0	V.N.A.[†]
18	1.70	65.0	65.0	15.0
19	1.70	14.0	14.0	19.5
20	1.80	40.0	40.0	12.0
Avg.	0.56	15.88	17.37	12.43
S.D.	0.576	19.36	19.60	13.88

*The subjects were ranked according to the preimmune serum antibody levels.
†Volunteer not available.

samples obtained from 19 volunteers three and a half years later.

Table 1 shows that all adults had detectable preimmunization anti-type b antibodies (0.04 to 1.8 μg Ab/ml). The three-weeks, three-months, and three-year levels were greater than the preimmune levels (P<0.0005). There was no statistically significant difference between the three-week postimmune levels and at three months and three years (P>0.5). There was a wide variation in the maximum level of the serum antibodies following immunization (1.1 - 65.0 μg Ab/ml). The postimmunization level seemed to be related to the preimmunization level of serum anti-type b antibodies as the average postimmune level of the five volunteers with the lowest preimmune levels was 2.86 and for the highest five was 22.1 μg Ab/ml.

Immunization of infants and children. The parents of patients infirmed at the Holy Angels Nursery, Belmont, North Carolina, were requested permission to have their children participate in the immunization program. Of 63 parents queried by a letter, 43 responded affirmatively. The first 40 affirmative letters were numbered consecutively and randomly assigned to one of four groups which received 10 or 50 micrograms of the polysaccharide injected subcutaneously or intradermally. All the patients in the nursery were examined by one of us (JCP). Nasopharyngeal and rectal cultures, urinalysis, complete blood count and blood for antibody assay was taken two days prior to immunization. Rectal temperatures were recorded before and six to eight hours following injection of the polysaccharide. A complete blood count and urinalysis including urine culture were taken in the afternoon and the following morning. A blood sample for antibody analysis was taken from all the children three weeks and two months following injection.

No toxic effects of injection of the *H. influenzae,* type b, polysaccharide were observed as measured by a febrile response, elevated peripheral white blood count or abnormal urinary sediment. One individual developed a temperature of 101° F. the following morning accompanied by signs and symptoms of an upper respiratory infection.

H. influenzae, type b, was not recovered from any of the cultures. Eight bacteria cross-reacting with *H. influenzae,* type b, were recovered from the stool cultures. Three of these were bacillus species, one was a streptococcus viridans, three were *Staphylococcus aureus,* coagulase positive, and one was an *E. coli* 075:Kf147:H5 (Strain Easter) (Bradshaw et al., 1971).

Table 2 summarizes the results of immunization of these infants and children. Not shown was a plot of the preimmune levels against age which showed significant curvature with a maximum at 5.7 years. The relationship between antibody level and age can be described by the equation

$$y = -3.528 + 0.956X - 0.0835X2$$

where y is the age in years and X is log (Ab). The controls differed slightly from the four experimental groups as their average age (5.75 years) was greater and their preimmune antibody level (0.90 μg Ab/ml) was higher than the controls. On the average, the controls showed an increase of 0.37 μg Ab/ml during the first three weeks (P<0.034). In view of this finding, the changes in the four

TABLE 2

SERUM ANTIBODY RESPONSE OF INFANTS AND CHILDREN
INJECTED WITH *H. INFLUENZAE*, type b, POLYSACCHARIDE

Group			Age	Micrograms Ab/Ml serum (± S.D.)		
Dose of Antigen μg	Route of Injection	No. of Subjects	(Years±S.D.)	Preimmune	3 weeks	2 months
50	I.C.	10	4.1±2.7	0.37±0.25	3.16±4.55	1.91±3.75
50	S.C.	8	4.3±3.1	0.17±0.21	3.91±4.63	3.09±3.40
10	I.C.	12	3.9±3.0	0.57±0.61	6.24±5.50	2.85±3.77
10	S.C.	10	4.9±1.7	0.34±0.41	3.52±3.54	2.43±3.72
Control		18	5.8±2.6	0.90±1.59	1.27±2.19	

NOTE: I.C. = Intracutaneous

S.S. = Subcutaneous

experimental groups were compared to the change in antibody levels of the controls.

All experimental groups responded with statistically significant antibody formation three weeks after immunization. The highest three weeks' level was in the 10 μg intracutaneous group (P<0.001). No consistent effect of the route of immunization was observed as the intracutaneous route was more effective at the 10-μg dose and the subcutaneous route was more effective at the 50-μg dose. The 10-μg dose seemed to be more effective in that only one out of 20 failed to respond with more than a twofold increase in serum antibody as compared to seven nonresponding subjects out of 20 injected with 50 μg.

Ten of the 40 injected infants and children had less than 0.04 μg Ab/ml prior to immunization. Only one of these children with undetectable preimmunization levels failed to respond with antibody formation. In contrast to the serum antibody response of the adults, the level in these infants and children declined within two months.

A slight increase in the serum anti-type b antibody levels was observed in the noninjected group (controls). Several of the children in this group had bacteria with cross-reacting antigen to the *H. influenzae,* type b, capsular polysaccharide which may have been the cause of their response.

Immunization of two-to-three-month-old infants. Based upon the previous results, an experiment was designed to test the effect of two antigen dosages, 5.0

and 10 micrograms, and the possible adjuvant effect of aluminum hydroxide upon the immune response of two-to-three-month-old infants. All the infants were born at Charlotte Memorial Hospital, Charlotte, North Carolina, and were examined at 4 days of age and during their visits to the well-baby clinic for physical examination and immunizations. During these visits, nasopharyngeal and rectal cultures were studied for *H. influenzae* and for bacteria with antigens cross-reactive with the type b capsular polysaccharide. The infants were injected at two to three months of age with 0.5 ml subcutaneously in the deltoid region. Blood samples were taken from the infants at each visit and from the mother at the time of immunization. No untoward effects of the immunization, such as fever, were reported to us by the parents. One infant developed a nonindurated erythematous reaction for two days at the site of the injection of 10 μg of the alum preparation.

The results from the 23 injected infants were compared to serum antibody levels of 90 infants, 3 to 10 months old, examined at the Charlotte Memorial Hospital for routine medical care. Their serum anti-type b antibodies and the results of the nasopharyngeal and rectal cultures of the immunized infants is shown in Figure 2. Whereas 87 of 90 nonimmunized infants had undetectable antibody, only three of the 23 continued to have undetectable antibody through 3, 10, and 11 months after immunization (T. J., D. F., and D. M., respectively). Of these three infants, the maternal level was 8.2 μg Ab/ml in one and 0.04 or less in the other two. Two of the five infants injected with 10 μg in saline did not develop detectable antibody.

The kinetics of the serum anti-type b antibody formation in the responding infants could be assessed only in a rough fashion. Thirteen of the immunized infants had increased serum anti-type b antibodies at the time of their next clinic visit. Six infants (A. A., L. W., D. B., A. P., L. A., and D. C.) responded only after two to three months. In two infants, A. P., and D. C., with high pre-existing serum antibodies, it was difficult to assess the onset of their serum antibody formation. In three infants, the serum anti-type b antibody level declined to below 0.1 μg Ab/ml (P. P., M. R., and A. W.). The maximum serum antibody levels observed in these three infants was higher than the average maximum titer.

The effects of dosage and aluminum hydroxide upon the serum anti-type b response were compared. The highest serum antibody levels were observed in individuals receiving 5.0 μg polysaccharide in saline. The group receiving 10 μg in saline included two nonresponding infants.

Five *E. coli* with cross-reacting antigens (CRA) to the capsular polysaccharide of *H. influenzae*, type b, were detected in the rectal cultures. All the *E. coli* were 075:H5 organisms. One infant (K. P., 10 μg alum) had *E. coli* with the CRA one month following immunization. The response of this individual was characterized by a rapid rise and sustained antibody level. One infant (A. W.)

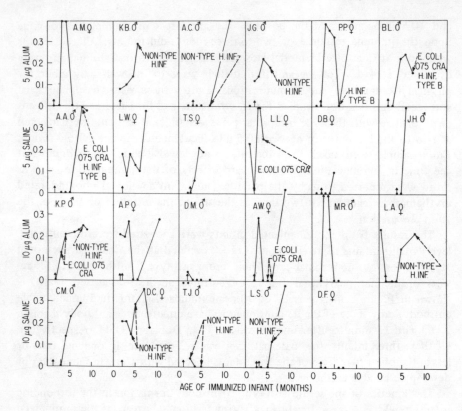

Fig. 2. Serum anti-type b antibody concentration and results of nasopharyngeal and rectal cultures of infants immunized at two to three months with *Hemophilus influenzae,* type b, capsular polysaccharide.

with an *E. coli* with the CRA after his level of immune serum anti-type b antibody had declined to less than 0.1 μg Ab/ml, showed a rise to 0.42 μg Ab/ml at the time of the next bleeding. One infant with nasopharyngeal *H. influenzae,* type b, two months after her level of immunization-induced anti-type b antibodies had declined, reacted with a high level of serum antibodies (0.58 μg Ab/ml) at her clinic visit one month later. These findings suggest that *E. coli* with CRA enhances the immune response to the *H. influenzae,* type b, polysaccharide (Myerowitz et al., 1972) and that injection of the *H. influenzae,* type b, polysaccharide does not inhibit the serum anticapsular antibody response to this bacterial antigen.

DISCUSSION

At least three differences contrast the serum type b polysaccharide antibody response of infants and children to that of adults. First, there is a longer interval to reach the maximum antibody concentration following the injection of the polysaccharide in the infants. Second, there are the lower levels of postimmunization anti-type b antibodies in the infants and children. Third, in contrast to the relatively constant level of anti-type b antibodies observed three to four years following immunization of the adults, a decline from the maximum level of serum antibodies was observed in most of the infants and children within several months. Similar results were recently observed in infants and adults injected with the meningococcal group C polysaccharide (Gotschlich et al., 1972) and in infants and children injected with whole encapsulated *D. pneumoniae*, types I and VI, and *Salmonellae* (Hodes, Ziegler, and Zepp, 1944; Smith et al., 1964).

The immune response elicited by the injection of the purified type b capsular polysaccharide differs from that elicited by intact *H. influenzae*, type b, antigen injected into animals (Schneerson et al., 1972). In rabbits, injection of the purified polysaccharide over a wide dosage range (0.1 to 100 μg) either as a saline solution or absorbed to aluminum hydroxide does not result in an increase in serum anti-type b antibodies (Hodes, Zeigler, and Zepp, 1944). In contrast, injection of live or formaldehyde-treated bacteria results in the rapid formation of serum anti-type b antibodies. A similar immune response to isolated capsular polysaccharides as contrasted to that of encapsulated bacteria has been observed for pneumococci and meningococci in laboratory animals (Heidelberger et al., 1946; Gotschlich, Goldschneider, and Artenstein, 1969). The immunogenic properties of the isolated type b polysaccharide may be compared to that of haptenic substance with the *H. influenzae* bacteria serving as a carrier molecule. Consistent with this explanation of the immunogenic properties of the type b polysaccharide are the observations that the serum antibody response to pneumococcal polysaccharides is thymus-independent and thus the increased immune reaction elicited by the whole encapsulated bacteria is related to the carrier portion of the immunogen (Humphrey, Parrot and East, 1964). The thymus-related system has been postulated to regulate the immune response to the carrier portion of the immunogen (Miller and Mitchell, 1969). The serum antibody response of adult humans elicited by the purified polysaccharide is similar to that elicited by pneumococcal, meningococcal, and other bacterial polysaccharides (Heidelberger, 1953; Heidelberger et al., 1946; Smith and Robbins, 1968; Anderson et al., 1972; and Myerowitz et al., 1972). The rapid and sustained serum antibody formation elicited by the type b polysaccharide may be due to direct stimulation of previously differentiated cells, perhaps induced

by *H. influenzae,* type b, as an asymptomatic infection by enteric or nasopharyngeal bacteria with antigens cross-reactive with the capsular polysaccharide. A continuous exposure to a microbial environment of a critical component of a two- or multi-cell biosynthetic pathway might explain the age-
related development to the isolated capsular polysaccharide. Thus, infants would
have only thymus-independent cells (carrier induced) which gradually develop following contact with whole bacteria. That these mechanisms may be operative is
suggested by the adult-type immune response of the three infants with fecal *E.
coli* containing the cross-reactive polysaccharide as contrasted to the immunized
infants and our experiments with neonatal rabbits colonized with cross-reacting
enteric bacteria (Myerowitz et al., 1972). This postulated direct stimulation of
previously differentiated antibody-producing cells by the purified polysaccharide
may also serve to explain the direct relation between the level of preimmune and
post immunization anti-type b antibodies in the adult volunteers. This explanation, that of a low level of bacteria-induced differentiated cells, may provide a
useful experimental model to study the age-related immune response observed
for protein, bacterial, erythrocyte as well as polysaccharide antigens in humans
and laboratory animals (Smith and Robbins, 1968). It has been suggested that
somatic antigens (lipopolysaccharides) may be an important stimulus for the
thymus cell system. Whether the somatic antigens of *H. influenzae*, type b, or
cross-reacting gram-negative enteric bacteria such as *E. coli* 075:H5:Kf147 induce the differentiation of cells capable of synthesizing type b polysaccharide
antibodies or whether this differentiation may be induced by some or all lipopolysaccharides is not known (Jones and Kind, 1968).

The results obtained in this experiment indicate that serum *H. influenzae,*
type b, antibodies may be elicited by injection of two-to-three-months-old infants with the purified capsular polysaccharide. Using two experimental ap-
proaches, an estimate of 0.04 to 0.1 µg anti-type b antibody/ml serum has been
postulated to be "protective." This level of antibodies was achieved in most of
the immunized infants. The exact dosage for optimum response, the mechanism
of antibody formation, and the protective effect of the injected purified polysaccharide requires further study.

SUMMARY

Hemophilus influenzae, type b, antibodies were measured quantitatively in
normal and immunized humans and in commercially available pooled immunoglobulin. A "protective" serum level was estimated to be 0.06 to 0.1 micrograms
antibody/ml based upon the anti-type b concentration in normal adult sera and
pooled immunoglobulin. An age-related difference characterized the adult and
infant serum antibody response to injection of the purified type b capsular

polysaccharide. The adults responded with higher and more sustained antibody levels than did the infants and children. An immunized infant reacted with type b antibody formation following nasopharyngeal carriage of *H. influenzae,* type b, and two infants reacted with type b antibodies following enteric carriage of *Escherichia coli* with a cross-reacting antigen.

Qualitative and quantitative differences characterize the adult versus the infant response to the capsular polysaccharide of *Hemophilus influenzae,* type b. This age-related difference in the serum antitype b antibody response may be due to the development of differentiated cells induced by whole bacteria, either as *H. influenzae,* type b, or by other organisms with cross-reacting antigens. The "protective" level of serum anti-type b antibodies, estimated by two methods, was achieved by immunization of infants, suggesting that this procedure may confer protective immunity.

REFERENCES

Alexander, H. E. 1965. In *Bacterial and Mycotic Infections of Man,* edited by R. J. Dubos and J. G. Hirsch, p. 724. Philadelphia: J. B. Lippincott.

Alexander, H. E.; M. Heidelberger; and G. Leidy. 1944. "The Protective or Curative Element in type b, *H. influenzae,* Rabbit Serum." *Yale J. Biol. Med.* 16:425.

Anderson, P.; R. B. Johnston; and D. H. Smith. 1972. "Human Serum Activities against *Hemophilus influenzae,* type b." *J. Clin. Invest.* 51:31.

Anderson, P.; G. Peter; R. B. Johnston; L. H. Wetterlow; and D. H. Smith. 1972. "Immunization of Humans with Polyribophosphate, the Capsular Antigen of *Hemophilus influenzae,* type b." *J. Clin. Invest.* 51:39.

Bradshaw, M. W.; R. Schneerson; J. C. Parke, Jr.; and J. B. Robbins. 1971. "Bacterial Antigens Cross-Reactive with the Capsular Polysaccharide of *Hemophilus influenzae,* type b." *Lancet* 1:1095.

Dawson, B., and K. Zinnemann. 1952. "Incidence and Type Distribution of Encapsulated *H. influenzae* Strains." *British Med. J.* 1:740.

Fothergill, L. D., and J. Wright. 1933. "Influenzae Meningitis: The Relation of Age-Incidence to the Bactericidal Power of Blood against the Casual Organism." *J. Immunol.* 24:273.

Gitlin, D., and C. A. Janeway. 1960. "Some Isotopic Studies on the Distributions and Metabolism of Plasma Proteins." *Adv. Biol. and Med. Phy.* 7:249.

Gotschlich, E. C.; I. Goldschneider; and M. S. Artenstein. 1969. "Human Immunity to the Meningococcus: IV. Immunogenicity of Group A and Group C Meningococcal Polysaccharides in Human Volunteers." *J. Exp. Med.* 129:1367.

Gotschlich, E. C.; M. Rey; R. Triau; and K. J. Sparks. 1972. "Quantitative Determination of the Human Immune Response to Immunization with Meningococcal Vaccines." *J. Clin. Invest.* 51:89.

Heidelberger, M. 1953. "Persistence of Antibodies in Men after Immunization." In *The Nature and Significance of the Antibody Response,* edited by A. M. Pappenheimer, p. 90. New York: Columbia University Press.

Heidelberger, M., and C. F. MacPherson. 1943. "Quantitative Micro-Estimation of Antibodies in the Sera of Man and Other Animals." *Sci.* 97:405.

Heidelberger, M.; C. M. Macleod; S. J. Kaiser; and B. Robinson. 1946. "Antibody Formation in Volunteers Following Injection of Pneumococci or Their Type-Specific Polysaccharides." *J. Exp. Med.* 82:303.

Hodes, H. L.; J. F. Zieger; and H. D. Zepp. 1944. "Development of Antibody Following Vaccination of Infants and Children against Pneumococci." *J. Ped.* 24:641.

Humphrey, J. H.; D. M. V. Parrot; and J. East. 1964. "Studies on Globulin and Antibody Production in Mice Thymectomized at birth." *Immunology* 7:419.

Jones, J. M., and P. Kind. 1968. "Enhancing Effect of Bacterial Endotoxins on Bone Marrow Cells in the Immune Response to SRBC." *J. Immun.* 108:1453.

McFarlane, A. S. 1958. "Effective Trace-Labelling of Proteins with Iodine." *Nature* 182:53.

Miller, J. F., and G. F. Mitchell. 1969. "Thymus and Antigen-Reacting Cells." *Transplant. Rev.* 1:3.

Myerowitz, R. L.; Z. T. Handzel; R. Schneerson; and J. B. Robbins. 1972. "Induction of Immunity to *Hemophilus influenzae*, type b, in Rabbits by Gastrointestinal Colonization with a Cross-Reacting *Escherichia coli.*" *Fed. Proc.* 31, No. 2 (March, April).

Nelson, J. D. 1972. "The Bacterial Etiology and Antibiotic Management of Septic Arthritis in Infants and Children." *Ped.* 50:437.

Norden, C. 1972. "Variable Susceptibility of *Hemophilus influenzae*, type b, Strains to Serum Bactericidal." *Proc. Soc. Exp. Bio. Med.* 139:59.

Norden, C. W.; M. Melish; J. C. Overall; J. Baum. 1972. "Immunologic Responses to *Hemophilus influenzae* Meningitis." *J. Ped.* 80:209.

Peter, G. S.; S. Greenfield; V. M. Howie; and D. H. Smith. 1971. "Acquisition of Type-Specific Antibodies Following Exposure to *Hemophilus influenzae* Meningitis." Abstract of the Society for Pediatric Research, 41st Annual Meeting.

Pittman, M. 1931. "Variation and Type Specificity in the Bacterial Species *Hemophilus influenzae,*" *J. Exp. Med.* 53:471.

Pittman, M. 1933. "The Actions of Type-Specific *Hemophilus influenzae* Antiserum." *J. Exp. Med.* 58:683.

Robbins, J. B. 1972. Unpublished observations.

Rodrigues, L. P.; R. Schneerson; and J. B. Robbins. 1972. "Immunity to *Hemophilus influenzae*, type b: I. The Isolation and Some Physiochemical, Serologic and Biologic Properties of the Capsular Polysaccharide of *Hemophilus influenzae*, type b." *J. Immunol.* 107:1071.

Rosen, F. S., and C. A. Janaway. 1966. "The Gamma Globulins." *N. Eng. J. Med.* 275:709.

Schneerson, R.; M. Bradshaw; J. K. Whisnant; R. L. Myerowitz; J. C. Parke; and J. B. Robbins. 1972. "An *Escherichia coli* Antigen Cross-Reactive with the Capsular Polysaccharide of *Hemophilus infuenzae,* type b: Occurrence Among Known Serotypes and Immunochemical and Biologic Properties of *E. coli* Antisera toward *H. influenzae,* type b." *J. Immun.* 108:1551.

Schneerson, R.; L. P. Rodrigues; J. C. Parke, Jr.; and J. B. Robbins. 1971. "Immunity to Disease Caused by *Hemophilus influenzae,* type b: II. Acquired and Immunization-Induced Antibodies to the Capsular Polysaccharide of *Hemophilus influenzae,* type b." *J. Immunol.* 107:1081.

Sinclair, S. E. 1941. "*Hemophilus influenzae,* type b, in Acute Laryngitis with Bacteremia." *JAMA* 117:170.

Smith, R. T; D. V. Eitzman; M. E. Catlin; E. O. Wirtz; and B. E. Miller. 1964. "The Development of the Immune Response. Characterization of the Response of the Human Infant and Adult to Immunization with *Salmonella* Vaccines." *Ped.* 33:163.

Smith, R. T., and J. B. Robbins. 1968. *Developmental Aspects of Immunity in the Biologic Basis of Pediatric Practice,* edited by R. Cooke, New York: McGraw-Hill.

Turk, D. C., and J. R. May. 1967. *Hemophilus influenzae: Its Clinical Importance,* p. 24. London: English Universities Press.

Waldman, T. A., and W. Strober. 1969. "Metabolism of Immunoglobulins." *Prog. Allergy* 13:1.

Discussion

John Witte, Presiding

David W. Fraser: I wonder why the incidence of *H. influenzae* meningitis is ten times higher in 6-month-olds than in 2-year-olds, even though the percentage of children with measurable antibody is not that different in the two groups.

John B. Robbins: I think the answer to your questions is an interpretation of data. First, because the 2-year-old does not have detectable antibodies does not mean that he is not actively sensitized. Actually, the Fothergill and Wright curve could be redrawn showing that it starts to ascend earlier than shown, with regard to development of antibodies. The second interpretation is derived from the experiments that we have done with neonatal rabbits fed cross-reacting *E. coli*. There is really little in the amount of detectable type b antibody that these animals synthesize as compared to what they will naturally synthesize months later. If one injects live *Hemophilus* intravenously into *E. coli* fed animals, the antibody response is of a greater magnitude than in unfed animals. I think the *E. coli* with cross-reacting antigens sensitizes so that an accelerated reaction to *H. influenzae,* type b, may be one explanation for the result. The development of natural immunity cannot always be measured.

Virgil M. Howie: There may be misinformation concerning the bactericidal test. In our data from patients with otitis, in the 2-to-5-months age group, only one of 28 had any detectable bactericidal power against *H. influenzae,* type b.

David H. Smith: Several aspects deserve further discussion. First, we are interested in nonimmune factors that may make a child 3 to 12 months of age more susceptible to meningitis. My thought, based on Dr. Janeway's tutoring, has been that maybe something such as the permeability barrier at the level of the central nervous system may affect the susceptibility of infants to meningitis. I would like to emphasize a point that did not come out in the discussion yesterday. We are in fact victims of thes sensitivity of the laboratory analysis of antibody. Interpretation of data like that of Fothergill and Wright should take into consideration the realization that the bactericidal test is not as sensitive as certain other methods. In fact, it is an order or two in magnitude above that which we can now detect by radioimmunoassay. Indeed, the amount of anti-PRP carried by many "immune" individuals is surprisingly

308

low; most healthy adults have nanogram levels as to aggammaglobulinemics on replacement therapy. Thirdly, to Dr. Fraser's question, I would emphasize that there is an age-related increase in RIA detectable antibody between six months and two years. In other words, below one year of age, there is X-amount and above a year of age there are two or three X-amounts. This immunological progression occurs even though all the sera have nondetectable bactericidal activity. More experience with the new serological systems is required to questions concerning the level of antibody that provides resistance to systemic infections.

Sarah H. Sell: I would like to make a plea, for some standarized methods. I feel frustrated that we have data derived from more than 2,000 observations that cannot be related to that of other laboratories because the methods are so different. There were children in our study who had *H. influenzae*, type b, in their nasopharynx at the time they had antibodies that were measureable by our crude methods. I hope that out of this discussion we can agree on some standarized methods that will make it possible to relate the experiences of multiple investigators in a meaningful manner. Dr. Anderson mentioned radioimmunodiffusion as a new method that is being developed. It promises to be the best yet. Each new method has been a bit better than the one before, and each time the results are more sensitive, but we have not yet achieved the zenith of what we all hope to reach.

Robbins: I would like to ask Dr. Anderson and Dr. Smith if they would comment about the values they obtained for the level of anti-type b antibody in the serum of hypogammaglobulinemics. We calculated that about 100 to 200 nanograms of antibody per milliliter are sufficient to protect against *H. influenzae* meningitis in these patients. Do you think that is a useful concept?

Smith: I think it may be a useful concept in that it is the amount of PRP which people have. We are also concerned about non-PRP antibodies and, in actual fact, we are not measuring the level of those antibodies by the present RIA method. I think antibodies to somatic antigens certainly play a role in the defense of individuals against this organism. Dr. Karzon asked yesterday for evidence that PRP is a critical immune factor, or that anti-PRP is protective. I think there is considerable evidence which led many of us to consider PRP as the critical antigen for *H. influenzae,* type b, and which also led us to think the presence of anti-PRP provides immunity. The best evidence was the rather substantial evaluation of passive serum therapy performed in New York. This mode of therapy worked, not only in experimental animals, but it was of clinical value with patients with meningitis. The active principal in the rabbit sera used in passive immunization was, in fact, the anti-PRP which could be absorbed out, with purified antigen. That information plus other data which are available from several laboratories in the past and at present would suggest that if one has anti-PRP, it is protective. I do not think, at present, that we are able to put a number on the critical concentration of anti-PRP. I think the level that aggammaglobulinemics carry, approximately 100 to 200 μg/ml, is an effective level to consider. It has been attractive to us and we have been doing some comparisons with our vaccine results relative to that value.

Robbins: I agree with everything that Dr. Smith has said. We would like to emphasize that we think PRP is a protective antigen of *H. influenzae,* type b. Out studies are directed toward the study of the host-parasite interaction by measuring the immune response to this one antigen. There certainly may be other factors in *H. influenzae* that will induce protective antibodies. But since this material has been isolated and characterized, it should be studied carefully to understand this one aspect of the host *H. influenzae* relationship.

Smith: I think it goes further than that. I think one can say that PRP is a protective antigen.

John Witte: I would like to bring up one factor that should be considered: the role of secretory antibody. It certainly may be important in pathogenesis, acquisition, and transmission of organisms. It is known from other models that parenteral administration of inactivated vaccines does not stimulate secretory antibody responses or does so poorly. It may explain some of the inconsistencies that cannot be explained at present.

Robbins: What are the inconsistencies you are talking about?

Witte: Well, one cannot explain frequency of infections in certain groups. One cannot explain protection in others.

Robbins: I can tell you about all the bad experiments we have done with secretory IgA. We have looked at pooled colostrum and we have looked at my nasopharyngeal mucous. We have looked at rabbit colostrum taken after prolonged immunization with the *H. influenzae,* type b, organisms. We have just not been able to demonstrate antibody activity, but that may be due to inadequate technique.

David T. Karzon: How much data on antibody response do you have in the age group in which we are most interested? What is the response to antigen in young immunological virgin individuals (that is PRP-virgin) when immunized with antigen, from any source, either *H. influenzae,* type b, or related antigens? I could not detect in the data how many children started out with no antibody by the radioimmunoassay, which could be most sensitive, and had a rise. What is the nature of the rise, its longevity, and so forth?

Smith: This is the kind of thing that keeps us up nights, because it is a key question. Actually, the radioimmunoassay is an extremely sensitive assay, so much so that I have chided Dr. Anderson that one can "hear the grass grow" with this method.

John K. Whisnant: In this regard, would you clarify Dr. Peter's criterion for response or nonresponse for those vaccine recipients?

Smith: Two standard deviations. Dr. Anderson has gone back and analyzed a larger number of specimens to see what the standard deviation of the technique is. Then we have said that this is the standard deviation of the error of technique. We now take two times that to define a significant result—we think it is a lot more accurate than using a conventional two- or fourfold increase as a significant titer rise.

Whisnant: Assuming a standard deviation of 10 to 20 micrograms per ml if the child went beyond the two standard deviations, is this, then a positive response?

Georges Peter: Yes. We can also say that the vast majority of responses were much greater than that.

Witte: Are you also saying, Dr. Smith, in answer to Dr. Sell's question, that it is a bit premature to agree on standarization of methodology for testing?

Smith: First of all, let me say that radioimmunoassay is now at the point where we can use it. Dr. Robbins and I have said that it would be good if there were a reference laboratory where we could check specimens of investigators doing the test. We are now doing tests on all specimens drawn during NIH-sponsored vaccine field trials wherever they may take place.

Sell: Are you using I^{125} tagged or tritium-labeled PRP?

Smith: It is a tritium label, internally labeled with glucose. If you want radioimmunoassays performed, we can do them now, as we are serving as the reference laboratory. I hope Dr. Anderson pointed out that we are all standardizing our results to one standard sera, which is a Mr. Klein, who resides somewhere in the Washington area. Thus I think we have come to a zenith in terms of co-operation in the field of antibody assays, in that we are all using one assay and one standard serum. Thus the results of the assays are in fact nanograms of antibodies compared with Klein serum per milliliter. As far as the PHA assay is concerned, I think our local philosophy is that, under the present conditions, we would like to abandon it. We know it is measuring only anti-PRP antibody, and we think that the radioimmunoassay does it better. Thus, we would suggest that it is obsolete, compared to the radioimmunoassay. Dr. Robbins is an immunologist, and we are trained as bacteriologists. It is not that we want to see bacteria die, but we are very comfortable doing bactericidal assays. I think there are some theoretical reasons, which Dr. Anderson pointed out yesterday, which lead us to think that we would still like to look at the bactericidal response. I would submit that with a single test, the bactericidal responses are measuring all of the antibody-antigen interactions that can be measured after an unknown number of antigens are purified and used in multiple RIA tests. Lastly, I would point out that Dr. Dave Feingold, who works across the street from us, has many times emphasized that, in terms of killing bacteria, it is possibly the complement that is really important. One can fix an antibody of any kind on a bacterium, then bring in complement activity, and the organism will be killed. If one can fix albumin on *E. coli* and then bring in antibodies to albumin, complement in the presence of this antialbumin interaction will kill the bacterium. I think that we can measure a myriad of antigen specificities in a single test. To answer the question of standardization, we are not yet to the point where I think we have a reproducible universal bactericidal test, but I think we would like to have a chance at it, and should be able to accomplish this in the next several months.

Robbins: It is very hard to raise calves that have not suckled colostrum for three weeks and keep them alive. It takes a great deal of effort and care. We will try to be in a position in two or three months to offer this precolostral calf serum, which may give everyone the same reference source of complement. It is a tremendous amount of work to keep those calves alive, but we think we can do it now. I would like to say something about the complement-bactericidal reaction, in theory. I would not want to discourage anyone from doing it. It is true that any antigen-antibody interaction which will activate the complement proteins next to a susceptible bacterial structure will give a bactericidal reaction. However, there are many instances in which antigen-antibody reaction with a bacterial substance does not result in a complement-dependent reaction. This failure to induce a bactericidal reaction may lead to misinterpretations. I would like to cite three examples so that the limitation of the tests can be apparent to everyone. There are many pneumococcal systems in which antibodies to pneumococci plus complement will not result in pneumococcal death. One would make the assumption from this test that antibodies to pneumococcus do not mediate immunity. In contrast, mycobacterium tuberculosis will be killed in the presence of antibody and complement. Yet one would not say that antibody to tuberculosis confers immunity. Thirdly, I would like to point out that, at least for *Salmonella typhi* and in the *E. coli* Easter experiment, enormous quantities of antibodies will not result in killing of the organisms. This is presumably due to the fact that the antigen which fixes the antibody is sufficiently far away from the susceptible bacterial structure that lysis does not occur.

On the other hand, we would think that antibodies to *E. coli* Easter will protect against disease. The complement-dependent reaction may be of an antibody unrelated to protective value. I would like to make a plea for one study many of us have avoided. I do not think we have looked at the bacteria carefully enough. I think it would be important to consider more closely the bacteria that cause epiglottitis and meningitis, to make sure that, by means other than serologic techniques, the capsular antigen is identical in these organims. More precise methods, such as chemical analysis, should be done. Yesterday, something that Dr. Anderson said touched me very much, that is, perhaps we are rushing too fast into the vaccine trials. We do not know enough about the pathology of the organism or the human immune response to it or to immunization. I think he is right. One never knows enough about human disease and certainly just this little flurry of activity about *Hemophilus* has unearthed so many new things that one realizes how little we know and how much more there is yet to be known.

Sell: On the other hand, consider the pertussis vaccine. Very little is fully understood about the dynamics of immunity; yet, we have enjoyed the protective benefits of the vaccine for three or four decades.

Witte: There are a number of issues we really did not have a chance to address ourselves to, such as directions for other field trials and numbers that are going to be needed to document evidence. I wonder if Dr. Karzon would summarize some the things we have come up with in the last day and a half.

Karzon: I would like to suggest that those investigators who are immunizing young infants and trying to determine whether it is a secondary or primary response should pursue this carefully. There are, again, analogies with virus systems. There are some children with no apparent antibody after live measles or rubella immunization or natural infection. When one reimmunizes them and looks at their antibody daily, one can detect a singular difference between those who were sensitized who have an antibody rise by five days versus those who were not sensitized and an antibody rise in 21 or more days. I think that looking at the kinetics of the antibody response may be unusually useful here. Do I gather some sense of unanimity in these areas that PRP is at least one and may be in itself sufficient antigenic mechanism for obtaining immunity in the human child against invasive *H. influenzae,* type b, infection? And that the radioimmunossay is a sensitive method of detecting that antibody and further, the cidal test should be run in parallel (at least this was my own impression) until we know more about the biology of the somatic antigens and what they mean in terms of protection? They can be looked at in parallel with the PRP antibody resposne. I am delighted to see the inter-laboratory co-operation which will permit standization of testing. This is a must for the work to go on and I hope the generous laboratories will continue to support the "have nots."

We have discussed where we are going, although mainly in terms of the antibody response systems. There are three parts to evaluating a potential vaccine or immunprophylaxis. One is a consideration of short-term and long-term dangers or toxicities; second is the measurement of some antibody that is a reflection of resistance, and we have discussed this a great deal during this conference. The third part we have not really tangled with very much. I think it is quite interesting and more complicated than in other disease-control issues: How do we measure vaccine efficacy in prevention of disease? Because serological response and efficacy still have a gap between them, studies of efficacy still have to be done. There are various ways one could look at this issue theoretically. One possibility is the determination of what it does to the flora in the community. There are examples of eradicating flora with immunoprophylaxis. Another possibility is documenting a decreased incidence of minor upper respiratory disease, including otitis media associated with *H. influenzae.* Yet another estimate of success is measurement of incidence of invasive disease such as meningitis, epiglottitis, or osteomyelitis. The incidence of the indicator becomes lower and lower, so that, if one restricts the efficacy trials to appearance of *H. influenzae,* type b, meningitis, one needs large denominators. A corollary question should be asked: Is it possible that one can prevent invasive disease and not mucosal respiratory diseases? This is theoretically possible and is exemplified in modified form with the Salk vaccine which has many analogies.

With *H. influenzae,* it is obviously easy to raise questions. The assembled conferences have probably done as much as in any time in history to probe into the answers. The stimulus has been the real prospect of an effective immunoprophylaxis.

CONFERENCE PARTICIPANTS

Robert H. Alford, M.D.
Assistant Professor of Medicine
Veterans Administration Hospital
Nashville, Tennessee

Porter Anderson, Ph.D.
Research Associate
Infectious Disease Division
Boston Children's Hospital
Assistant Professor of Microbiology
    and Molecular Genetics
Harvard School of Medicine
Boston, Massachusetts

Meir Argaman, M.D.
Visiting Associate
Developmental Immunology Branch
National Institute of Child
    Health and Human Development
National Institutes of Health
Bethesda, Maryland

Robert Baker, Ph.D.
Immunizing Biologicals Research
    and Development
Lilly Research Laboratories
Indianapolis, Indiana

John G. Buddingh, M.D.
Professor and Chairman
    Department of Microbiology
Louisiana State University School
    of Medicine
New Orleans, Louisiana

William J. Cheatham, M.D.
Professor, Department of Pathology
Vanderbilt University
School of Medicine
Nashville, Tennessee

William D. Donald, M.D.
Associate Professor of Pediatrics
Director, Pediatric Outpatient
    Department
Vanderbilt University
School of Medicine
Nashville, Tennessee

Gordon Douglas, M.D.
Head, Infectious Disease Unit
University of Rochester
School of Medicine & Dentistry
Rochester, New York

Linda J. Duke, Ph.D.
Research Associate
Department of Pediatrics
Research Associate
Department of Microbiology
Vanderbilt University
School of Medicine
Nashville, Tennessee

Charles F. Federspiel, Ph.D.
Associate Professor of Biostatistics
Vanderbilt University
School of Medicine
Nashville, Tennessee

315

Roger A. Feldman, M.D.
Chief, Special Pathogens Section
Bacterial Diseases Branch
Center for Disease Control
Atlanta, Georgia

Douglas P. Fine, M.D.
Clinical Associate
Infectious Diseases
Veterans Administration Hospital
Nashville, Tennessee

William F. Fleet, M.D.
Associate Professor
Department of Pediatrics
Vanderbilt University
School of Medicine
Nashville, Tennessee

David W. Fraser, M.D.
Medical Epidemiologist
Special Pathogens Section
Bacterial Diseases Branch
Center for Disease Control
Atlanta, Georgia

Zeev Handzel, M.D.
Visiting Fellow
Developmental Immunology Branch
National Institute of Child
    Health and Human Development
National Institutes of Health
Bethesda, Maryland

A. Lynn Harding
Research Associate
Boston Children's Hospital
Infectious Disease Division
Boston, Massachusetts

Richard Horton, M.D.
Medical Officer
Infectious Disease Branch
National Institutes of Health
Antiviral Substances Program
Bethesda, Maryland

Virgil M. Howie, M.D.
2345 Whitesburg Drive, South
Huntsville, Alabama

Richard B. Johnston, Jr., M.D.
Assistant Professor of Pediatrics
    and Microbiology
University of Alabama in Birmingham
Birmingham, Alabama

David T. Karzon, M.D.
Professor-Chairman,
Department of Pediatrics
Vanderbilt University
School of Medicine
Nashville, Tennessee

Grace Leidy
Columbia University
    College of Physicians and Surgeons
New York, New York

Samuel R. Marney, M.D.
Assistant Professor of Medical Research
Veterans Administration Hospital
Nashville, Tennessee

Martha Mattheis
Microbiologist
Antiviral Substances Program
National Institute of Allergy and
    Infectious Disease
National Institutes of Health
Bethesda, Maryland

Kenneth McIntosh, M.D.
Assistant Professor, Pediatrics
Pediatric Infectious Disease
University of Colorado
Medical Center
Denver, Colorado

Richard H. Michaels, M.D.
Children's Hospital of Pittsburgh
Pittsburgh, Pennsylvania

Richard L. Myerowitz, M.D.
Clinical Associate
National Institute of Child Health and
   Human Development
Bethesda, Maryland

Carl W. Norden, M.D.
Department of Medicine
Montefiore Hospital
Pittsburgh, Pennsylvania

James C. Parke, Jr., M.D.
Associate Chairman, Department
   of Pediatrics
Charlotte Memorial Hospital
Charlotte, North Carolina

F. B. Peck, Jr., M.D.
Director, Medical Plans and
   Regulatory Affairs
Lilly Research Laboratories
Indianapolis, Indiana

Georges Peter, M.D.
Assistant Professor of Medical
   Science (Pediatrics)
Division of Biological and Medical
   Sciences
Brown University
Providence, Rhode Island

John B. Robbins, M.D.
Clinical Director
National Institute of Child
   Health and Human Development
National Institutes of Health
Bethesda, Maryland

John P. Robinson, Ph.D.
Associate Professor
Department of Microbiology
Vanderbilt University
School of Medicine
Nashville, Tennessee

William Schaffner, M.D.
Assistant Professor
Department of Medicine
Vanderbilt University
Nashville, Tennessee

Rachel Schneerson, M.D.
Visiting Associate
Developmental Immunology Branch
National Institutes of Health
Bethesda, Maryland

Sarah H. Sell, M.D.
Associate Professor
Department of Pediatrics
Vanderbilt University
Nashville, Tennessee

David H. Smith, M.D.
Chief, Infectious Disease Division
Boston Children's Hospital
Associate Professor, Pediatrics
Harvard University
Boston, Massachusetts

Thomas H. Stoudt, Ph.D.
Director, Applied Microbiology
    Department
Merck Sharp and Dohme
Rahway, New Jersey

John K. Whisnant, M.D.
Clinical Associate
National Institute of Child
    Health and Human Development
National Institutes of Health
Bethesda, Maryland

Jeannette Wilkins, M.D.
Assistant Professor of Pediatrics
University of Southern California
Los Angeles, California

John Witte, M.D.
Chief, Immunization Branch
State and Community Services Division
Center for Disease Control
Atlanta, Georgia

Shelby Wyll, M.D.
Medical Epidemiologist
Immunization Branch
Center for Disease Control
Atlanta, Georgia

CO-AUTHORS NOT PARTICIPATING

Damon E. Averill
Boston Children's Hospital
Division of Infectious Diseases
Boston, Massachusetts

Daniel G. Colley, M.D.
Assistant Professor, Microbiology
Veterans Administration Hospital
Nashville, Tennessee

Charles P. Darby, M.D.
Assistant Professor of Pediatrics
Medical University of South Carolina
Charleston, South Carolina

Roger M. DesPrez, M.D.
Professor of Medicine
Cheif, Medical Service
Veterans Administration Hospital
Nashville, Tennessee

Emil C. Gotschlich, M.D.
Associate Professor
The Rockefeller University
New York, New York

David Ingram, M.D.
Research Fellow
Boston Children's Hospital
Division of Infectious Diseases
Boston, Massachusetts

Cecil F. Jacobs, M.D., M.P.H.
Director, Charleston County
    Health Services
Charleston, South Carolina

Robert E. Koehler, M.D.
Medical Epidemiologist
Center for Disease Control
Atlanta, Georgia

Darrell T. Liu, Ph.D.
Biochemist, Department of
    Biochemistry
Brookhaven National Laboratories
Upton, New York

Joseph Marino
Predoctoral Student
Harvard University
(Boston Children's Hospital)
Boston, Massachusetts

Richard E. Moxon, M.D.
Research Fellow
Boston Children's Hospital
Boston, Massachusetts

Simon L. Newman
Boston Children's Hospital
Division of Infectious Diseases
Boston, Massachusetts

Richard O'Reilly, M.D.
Research Fellow
Boston Children's Hospital
Boston, Massachusetts

John H. Ploussard
2345 Whitesburg Drive
Huntsville, Alabama

G. Nicholas Rogentine, M.D.
Senior Investigator
Immunology Branch
National Cancer Institute
National Institutes of Health
Bethesda, Maryland

Shirley S. Schuffman
Instructor, Department of Pathology
Vanderbilt University
School of Medicine
Nashville, Tennessee

William F. Schultz, B.S.
Children's Hospital of Pittsburgh
Pittsburgh, Pennsylvania

Russell P. Sherwin
Hastings Professor of Pathology
University of Southern California
Los Angeles, California

Arnold L. Smith, M.D.
Associate, Infectious Disease Division
Assistant Professor, Harvard University
Boston Children's Hospital
Boston, Massachusetts

Dorothy Turner, M.D.
Pediatric Program Co-ordinator
Child Health and Development
State of Tennessee
Nashville, Tennessee

Roger Vander Zwaag
Assistant Professor of Biostatistics
Vanderbilt University
School of Medicine
Nashville, Tennessee

Peter F. Weller
Predoctoral Student
Harvard University
(Boston Children's Hospital)
Boston, Massachusetts

CHAIRMEN OF THE MEETINGS

Sarah H. Sell, M.D.
Associate Professor of Pediatrics
Vanderbilt University
Nashville, Tennessee

David T. Karzon, M.D.
Professor and Chairman, Department of Pediatrics
Vanderbilt University
Nashville, Tennessee

John Witte, M.D.
Chief, Immunization Branch
State and Community Services Division
Center for Disease Control
Atlanta, Georgia

CO-ORDINATOR

Sarah H. Sell, M.D.
Associate Professor of Pediatrics
Vanderbilt University
Nashville, Tennessee

Index

Acute-sudden-death syndrome, 263-264
Agammaglobulinemia: serum used for complement, 100, 102, 176, 188; and *H. influenzae,* type b, meningitis, 154; gamma globulin prophylaxis, 281; protective level of PRP in children, 282, 285-290, 297; individual susceptibility to *H. influenzae,* type b, 294; antibody in serum of hypogammaglobulinemics, 309
Antibiotics, 189
Antibodies: age-related differences following *H. influenzae,* type b, meningitis, 95-98; bactericidal activity, *H. influenzae,* type b, 96; hemagglutination assay, *H. influenzae,* type b, 96; opsonization, 104; complement, 118-119; "natural," 118, 269-270, 275-278; heating at 56° C for 30 minutes, 120; serum antibody activity against *H. influenzae,* type b, age relation, 122; in otitis media, 122; electron microscopy studies in *H. influenzae,* type b, 135-139; hybrid technique, 152; produced at age two, 154; passive hemagglutination, 163, 169, 170, 177-183; need for standardization of assays, 172; serum antibody levels accumulate with age, 172; age relationship, 177-183; bactericidal assay (BC), 177-183; reduced by heating, 187; research and antigens, 190; response in *H. influenzae,* type b, immunization, 286-287, 297-305; anticapsular, protective nature, 293-294; reference standard (Stan Klein's serum), 295; age-related increase in RAI detectable antibody, 309; in children who had *H. influenzae,* type b, 309; in serum of hypogammaglobulinemics, 309; serologic techniques, 309, 313; limitation of tests, 312. *See* Radioimmunoassay (RIA)
Antigenemia, 45

Antigens: cross-reacting, 49-55; and antiserum-agar techniques, 59, 61; cross-reacting from *E. coli,* 59, 60, 61; somatic, 176; cross-reacting with *H. influenzae,* type b, 269-278; with Neisseria meningitidis, Group A, 270, 272-278; with Neisseria meningitidis, Group C, 270, 272-278; with Diplococcus pneumoniae, types I and III, 275-278. *See also* Polyribophosphate
Arizona, 270-278

Bacillus strains, 270-278
Bacillus subtilis, 49-55
Bactericidal assays, 93-94, 100, 118-119, 188, 311-312
Bacterial inhibitory substance (BIS): assay, 160-164, 169; indication of antibody activity, 164-173; inhibition difference and noninhibitory control, 163, 164-165; assays after adsorption, 165; results-percentage inhibition, 164, 165; in cord serum, 166; heating serum, 187
BIS. *See* Bacterial inhibitory substance (BIS)
Blacks: *H. influenzae* meningitis, mortality, 223-229; coded, birth and death records, California, 225-226, 229; and incidence of *H. influenzae* meningitis, Charleston Co., S.C., 232-239; incidence of *Hemophilus* meningitis patients, 245-249; *H. influenzae,* type b, meningitis, 254-259
Bleb formation, 146-150
Boston, Mass., 264-265
Brain Heart Infusion (BHI). *See under Hemophilus influenzae*
Bronchiectasis, 127

C2, 100, 105, 106
C3, 101, 105-110, 113-117
C5, 107, 108, 109

321